Annual Review

of

REHABILITATION

VOLUME 1 • 1980

Annual Review of REHABILITATION

Co-Editors

Advisory Board

Annual Review of REHABILITATION

VOLUME 1 • 1980

Edited by

Elizabeth L. Pan, Ph.D.

Thomas E. Backer, Ph.D.

Carolyn L. Vash, Ph.D.

SPRINGER PUBLISHING COMPANY
NEW YORK

Springer Publishing Company, Inc.
200 Park Avenue South
New York, New York 10003

80 81 82 83 84 / 10 9 8 7 6 5 4 3 2 1

ISBN 0-8261-3090-9
ISSN 0197-2251

Printed in the United States of America

CONTENTS

FOREWORD

HOWARD A. RUSK, M.D.

Much of the knowledge in the field of rehabilitation is in the form of uncodified wisdom based on experience and time and learned primarily on an informal basis. Communication of that knowledge rests primarily upon a colleague relationship, which is often a costly trial-and-error process. In a sense, this book is an attempt to get on paper what has been learned the hard way by experienced researchers and clinicians. More than that, it represents a sincere effort to arrive at syntheses—no small task.

It has been variously observed that social research is an activity whose problems and methods are affected by the milieu in which it takes place, and that disability is a social problem often with complicating medical overtones. This quite accurately reflects the status of rehabilitation today. The pendulum has swung from the totally medical and the totally vocational to a concern for the severely handicapped who may not have vocational goals. With the work ethic so strong in our society, how do we bring about a satisfactory synthesis?

In reality, rehabilitation, like society as a whole, is deeply involved in the process of social change and even changing value systems. Its research can no longer be the avocation for a few but must be a basic part of service program planning and development.

This change does not relate solely to so-called independent living services. We must face up to a greater concern for those with mental handicaps, and this is not easy to do. The very nature of the disability may well be an impediment to success in work or daily living; or conversely, with new knowledge, new opportunities may well be developed for these individuals. This is a relatively unexplored area, with meager and vicarious experience.

The question has arisen as to who is "captain" of the rehabilitation team. There is no easy answer. Different problems will require different types of leadership at different times. In seeking solutions to specific problems in the future, the issue of who should be the leader at a specific time should become self-evident as the problems evolve.

Today we are deeply concerned with the role of the consumers—their rights and advocacy. We are ill prepared without time, study, and experience to give definite answers to these important questions. This should be a primary area in the future.

This becomes the challenge of the *Annual Review of Rehabilitation.*

To place what we know in reasonable perspective and see the unified nature of that knowledge is difficult enough. To utilize this knowledge to effect changes is still more difficult. To attempt to anticipate the need for change is the great challenge to which the *Review* is dedicated.

INTRODUCTION

ELIZABETH L. PAN, PH.D.
THOMAS E. BACKER, PH.D.
CAROLYN L. VASH, PH.D.

Knowledge about developments in theory, practice, and technology of rehabilitation is growing rapidly, and this volume represents one way professionals in the field can have ready access to this accumulating body of information. The *Annual Review of Rehabilitation* follows the tradition long established by yearly review volumes in other fields (e.g., psychology, sociology, information science, chemistry) in its overall design:

- We have attempted to define the major topic areas of interest that fall within the scope of both research and practice related to rehabilitation of disabled persons.
- A master plan for periodic coverage of these topics has been established, since the field is far too broad for any one hardcover book to include chapters on all relevant subjects.
- Respected authorities in the given subject areas have been selected to write the review chapters.
- The editors have attempted to provide a general structure, so that there is some regularity in the focus of the various chapters, despite necessary (and desirable) differences depending upon the subject and the individual author's point of view.
- Our editorial work with each author has also included the traditional functions of critique in order to maintain a high quality of writing style, scientific accuracy, and comprehensiveness in scope.

In this introduction we will highlight the contents of our first edition; present the master plan that will guide future volumes of the *Annual Review;* give a preview of the upcoming Volume 2; and describe how this volume came to be. Along the way, we will share some of our philosophy about *Annual Review* volumes, which we believe has resulted in some distinctive features of the *Annual Review of Rehabilitation.*

This philosophy hinges on the longstanding involvement of all three editors in efforts to promote effective knowledge utilization in the rehabilitation field. Research findings, or promising innovations developed by practitioners, are of value only if they are actually *used* to improve service delivery and its ultimate goal—the well-being of disabled individuals. The Rehabilitation Services Administration (RSA), the principal federal funding agency for rehabilitation services, has long recognized this, and has since 1967 supported a program of research utilization activities in its R&D division (now part of the National Institute of Handicapped Research). Much of this work has proceeded on the assumption, now well validated by research on the knowledge utilization process, that use of information in print formats is greatly influenced by effective formating of the communication—particularly on the basis of *user involvement* in determining what information is needed and how it should be presented to the target audience.

It is in the area of format, and particularly in the matter of user involvement in designing the volume, that our *Annual Review of Rehabilitation* differs somewhat from most other review volumes in various professional fields. As will be described further below, we have made an intensive effort to seek input from representatives of the major audiences for this book about what subjects are of most urgent concern, and about how information should be presented in the *Annual Review.* While virtually all annual review volumes in various subject areas have editorial advisory boards, most of these boards are composed entirely of leading scholars and researchers in the field. The advisory board for the *Annual Review of Rehabilitation,* on the other hand, includes not only a senior research scientist in the rehabilitation field but also representatives of our other main readership groups: rehabilitation administrators in state Vocational Rehabilitation agencies and private facilities, rehabilitation counselors, legislators concerned with rehabilitation services, and the consumers of these services—disabled people. Moreover, we have sought and received input from these advisors not only about what subjects should be covered by the *Annual Review* but also *how* we should cover them. As a result, the editors and authors have been able to work closely together to establish a high level of readability and ease of communication for our various chapters, moving away from the dry, scholarly tone of many other annual review volumes. Our emphasis is on major knowledge developments with implications for practice, on needed directions for future work, and on integrating the present state of knowledge in a given field in a way that will be at least partly relevant to the concerns of administrators, practitioners, policy makers, and consumers simultaneously.

HOW THE ANNUAL REVIEW DEVELOPED

Our colleagues tell us that efforts to develop an *Annual Review of Rehabilitation* date back as early as the 1950s. The need for such a knowledge-integrating mechanism is evident: The history of physical rehabilitation is long (and, of course, documented in part by various efforts within the field of medicine), and psychosocial/vocational rehabilitation* has been an organized field of practice since the 1920s. Drawing together the diverse threads from these areas is even more important now, since the focus of rehabilitation services in the United States is changing—from an earlier emphasis in PSV rehabilitation on vocational goals alone (a decade ago this volume would surely have been titled "Annual Review of *Vocational* Rehabilitation") to providing services aimed at helping more severely disabled individuals who may never be able to participate fully in work activities, and to promoting independent living for all disabled persons. With such changes, available knowledge has to be reappraised and adapted for use as we move into the 1980s.

The *Annual Review of Rehabilitation* began with a special effort to reappraise and adapt knowledge in the rehabilitation field. The Rehabilitation Services Administration funded a project in which all three editors participated (the first author of this introduction as principal investigator) in a project designed to develop monographs on topics of urgent concern in rehabilitation. A consumer panel representing rehabilitation counselors, administrators, researchers, RSA, and disabled consumers worked to select the topics addressed in this project, concentrating on particularly visible issues of concern to the rehabilitation field nationally.

At the end of the project, it seemed apparent that a highly useful mechanism for identifying topics of real relevance to rehabilitation professionals, and then developing information packages about them, had been created. We decided to use this already-existing mechanism as a springboard for creating the *Annual Review of Rehabilitation.* The four monographs prepared for the project were condensed into chapters for this volume, and the consumer panel was expanded and turned into the *Review's* advisory board. Once a publisher was found, we were on our way.

**Psychosocial/vocational rehabilitation* (PSV), a relatively new term promoted by such organizations as the American Psychological Association's Division of Rehabilitation Psychology, is used to distinguish all other types of rehabilitation services from medically based physical restoration. This volume will concentrate mainly on developments in PSV rehabilitation, although there will also be selected coverage of physical rehabilitation (e.g., major parts of the chapter on rehabilitation of burn patients).

Why did an annual review volume in rehabilitation take such a circuitous path? It is perhaps significant that this effort sprang from a project funded under the RSA's research utilization program, which also sponsors a number of other efforts to accumulate knowledge and make it more accessible, such as the *Research Indexes, Research Abstracts, R&D Briefs,* and the National Rehabilitation Information Center (NARIC). These publications, in conjunction with NARIC and other support systems for knowledge utilization, make it possible for the first time to achieve a truly broad overview of what knowledge in fact exists in the rehabilitation field. Perhaps these efforts, plus the changing focus in rehabilitation services, were necessary events before the *Annual Review* could fruitfully develop.*

OVERVIEW OF VOLUME 1

Our first volume begins, appropriately enough, with an overall perspective on rehabilitation services. Although not a review of literature like our other chapters, Robert Humphreys' chapter gives us the long view of rehabilitation moving into the 1980s. Humphreys' chapter highlights some of the concepts that will guide RSA's efforts over the next decade and provides one way of looking at many of the individual contributions to this volume.

Herbert Dorken's chapter on national health insurance focuses on another prime moving force that will have much impact on rehabilitation in the 1980s. Similarly, James Reswick's treatment of rehabilitation engineering and Frank Bowe, Frederick Fay, and Janet Minch's chapter on consumer involvement and advocacy identify major new trends in the rehabilitation field that will be of major importance throughout the coming years. And Susan Stoddard's chapter on independent living uses as its title what will doubtless be one of the principal catch phrases in rehabilitation for the immediate future. Closer to the domain of rehabilitation research, but still dealing with subjects that very closely touch the lives of practitioners and clients, are the chapters on outcome measurement by Thomas E. Backer, on performance measures by Linda Barrett and Susan Shea, and on the impact of psychosocial research by Jerold Bozarth and John Barry. Carolyn Vash's review of sheltered industrial employment is more directly in the practice area, and perhaps the most practitioner-oriented of all are the reviews on sensory disabilities by Hilde Schlesinger and Margaret Lee, on severe burns by Garry Brody and Mark Johnson, on spinal cord injury by

*The *Annual Review* is not now, nor was it in the past, supported financially by RSA, but the project mentioned above did provide a helpful start.

Roberta Trieschmann, and on pulmonary disease by William Miller. Yet these too contain information that will be relevant to researchers attempting to find new solutions for some of the many problems faced by persons with various disabling conditions.

Thus, there is in this volume a balance among concerns and issues relevant to practitioners, administrators, and researchers. We hope to maintain this healthy balance in future editions of the *Annual Review of Rehabilitation.*

MASTER PLAN

The key mechanism by which balance and comprehensiveness in coverage will be attempted is the master plan. This plan was developed in collaboration with our advisory committee, and is an effort to delineate the boundaries of the field of rehabilitation as covered in this and succeeding volumes of the *Annual Review.* In the list that follows, we present the master plan, along with notations concerning the time frame for coverage of each topic. We will, of course, be open to some variation in the structure imposed by the plan, depending upon future developments in the rehabilitation field. The plan is intended only to provide guidance, not to rigidly limit what can be included in subsequent volumes of the *Annual Review.*

	*Time Coverage**
ADMINISTRATION	
Economics of Rehabilitation	I
Management of Rehabilitation Organizations	I
REHABILITATION PROCESS	
Case Management	3
Counseling	3
Work Preparation	5
Placement	3
Medical Rehabilitation	3
Rehabilitation Engineering	3
Referral	5
Intake	5
Outreach	5

*3 = articles in this area every three years; 5 = every five years; I = articles in this area intermittently.

Follow-up Research	5
Client Evaluation	5

HUMAN RESOURCES DEVELOPMENT

Education and Training	3
In-service Training	5

SERVICES DEVELOPMENT

Research Methods	5
Program Evaluation	5
Knowledge Transfer and Organizational Change	5

TOTAL REHABILITATION

Deinstitutionalization	5
Independent Living	3
The Family and Rehabilitation	3
Sexual Aspects of Rehabilitation	5
Consumer Advocacy	5
Barriers	3
Recreation	5
Social Aspects of Disability	3

DEMOGRAPHIC GROUPS

Aging and Chronically Ill	5
Homebound	5
Rural	5
Children	5
Severely Disabled	3

DISABILITY TYPES

Spinal Cord	5
Cardiovascular	5
Neurological	5
Neuromuscular	5
Emotional Impairment	5
Pulmonary	5
Sensory	5
End-state Renal	5
Mental Retardation	5
Head Trauma	5
Severe Burns	5

SETTINGS

State VR Agencies	I
Facilities	I
International	I

The direction in which we are moving to implement this master plan can be seen in the tentative topic list for Volume 2 of the *Annual Review.*

Work Disincentives	*Monroe Berkowitz*
Program Evaluation in Vocational Rehabilitation	*Robert Struthers*
Job Placement	*Dennis Dunn*
Sex and Disability	*Susan Daniels*
Follow-up Research	*Brian Bolton*
Private Facilities	*Keith Gardner*
Comprehensive Client Evaluation	*Fred McFarlane*
Information Delivery in Rehabilitation	*Judy Senkevitch and Helga Roth*
Case Management	*Bryan Kemp*
Epilepsy	*Robert Fraser*
Mental Retardation	*Tony Appoloni*
Cerebral Palsy	*Jack Jonas*

We already are making plans for Volume 3 as well, after which some revisions in our master plan are anticipated (on the basis of experiences with the first two volumes).

SUGGESTIONS FOR USING THE ANNUAL REVIEW

An annual review volume can be seen as something of a hybrid between an encyclopedia and a newspaper of record such as the *New York Times;* we also want our *Annual Review of Rehabilitation* to provide a perspective on the various topics we cover in each volume, including the personal viewpoint of the authors who prepare our chapters. In achieving this multiplicity of purposes, we have attempted to minimize the number of structural constraints on authors, but there are a few common features of each chapter that should make the *Annual Review* somewhat easier to use. An introductory portion indicates the scope of coverage, the general orientation of the chapter, and, if appropriate, the mechanism used to develop the chapter. It also provides any needed definitions of terms. This is followed by the main body of the chapter, which is a review of current literature and practices in the area covered. Next is a discussion section that highlights the critical elements of the chapter and gives implications for policy, research, and practice. Finally, a list of references cited in the chapter is presented.

We have also provided an overall index of subjects and authors for the *Annual Review,* and some readers may want to use these indexes selectively as a supplement to reading given chapters. Reference citations can be used as a starting point for a literature search in any area of interest to the reader, and the RSA-sponsored publications mentioned earlier may be helpful in tracking down desired articles, books, or research reports. Inquiries to the National Rehabilitation Information Center,* or to other clearinghouses for information in the social sciences and human services, may also be of value. And readers may well want to enlarge their knowledge in given subject areas by direct interactions with their professional colleagues, including the authors in this volume. The best-validated principle in research on the knowledge utilization process is that knowledge useful in stimulating significant change comes primarily through *personal contact.*

Since this is the first volume of the *Annual Review of Rehabilitation,* the editors regard themselves very much as students of the process by which useful annual review volumes can be developed and brought to fruition. Feedback on how future volumes could be improved in any aspect—structure, writing style, content, cycling, and so forth—will be welcomed. Through such communication with our readership, each succeeding volume should be superior to its predecessors in usefulness and readability. Your comments may be addressed to: Elizabeth L. Pan, Ph.D., President, Institute for Information Studies, 200 Little Falls Street, Suite 202, Falls Church, Virginia 22406.

*National Rehabilitation Information Center, Eighth and Varnum Streets, N.E., The Catholic University of America, Washington, D.C. 20064.

1

Disability in America: 1980 and Beyond

ROBERT R. HUMPHREYS, LL.B.

In this paper, Commissioner Robert R. Humphreys presents his concepts for the development of a national policy on disability which offers a rational basis for more effective and more comprehensive service delivery. He views the need for such a policy as critical in an era of limited resources. After reviewing the major legislation related to handicapped people as opportunities for new initiatives, the author describes his basic framework for future action.

Disabled individuals represent a sizable minority of the nation's population. Despite recent substantial advances, the needs of this population are still addressed in an ad hoc, piecemeal fashion, without an overall strategy, policy, or plan to use as the basis for service delivery which meets all, or a large percentage of, those needs. As a result, there are service gaps and unmet needs, and there is no coordinated, comprehensive network for the provision of services.

Our country cannot afford the enormous social and economic costs —the waste of human talents—that accrue from allowing, and even forcing, millions of disabled people to live in a state of dependency. Nor can we as professional people, service providers, and consumers afford to be lulled by the successes of the current decade into a belief that the "revolution" in expanding opportunities for handicapped people will have an inevitable and positive outcome. If such an outcome is to result, it must be carefully planned and developed.

This paper proposes that a national policy on disability be constructed which offers a rational basis for more effective and more comprehensive service delivery. The creation of such a policy becomes a critical necessity in an era of limited federal, state, and local resources. These resources must be marshaled in such a way as to ensure the maximum efficiency in their use and the minimum waste, duplication, and overlap in their distribution. This short treatise does not purport to address all of the needs of this important segment of our society, for the needs are many and complex. But it does focus on the *scope* of the issues involved and offers the beginning of a conceptual framework for future action. Further, it strongly recommends the exploration of bold new approaches in order to ensure more rationality, coherence, and efficiency in the nation's efforts to help citizens with disabilities.

MAGNITUDE OF THE PROBLEM

Statistical descriptions are limited in their ability to portray the human condition. To say that there are millions of disabled individuals does not tell us how these individuals are coping. Statistics, however, do provide some measure of the size of problems and extent of needs. The following figures[1] provide us with a picture of the magnitude of these needs.

- About 24 million Americans have arthritis. Of these, some 5 million are handicapped by it and 475 thousand are receiving Social Security disability benefits (SSDI).
- There are 250,000 to 500,000 adult Americans with multiple sclerosis.
- According to a survey conducted by the National Association of the Deaf, some 13 million Americans are hard of hearing. Of these, a little over 1½ million are severely disabled by deafness and an estimated 100,000 are "low-functioning" deaf.
- Over 5½ million people are mentally retarded. Of these, about 3½ million are substantially handicapped.
- More than 4 million Americans have epilepsy, of whom almost 1½ million are substantially handicapped by this condition.
- At least 2 million adults with severe, persistent psychiatric disabilities reside in local communities outside of an institutional support environment.
- The following ratios, provided by the Social Security Administration, apply to totally disabled people in relation to nondisabled people:

Hospitalization (men)	*four times* as often as nondisabled.
Days hospitalized	*three times* longer than nondisabled.
Cost of medical care	*three times* higher than nondisabled.

Median cost of care as a percentage of income	*five times* as high as nondisabled.
Average income	*half* that of nondisabled.

- Only 50 percent of totally disabled men and 60 percent of totally disabled women have health insurance protection, compared with 90 percent of those who are not disabled.
- Over 37 percent of totally disabled people have incomes, earned and unearned, below the poverty level.
- Fully 76 percent of totally disabled men and 87 percent of totally disabled women are not in the labor force; only 12 percent and 2 percent, respectively, work full-time.
- Educational achievement and disability are inversely related. That is, 9 percent of totally disabled people have attended college, as opposed to 30 percent of those who are not disabled. Further, 44 percent of the totally disabled population have no more than an elementary school education, compared to only 13 percent of the nondisabled.
- Although rates of marriage are comparable for totally disabled and nondisabled people, the totally disabled are twice as likely as their nondisabled counterparts to be divorced or separated.

There are also extraordinary expenses faced by disabled people that the able-bodied do not have. An electric wheelchair costs from $3,000 to $4,000, with *annual* maintenance costs of $1,200 to $1,600—more than most automobiles. Interpreters for deaf people, readers for blind people, attendants for people with severe physical disabilities, and home health care all represent continuing expenses for disabled people. Adding to the complexity and the challenge of these factors is the phenomenon of a steadily increasing number of handicapped people. Estimates place the annual incidence of disability for persons who may be eligible for vocational rehabilitation at between 500,000 and 800,000.

The total incidence of disability is far higher, and there are many reasons for this. A major reason is the constantly accelerating advance in medical and biomedical knowledge and technology. People with congenital defects, traumatic injuries, or disabling diseases who would have died a generation or two ago are, through these advances, being sustained. Another reason is the increasing number of people who live longer and who consequently suffer diseases of old age, such as arthritis, renal disease, retinitis pigmentosa, and many others. Recreational, automobile, and motorcycle accidents contribute substantial numbers of people with spinal cord injuries and traumatic brain damage. Cancer, stroke, and heart disease continue, inexorably, to add to the list of disabled people.

ON THE THRESHOLD OF CHANGE

The period just ahead is a time of unparalleled opportunity for federal, state, and local governments, voluntary agencies, business and labor, and private citizens to advance the quality of life for people with disabilities. Most especially, it is a time of opportunity for disabled people to help themselves achieve a fuller life. It is a time to build upon the increased awareness of, and sensitivity to, the rights, problems, needs, and concerns of disabled persons that have been manifested in a wide variety of developments, particularly of a legislative nature, over the past five years.

The Rehabilitation Act of 1973,[2] which called for a major revamping of the vocational rehabilitation (VR) program, was a giant step in this direction. Priority was given to severely handicapped people. A new program of client assistance projects, designed to aid disabled participants in coping with the VR system, was established. An Office for Handicapped Individuals was created to serve as an information clearinghouse and coordinator for HEW programs that serve disabled people. An individualized written rehabilitation program was required for all vocational rehabilitation clients. The latter assured a partnership between the agency (in the person of the counselor) and the handicapped person.

The most dramatic innovations in this law were the provisions of Title V, which have often been characterized as the Civil Rights Act for handicapped people. These include the antidiscrimination mandate of Section 504, requirements for affirmative action by the federal government and government contractors under Sections 501 and 503, and the Architectural and Transportation Barriers Compliance Board in Section 502. When fully implemented, these provisions will have profound and lasting effects on the very fabric of American society. They will mean opportunity for a long neglected but important part of our population in the areas of employment, health care, transportation, housing, education, legal rights, voting, and recreation, among others.

In 1975, the Developmentally Disabled Assistance and Bill of Rights Act[3] was aimed at improving services to people who are mentally retarded, epileptic, cerebral palsied, or autistic. It set forth guidelines for the treatment and care of institutionalized mentally retarded people in an effort to correct frequently deplorable conditions that had existed in many institutions. Protection and advocacy systems were required to be instituted in all states. Emphasis was placed on plans and projects which would result in appropriate deinstitutionalization.

Public Law 94–142, the Education for All Handicapped Children Act,[4] is yet another major legislative milestone in the national effort to bring about changes that will benefit handicapped people. Under that law, all disabled children must be provided a free, appropriate, public education. As with the Rehabilitation Act, an individual education plan must be written—in this case, for each handicapped child, with participation by the child's parents or guardian.

The White House Conference on Handicapped Individuals, another legislatively mandated effort of the amendments to the Rehabilitation Act of 1973, was held in May 1977.[5] Thousands of disabled and professional people and providers of services participated. Just as important, numerous state and regional conferences were held in preparation for the national conference, in which thousands more took part. Hundreds of recommendations for action to be taken by various Federal Executive Branch agencies, the Congress, states, and communities emanated from that momentous gathering.

On November 6, 1978, President Jimmy Carter signed the Rehabilitation, Comprehensive Services and Developmental Disabilities Amendments of 1978.[6] The new law contains many innovations. For the first time, independent living services are specifically authorized for people who are severely disabled and have little, if any, employment potential. A new National Council on the Handicapped is to be established which will significantly increase the involvement of disabled consumers and professionals in the field of disability in the development of federal policy. A National Institute of Handicapped Research is to be created. A Community Service Employment Program is authorized to provide full and part-time employment opportunities to handicapped people. The new Act includes other expansions and refinements of many elements contained in the Rehabilitation Act of 1973. In the developmental disabilities amendments, an expanded definition of the target population creates a broader base for that program.

Finally, the Rehabilitation Services Administration (RSA), which is the principal federal agency concerned with the delivery of services to disabled people, has recently undergone a major reorganization. The purpose of that effort is to improve the agency's capacity to respond to the emerging problems and opportunities in service delivery and to give the agency some new areas of emphasis so that it may assert a leadership role in policy, planning, coordination, and advocacy.

The new RSA has four major offices: two line offices—Program Operations and Program Development; and two staff offices—Policy Management and Advocacy and Coordination.

Program Operations is the "hub" of the agency, to use an analogy to the wheel, while Program Development represents the spokes of the wheel. Operations include VR program administration, the Social Security rehabilitation programs, facilities, Developmental Disabilities, and the Randolph-Sheppard program.

Program Development includes all of RSA's discretionary grant activities in research, engineering, training, special projects, evaluation, utilization, and international projects.

The new Office of Advocacy and Coordination will have day-to-day contact with groups, organizations, and individuals in order to be more responsive to the needs of the populations served. A consumer communication system will be established to bring federal, state, and local agency response quickly to the problems and needs of disabled citizens.

"Disability desks" are planned, which will be staffed with people who have broad and extensive knowledge of specific disabilities and the various programs serving those disabilities. A White House Conference Implementation Action Unit has been established to guide HEW and other federal agencies in focusing attention on the White House Conference recommendations.

Coordination with other federal agencies and programs will be of vital importance in this era of scarce resources. We must develop the capacity to marshal the resources that *are* available in the most efficient and effective manner possible. This means maximum coordination and elimination of expensive duplication and overlapping of efforts.

We need, for example, to establish cooperative program relationships with public education, social services, mental health, the Labor Department, the Social Security Administration, HUD, the Department of Transportation, and other agencies. We need to accelerate our interaction with private organizations, labor, and industry.

The Deafness and Communicative Disorders Office, part of Advocacy and Coordination, will aid in bringing new emphasis to programs for a seriously underserved handicapped population.

Finally, to ensure that research, engineering, and utilization efforts have maximum impact through our own efforts and those of the Veterans Administration, NASA, the National Science Foundation, and the National Academy of Sciences, RSA will work on disability prevention in conjunction with the National Institutes of Health and other agencies of the Public Health Service.

The Office of Policy Management, through policy analysis and development and planning, will give us the capability of focusing on broad and long-term policy issues and giving attention to long and short-term planning needs. The office gives us the capacity to propose courses of action rather than merely reacting, on an ad hoc basis, to short-term events.

Given this progress on conceptual, legislative, and administrative fronts, the challenge that faces us now is to seize the opportunity to expand the quality of services, and indeed, the quality of life for disabled people by moving toward a more rational and comprehensive approach to service delivery.

TOWARD A COMPREHENSIVE SERVICE SYSTEM

Although numerous programs are designed to provide services to disabled people, and although many of these programs are eminently successful in addressing a portion of the total need, there is as yet no overall direction or plan to meet the complex and interrelated needs of the disabled person as a total individual. There are many reasons for this deficiency, including the highly specialized nature of our society and the political realities involved in establishing and maintaining service programs. We must move toward developing a national policy on disability which looks at the total spectrum of needs of handicapped persons if we are to take full advantage of recent legislative developments and attitudinal improvements.

A system is needed for the delivery of a full range of services to disabled people in America. There are now many scattered programs which, with varying levels of adequacy, address different needs of these people. Some of these are directed to the special needs of this population, such as rehabilitation services and Social Security Income Assistance. Others are not specifically directed to disability, such as the Social Security Act's Title XX, food stamps, the Comprehensive Employment and Training Act, and Head Start. Since there is no coherence, pattern, or plan relating to the provision of services, the needs of the *whole person* are nowhere considered. As a result, there are major gaps in services and, as a result, pervasive unmet needs.

In the absence of comprehensive plans and policies to meet those needs, it is a logical consequence that *capacity* is also lacking on the part of federal, state, and local governments, and in the private sector, to provide a full range of services. In addition, government and private funds in past years have been spent on facilities and services that are now perceived to be inappropriate.

These deficiencies in policy, planning, services, and facilities all represent barriers to the full integration of people with disabilities into the mainstream of American society. Since these deficiencies have existed since the beginning of our nation, disabled people, for the most part, have been hidden, sheltered, and institutionalized. Because they are perceived as being "different" from the able-bodied, and because they have not been visible in our society, they are all too often misunderstood and even feared.

Fear, misunderstanding, and a sheltered environment have resulted in a society that either ignores the needs of this population or abuses it. Barriers, not only physical but also attitudinal, are the legacy of long generations of neglect.

The task for society, then, is to correct its errors. The Rehabilitation Services Administration is working to provide a conceptual framework for the accomplishment of this through a planned, comprehensive network for service delivery, to begin to fill some of the gaps in services and service delivery capacity, and to improve public awareness and attitudes.

The following assumptions are offered as the basis for evolving a national policy on disability. They are presented as the starting points which, hopefully, will grow and mature through the process of informed debate and rational deliberation.

The ideal structure for comprehensive service delivery would ensure a continuum of service for all disabled people ranging from preconception through senescence. This implies the coordinated development of a capacity to provide five levels of care and service: prevention, maintenance, amelioration, habilitation, and rehabilitation.

In order to ensure continuity of services in a holistic framework—one that views the whole individual—it is necessary to provide a focal point in government to coordinate both the activities of service providers and the programs under which services are provided. RSA is responsible for administering the vocational rehabilitation program and the developmental disabilities program, staffing the President's Committee on Mental Retardation, following up on the recommendations from the White House Conference on Handicapped Individuals; and planning U.S. participation in the United Nations' International Year for Disabled Persons. Under the new law it has also been charged with important new responsibilities in independent living and other areas. The new National Council on the Handicapped, possibly utilizing the recommendations of the White House Conference as a base, could be a partner with RSA in the formulation of such a policy.

Pending the development of a national policy, a conceptual framework for building a comprehensive service delivery network for people with disabilities should be developed. Such a network would necessarily include (1) institutionalization for those who are so profoundly disabled that no alternative living arrangements are feasible; (2) independent living rehabilitation, including transitional living, and halfway house accommodations, and a broad range of services to help disabled people who have no vocational goal to develop the capacity to live independently and normally in their homes and communities; (3) vocational rehabilitation for persons, both severely and less severely disabled, who reasonably can be expected to develop vocational goals; (4) community-based services to ensure that a continuum of services is available at the local level for all disabled people who are not in institutions. The level of services and their intensiveness would depend on the needs of the person. Many disabled people will need some services throughout their lifetime, which may not be directly proportional to the level of their disabilities. The schematic in Figure 1 portrays, in broad terms, the scope of this network.

Examples of the range of services under these existing and proposed programs include:

- *Community-based services (all disability levels, all ages):* equal employment; affirmative action; architectural barrier removal; tax abatement; financial incentives; local information, referral, and outreach; public health—prenatal and postpartum testing, immunization; integrative government social service agency programs; technical assistance to school systems; appropriate education assurance; transportation; recreation; public safety; and public awareness and education.
- *Vocational rehabilitation services (working-age population, vocational goals):* counseling and guidance; evaluation of rehabilita-

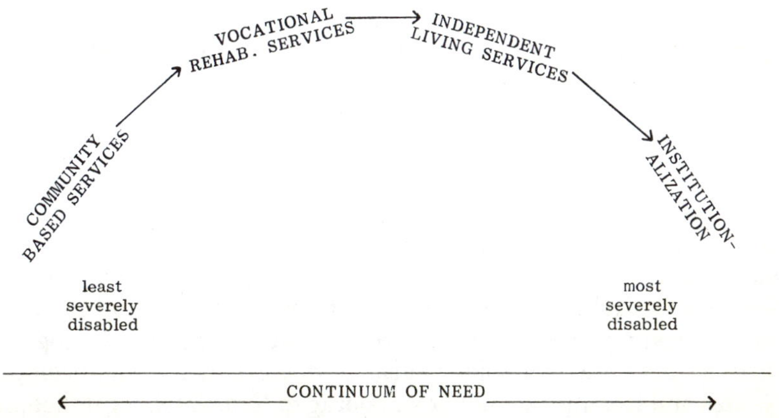

FIGURE 1

tion potential; provision of aids and devices; maintenance during rehabilitation; interpreter and reader services; vocational and other training services and materials; transportation related to vocational rehabilitation services; restoration services; extended evaluation; family services; job development; placement and follow-up; and recruitment and training services.

- *Independent living services:* attendant management and attendant care; financial management; mobility and transportation; home management and chore services; medical maintenance and self-care; transitional living arrangement; recreation; peer counseling and self-advocacy training; sexual and personal adjustment; social skills and problem solving.
- *Institutional services (all ages, most severely disabled):* activities of daily living; educational development; medical care and other life-sustaining services; physical exercise; and social development.

A nationwide network of comprehensive services to disabled people incorporating mechanisms, delivery systems, and coordination points must be established. Greater stress should be placed on community-based services. As a first step, local capacity needs to be developed through regional, intergovernmental resource centers which will provide technical assistance, guidance on integrative programing, model ordinances, and public information materials. Such centers would aid communities in their regions in developing community service mechanisms.

For independent living rehabilitation, grants should be provided to state vocational rehabilitation agencies, community-based organizations, private nonprofit and possibly profit-making organizations, and consumer organizations and cooperatives of disabled consumers. Close coordination with vocational rehabilitation agencies is essential so that people who develop vocational goals as a result of independent living rehabilitation can easily be transferred to the vocational rehabilitation program.

A much stronger link between vocational rehabilitation and employment should be forged through a major new cooperative effort with business and labor. Vocational rehabilitation agencies should work on a continuing basis with industry councils in major cities and industrial areas to match jobs and vocational rehabilitation clients and to modify jobs to accommodate individual needs. Field testing, marketing, and distribution of new technology aids and devices should be developed.

States and localities should be encouraged to develop a gatekeeping capacity to prevent institutionalization of people and to remove people from institutional settings where such placement is inappropriate, and to ensure, for people for whom institutionalization is required, provision for adequate community alternatives for persons who are kept out of or removed from institutions, so that the best possible conditions are maintained.

To ensure that the rights of disabled people are safeguarded and that voluntary compliance with laws protecting those rights is fully accomplished, technical assistance to states, government contractors, and recipients of federal financial assistance should be increased. To do so, protection and advocacy systems should be expanded in each state; community-based offices should provide counseling to disabled people on their rights under law and on means to break down barriers that confront them in the environment; and a nationwide client assistance program should provide ombudsmen for ensuring that vocational rehabilitation and other service system clients receive appropriate attention to their needs.

To eliminate fear, mistrust, and misunderstanding in the community so that attitudinal barriers and impediments to community support can be removed, community advocacy and information functions should be established through the regional centers described above. Public forums and discussions should also be encouraged.

Some additional new directions to be explored include:

- Working toward a fully coordinated home start—Head Start—special education—vocational education—vocational rehabilitation program, nationwide.
- Conducting a comprehensive national survey of disability and service needs, with consequent development of a national data system on disability.
- Mounting a major outreach and referral program with respect to disabled people who are most egregiously underserved—those with multiple physical or mental disabilities combined with cultural and economic deprivation.
- Creating a coordinated program of deinstitutionalization involving transitional living, group homes, and habilitation and rehabilitation services.
- Eliminating work disincentives now inherent in the Social Security rehabilitation programs.
- Supporting legal assistance centers for people with disabilities to protect their rights under Title V of the Rehabilitation Act.

- Establishing a nationwide system of client assistance programs so that through ombudsmen, disabled individuals will be able to cope with "the system" to obtain the fullest possible service benefits appropriate to their individual needs, delivered in the most expeditious and efficient manner possible.
- Demonstrating new approaches to meeting the transportation and residential needs of disabled people, including new joint initiatives with the Department of Transportation and the Department of Housing and Urban Development.
- Initiating cooperative, focused research efforts in central nervous system (spinal cord) regeneration and in other high-priority areas of disability prevention, amelioration, and treatment.
- Adopting a new focus for international rehabilitation interchanges to take advantage of technological and service delivery innovations of developed nations.
- Exploring ways to meet the need for new or renovated rehabilitation facilities and physical improvements in institutions which house physically and mentally disabled people.

CONCLUSION

These are exciting times for disabled Americans because the potential exists for dramatic breakthroughs for their well-being. We must have the will and the determination to see to it that being disabled in America is not a continuation of that which has gone on before. We must, as a government and as a society, reinforce our commitment to meet head-on one of the major challenges of our day: bringing into the mainstream of American society a vulnerable and precious human resource—the millions of disabled citizens in our land.

NOTES

[1]DHEW, Social Security Administration, Office of Research and Statistics, "Work Disability in the U.S.: A Chartbook", Washington, D.C., June 1977.

[2]Public Law 93–112, 93rd Congress, H. R. 8070, September 26, 1973.

[3]Public Law 94–103, 94th Congress, H. R. 4005, October 4, 1975.

[4]Public Law 94–142, 94th Congress, S6, November 29, 1975.

[5]Public Law 93–516, 93rd Congress, H. R. 17503, December 7, 1974.

[6]Public Law 95–602, 95th Congress, H. R. 12467, November 6, 1978.

2

Perspectives on National Health Insurance and Rehabilitation*

HERBERT DORKEN, PH.D.
With a Commentary by Joseph La Rocca

From 1969, a succession of bills on national health insurance programs has been introduced before Congress. The United States is now the only industrialized nation in the Western world which does not have a comprehensive national health service or insurance plan. If national health insurance (NHI) is enacted, what effect will it have on related programs such as vocational rehabilitation?

"PERSPECTIVES ON NATIONAL HEALTH INSURANCE AND REHABILITATION" *considers this question and others of importance to vocational rehabilitation administrators and planners in the public and private sectors as they engage in future program planning and speculate about their own professional futures.*

This chapter describes the concepts and forms of health insurance, reviews pending legislation and existing programs, and discusses the major issues and implications of a nationally legislated program. Current experience with comprehensive health care programs in Connecticut, Canada, and the Civilian Health and Medical Program of the Uniformed Services (CHAMPUS) are examined and the implications of this experience for U.S. vocational rehabilitation programs discussed.

In its bibliography, more than eighty selected references are listed, adding perspective to the social, economic, and health care principles involved, together with data on the utilization of health services. A commentary by Joseph

*This chapter is based on a monograph of the same title that appeared as one of a series called "Emerging Issues in Rehabilitation," published by the Institute for Research Utilization (Washington, D.C., 1977) with funding support by the Rehabilitation Services Administration. The author wishes to thank the following individuals who contributed to the preparation of the earlier monograph: Mr. Clarence Martin, Dr. Charles A. Roberts, Mr. A. T. Blue, Mrs. Ann Steele, Dr. Steven Mogul, Dr. James Peters, Dr. Gordon H. Cumming, Dr. Thomas E. Backer, Dr. Elizabeth Pan, Ms. Susan Stoddard, and Dr. Carolyn L. Vash.

La Rocca, rehabilitation consultant, provides special insight into the concerns of vocational rehabilitation professionals about the issues surrounding national health insurance legislation and vocational rehabilitation.

INTRODUCTION

Implementation of the Rehabilitation Act of 1973, which places priority on services to the severely handicapped individuals, will change the clientele of state Rehabilitation Programs. Persons more disabled physically or mentally, including those with more severe sensory, locomotion, speech, and cognitive handicaps, will now be demanding services. It follows that the need for restorative services or remedial health care, to restore function or offset handicap, will be heightened. Will this require state vocational rehabilitation (VR) agencies to give increased emphasis and a higher proportion of limited fiscal resources to restorative services? Would this alter the character of state VR programs? If health care becomes increasingly important, will there be an increased medical direction to the rehabilitation process? If national health insurance (NHI) is enacted, will it control health/disability care and will this control spread to related programs such as rehabilitation?

The answers to these questions are of importance not only to the VR client but to agency staff as they attempt future program planning and speculate about their own professional future. There are as yet no absolute answers, but the purpose of this chapter is to review "insured" or prepaid health care, provide a perspective on this dialogue, and describe outcomes which seem desirable and probable.

From 1969, a succession and increasing number of NHI bills have been introduced before each session of Congress. The United States is now the only industrialized nation in the Western world which does not have a comprehensive national health service or insurance plan. In 1966 new Social Security programs were introduced: Medicare (Title XVIII) to provide health services to the elderly and certain disabled persons, and Medicaid (Title XIX) to provide medical assistance to the categorically needy, those on public welfare. The health and restorative services available to job-injured workers under workers' compensation laws are currently quite extensive. Health care is provided for military personnel and extensive health plans. Indeed, in periods of wage stabilization, more comprehensive health plan coverage is a typically negotiated fringe benefit. These programs and plans have different administrations, different sources of revenue, provide different benefits, and make different fiscal demands upon those eligible for service.

Both the privately and publicly financed programs now entitle about

90 percent of all residents of the country to some plan of health services. There may be a substantial gap, however, between the services available through a particular health plan and the actual need of the consumer for health care. A number of persons, for example, only have hospital insurance. And none of the insurance plans are designed for long-term care. The minority without any health insurance include some persons recently unemployed, many migrant workers, others who are marginally employed or are employed by small employers with a marginal business, and some self-employed persons.

Each of the major forms of health care plans has its proponents and opponents. Deriving some form of national consolidation will be a complex task. To better orient the reader to the concept of insurance and the different major forms of health insurance, a working definition of terms common to this field follows.

Premium payment, payroll deduction, and taxation are three common methods by which health/disability insurance or health service plans are *prepaid.* The price charged is based upon the predicted cost of the services that will be used/provided. Stated otherwise, the prediction is a financial calculation of the *risk* expected in terms of services to be provided and the charges for them. When the premium is the same for all persons or family groups in an area, the plan is *community rated.* If, however, a special premium is set either because of a favorable or a high-risk expectancy for a particular group of people, then it is *experience rated.*

Most plans allow the client/patient/consumer direct access and personal choice (freedom of choice) among qualified *providers* (practitioners) of named professions. Since the client or *user* has prepaid for the services to a *third party,* the insurance carrier, health care organization, or government agency, as the case may be, will make a *reimbursement* or payment for the charges billed. The charge paid for any service may be: an amount not to exceed rate limits; a *schedule of maximum allowances;* on a *UCR* basis, meaning that it is the provider's Usual charge for the particular service, is Customary in the area, and is Reasonable for the service; or on a preset or *prospective rate-setting* basis.

The services covered by the plan comprise a *benefit package,* while those not covered are *exclusions.* In all plans, the *entitlement* of the *beneficiary* will carry *limitations.* The limitations can be in terms of a dollar limit or duration of services, or the consumer may be obliged to pay a certain dollar amount of the costs first, *the deductible,* before the plan makes any reimbursement, or the consumer may have to pay a proportion of the costs, a *co-insurance.* Most plans do not allow duplication of benefits. When other coverage must be used first (e.g., workers' compensation), the plan provides only supplemental or *second-dollar coverage.* When other plans supplement, the plan benefits are *first-dollar coverage.* When it is possible to send on or accumulate all the charges to be forwarded to the third party for payment, the process is one of *pass-through costs.*

Some providers may agree with a particular plan not to charge more than a certain fee, so that it may be to the consumer's advantage to seek the services of such a *participating provider.* Typically, such plans will not pay extra for the services of nonparticipating providers, the user being billed the difference. When the user may select only from among providers in a specific group practice or health care organization, it is described as a *closed panel. Fee for service,* a piece-rate method of billing, is the traditional form of billing and paying for health care in private practice. In health plans where potential users subscribe to or enroll in the plan, the professional staff may be paid a salary on contract, with or without profit sharing, which does not vary by the amount of service/visits rendered but by professional standing (specialty credentials), seniority, and whether full- or part-time. Or providers in such plans may be paid on a *capitation* basis, a fixed amount for each subscriber/user for whom the provider is responsible, regardless of the visits made. Or the providers may charge the plan on a fee-for-service basis up to the funds available and be responsible for additional services, if any, that may be needed. Providers may also contract to render a block of services to a particular plan.

THE CONCEPT OF INSURANCE

Health insurance has become a popularized term. The insurance principle involves risk spreading and is at its best when it protects against a large loss that is unlikely to happen. Given that the average person makes just over five doctor visits a year, and the elderly three times this number, it is obvious that we are not dealing with an unlikely event. What is commonly called health insurance is really prepayment of expenditures. Some generalizing of cost does occur. But for those with preexisting conditions, who are in hazardous occupations or who are unemployed, health insurance may be impossible to acquire.

In marketing experience, select individuals of low risk and apparent good health can be insured for less than the general community. In a competitive market, those who can buy better coverage at less cost typically do. As the balance of uninsured persons shrinks, the cost progressively rises. From this perspective, those who need coverage the most become those who can least afford it or even acquire it. And if we averaged out the costs for everyone, those with favorable experience plans would have to pay more, perhaps double.

The indigent, the chronically sick, and the handicapped, on the other hand, cannot, for the most part, afford to prepurchase health care. To the extent that they are to have health care, it must be publicly funded —funding which comes from those with earnings who can pay. The more closely we address the broad financing problems of health insurance, the more evident it becomes that national health insurance, like other social legislation, for whatever else it accomplishes, also involves a measure of income redistribution.

Insurance coverage can be viewed in four layers: minor expenses, such as doctor visits, preventive, and ambulatory care; basic protection, generally hospitalization and associated expenses; major medical plans which extend hospital benefits and provide some out-of-hospital costs; and catastrophic plans with high expense ceilings. The increasingly popular comprehensive plans are essentially a combination of the middle two levels. Whether derived from a collective bargaining agreement or as a fringe benefit of employment, in large part employer paid, these plans are attractive. Such group plans typically return more than 95 percent of the premium in benefits. For individual insurance, the return is generally little more than 55 percent.

With the exception of health maintenance organizations (HMO), foundations for medical care (FMC), and some individual practice associations (IPA), health insurance plans are essentially illness insurance. A common exclusion, for example, is general maternity coverage, since maternity is not seen as an illness or a traumatic accident. But the more widespread coverage for hospitalization leads to greater than necessary hospital use and higher expenses. Aggravating this is the pass-through cost mechanism of the third-party payer. The general focus, then, is not on the health care of the many but on illness care of the few. The providers, the hospitals, and the pharmaceutical industry are well covered. Not so the generally healthy consumer, whose basic need is for early intervention, prevention of illness, and health maintenance.

Rising health care costs are generating increasing public and political resistance. Adding on to the current system will hardly reduce or control costs. Nor would turning over service responsibility to a federal bureaucracy imbue the plan with a better sense of public access, to say nothing of the tremendous dislocation problems. Blue Cross-Blue Shield and all the commercial health insurers would no longer be in business for the design of prepaid plans; the marketing and sales and service as third-party intermediaries would be their business. Rather than augmenting or transfering existing health resources, perhaps the easier solution—the introduction of national health insurance—offers the potential for major reorganization of health care delivery—for systemic change.

FORMS OF HEALTH INSURANCE

Private health insurance may be grouped into five types. First are the stock or mutual health *insurance companies,* the commercial carriers such as Aetna, Metropolitan, Travelers, Prudential, Occidental, and hundreds of other companies, some 320 of which are members of the Health Insurance Association of America. The five companies cited are the largest underwriters of health/disability insurance which indemnifies against the costs of illness or injury.

Second are the "nonprofit" open-panel *hospital-medical service plan* corporations, such as Blue Cross or Blue Shield. Typically, they have a physician majority in the membership of their boards. The Blue Cross and Blue Shield corporations, which are registered in all states, collectively have a premium subscription volume which very closely approaches that of the insurance industry.

Third, there are the *health maintenance organizations* (HMO) like Kaiser-Permanente, which function with a closed panel of salaried practitioners who own and control their facilities. They are community-based and service radius restricted. In the few cities where they are well established, they are a major health resource. Nationally, their enrollment represents 8 percent of the population.

Somewhat related are the *foundations for medical care* (FMC). This newly emerging fourth model, pioneered in California, is beginning to receive close attention among county medical societies. Strong advocates of peer review, the foundations will contract for health service delivery on a prepaid at risk basis. Essentially each one is a federation of fee-service practitioners in a competitive health care organization. With the exception of the commercial carriers, the latter insurance plans are generally not regulated by the State Insurance Code but by the Business and Professions Code, Health and Safety Code, or the Government Code, depending on the state.

Finally, there are the self-insured *employee welfare benefit plans* of some unions and some large corporations, and several fraternal benefit societies.

Health insurance, broadly stated, has traditionally been a matter of state jurisdiction—and there are some strong pressures to keep it that way. However, in passing the HMO Development Act, Public Law

93–363, Congress made explicit provision that this federal law would supersede any state law which precluded the formation of an HMO or otherwise prevented this type of organized group practice. In more definitive fashion, the Employee Retirement Income Security Act, Public Law 93–406, brings all employee welfare benefit plans under federal jurisdiction.

The wide interstate variance in workers' compensation laws has brought National Commission inquiries, and there is now mounting pressure for passage of Section 2018 (Williams, N.J.) of the National Workers' Compensation Act, to set minimum national standards, among other things. Other far-reaching and significant health legislation is in place and is intended to break and set ground for national health insurance. The Social Security Amendments of 1972 created the multidisciplinary Professional Standards Review Organizations, first to review hospital services under Medicare but with the intent to progress throughout all phases of clinical services.

Placing controls upon the provider has implications not simply for quality assurance but also for cost control. It is the provider essentially who makes the treatment and care decisions which can be cost effective or lead to overutilization or unnecessary services. In January 4, 1975, Public Law 93–641, The Health Services Planning and Resources Act, a sleeper bill, was enacted. This totally revises health planning, requires the creation of health service areas within each state, and will control the allocation and use of various categories of federal funds and assure consumer representation in the planning process. Thus, while it may seem that we have been holding an endless debate on national health insurance without progress, the foundations for change are being laid.

THE DIALOGUE ON NATIONAL HEALTH INSURANCE

Various committees of the House of Representatives and the Senate have held scores of public hearings on the subject of national health insurance (NHI). The purposes of these hearings are many: to measure dissatisfaction with the present system—some would say nonsystem; to entertain innovative proposals for change; and basically to assess the public mood on this topic. Every major health profession has testified. So, too, have hospital organizations, the pharmaceutical industry, employer organizations, unions, and consumer groups.

As the dialogue continues, there appears to be a concurrent move by the insurance industry and by health (medical) care service plans to become more comprehensive in their coverage for those they insure—

those who have prepaid their care. They are also attempting to narrow, or at least theoretically close, the gap so that no self-responsible, independent person is not eligible to purchase a policy. Provider groups, for their part, are subtly, and sometimes not too subtly, attempting to guarantee their professional future. Hospitals are sectionalizing components to convalescent care facilities and ambulatory health care centers, and further developing a working/training relationship with schools of the health professions.

The federal and state agencies are also making efforts to reorganize health care administration and health planning, and to exert cost controls. This is yet another measure of responsiveness.

If there has been such extended consideration of NHI, then why don't we have it? Because on almost every issue there is a core of fundamental disagreement. Concepts or principles in the abstract are one thing, but when implemented may be quite another.

Some Questions

Prevention is a great public health concept. The scientific evidence that fluorides assist in the prevention of tooth decay is clear. But many communities that have tried to fluoridate the public water system have run into a storm of public protest. The evidence on the association of increased risk of lung cancer and heart disease with cigarette smoking is also clear. Yet the growing of tobacco is not only subsidized by public funds, cigarettes are widely advertised and available. How about sex education, family planning, or abortions? Blood transfusions and inoculations, however beneficial, are contrary to some religious beliefs. Unnecessary malnutrition and overnutrition are widespread. So is the use of alcohol. Moreover, trends in the American life style seem to make life for many more precarious and less stable: the increased divorce rate; greater job and residential mobility; pressures for earlier retirement; and high rates of inflation and unemployment. Now, where do we draw the line on preventive endeavors? For all? For whom? Which aspects?

If there is to be NHI, how will it be financed? By premiums, by payroll taxes or deductions, by general revenue or "earmarked" revenue, or by some combination? Will it be a set rate for all, or graded or taxed by income? Will it include unearned as well as earned income, or only a certain level? The result of set rates would be that coverage for the needy would come from general revenue, as now, and the nation would be community rated. Health care costs substantially more in some areas than others. How you react to "leveling" probably depends on where you live. If some form of assessment is tied to income, then those earning more would find their health care costing more, perhaps a good deal more, and irrespective of their health status. Would those in the upper income brackets tolerate such a direct subsidy against their resources? Almost all variants have been proposed and there are proponents for each method, but no consensus by far.

Once the revenue has been secured, how will services be paid for? Will providers continue to receive their usual, customary, and reasonable (UCR) fee, or will fee schedules be adopted—mandated or negotiated—at rates typical of public service or private practice? Or will they receive a capitation amount—so much for each person in their care, whether well, sick, or very sick? Will providers become salaried? When providers are paid cash, whether directly or via health insurance, only those who pay gain access to care. Decisions to seek health care are, to an extent, economic decisions. If NHI carried universal entitlement, would the care resources be sufficient and would those who now have the access concur that access be equally shared? And who are the recognized providers anyway? Would medicine be the gatekeeper controlling entry to the health care system, designating the services to be provided and holding general supervision over the other professions? Dentists, podiatrists, optometrists, psychologists, nurses, social workers, and others have views on that! Or would consumers be given freedom of choice, and have direct access to the provider of their choice and of any discipline? Will brand name or generic drugs be covered? How much of the range of medical devices and health appliances should be included? Should it vary by age?

Now, with so much undecided, how will the program be administered? Will the only intrusion of government be to pay for the care of the needy? Should the revenue be collected by the federal government, with the administration by private enterprise or by local or state government? Should health be viewed as a natural resource and health care services established in a manner similar to a public utility? A cynical view is that we have the choice of being ripped off by the private sector or having our lives further controlled by government.

There is a serious concern about assuring access to health care for the handicapped, the unemployed, the needy, and the self-employed. Questions are being raised about escalating, inflationary costs, widespread fraud, and gross variance in level of benefits among state Medicaid programs. If NHI were federalized, would we want to see it tied to Medicare and Social Security? Will Social Security be solvent down the road? Does it provide an equitable return for the taxes collected? Do we even want the return to be equitable? Do we have assurance of stability from general revenue funding, knowing that it is subject to political decisions and incursions? For purposes of NHI, do we amalgamate all health care programs and render health care on a no-fault basis? Should NHI subsume Medicare and/or Medicaid? Should it include all or some of the following: the health/restorative services of Workers' Compensation; Vocational Rehabilitation; the Veterans Administration; the Public Health Service; the CHAMPUS; student health services; state hospitals; county mental health services; and others? Should NHI go beyond administering direct health care services and include: health research—basic and/or applied; the training of health professionals, indentured or with free choice of subsequent location; and public health regulations, such as air pollution, waste disposal, water standards, food inspection, and communicable disease control?

Hopefully this will suffice to illustrate that we are far from a consensus on major questions. We may not even have a majority agreement on most. It is obvious that important compromises will have to be reached or there will be no NHI. A lagging national economy adds further hesitancy in the face of uncertainty. An administration committed to NHI, however, might well catalyze public demand and achieve major change on fairly short notice.

Health insurance as we know it today seems designed to evade the clients of state Vocational Rehabilitation agencies. Many plans, especially individual policies, eliminate health care for prior existing conditions, do not provide for comprehensive rehabilitation coverage on either an inpatient or outpatient basis, or have a waiting period, perhaps two years, before care is provided for a prior health disability. The unemployed and marginally employed typically do not have access to health insurance. In any event, the objective of most plans is to enable active treatment but not long-term care.

Most of the NHI proposals to date, while making substantial modifications or provision for acute health services, retain the federal-state Medicaid plan for long-term care for those on categorical assistance and for the indigent. To the extent that acute health services will be beneficial to the VR client, particularly the more severely disabled client, access to NHI will be a decided asset not only to the client but also to the VR program. To the extent that long-term care, a network of social services, or an income maintenance program are essential, these resources will probably have to come from a source other than NHI.

There are fifteen Vocational Rehabilitation Services which are provided within the scope of a state agency's program. While the diagnostic services required in Evaluation of Rehabilitation Potential might to some extent be indirectly covered by a health plan as well as some counseling relative to personal adjustment and needed referrals, it is the Physical and Mental Restoration Services (CFR, Ch. XII, Title 45, Section 1361.1(2)) which could be subsumed in major part or at least enhanced by NHI. Not all fifteen Physical and Mental Restoration services are covered by any of the bills, so some gaps can be expected.

PERSPECTIVES OF CONGRESSIONAL STAFF

What follows represents the consolidated views and comments of five influential staff persons regarding the probable interface between national health insurance and Vocational Rehabilitation Services. Because the exchanges were informal, no one is identified. Interviewed in their Washington offices, early in June 1977, were staff to the Workers' Compensation Committee of Senate Labor and Public Welfare, the Subcommittee of Senate Finance, and Health Professions Educational Assistance programs in the Senate.

One clear consensus is that there are other priorities more pressing than NHI. These include the resolution of energy problems, tax reform, welfare reform, Social Security financing, and mechanisms for cost containment of health services. From this perspective, the view is that these issues need to be resolved before it becomes feasible to address NHI. But obviously these are major issues for which a current, but hardly a permanent, solution can be achieved. Compromises are likely, and the pressure of other issues will bring new priorities. There is a surplus of human needs but not of fiscal resources.

Any changes in Social Security and welfare reform could have major implications for those requiring long-term care. Any broadening of these programs—indeed, putting the Social Security Trust Fund on a self-sustaining basis—will likely require increased taxation unless the recipient population is narrowed as to age or eligible categories. To the extent that taxes are increased, the financing of NHI from new taxation may have less and, perhaps, no appeal. The current thrust of NHI is that it would be a national program. Another resolution would simply have federal law set standards and leave actual implementation to states. The state jurisdiction perspective is well entrenched throughout the insurance industry, whether in the areas of health, life, casualty, fire, auto, or workers' compensation insurance. The age and occupational mix vary among states. So too do population density, climate, and economic conditions, all factors which can have a bearing on health.

Generally, the state-administered VR programs, despite wide interstate variations, have broad congressional support. They are, of course, funded on a grant basis, leaving allocation and selection of clients to state administration. Service is not based on dollars prepaid or a reimbursement for approved services rendered. Most people, however, look upon their health insurance as a benefit package bought for use when they need it. Some of this attitude carries over to Social Security pensions, but the pensions are not an annuity bearing a direct relation to taxes invested. Other services may be provided to some but not to all. Public dissatisfaction with Medicaid is partly because of widespread interstate variance on services provided. There is also mounting concern about dramatically escalating costs—as in public welfare—while those paying are not benefiting.

The political dilemma is to simultaneously grasp the taxpayers' concern for public welfare, the public's tolerance/demand for new services, the taxes involved, and the degree to which government must administer a direct (clinical) health care service. President Franklin D. Roosevelt came within an ace of combining health insurance with Social Security in 1935. Later, President Harry S. Truman made an ill-fated attempt to introduce an NHI bill. In 1965, The Johnson administration settled for Medicare and Medicaid as additions to the Social Security Act. More recently, Representative Wilbur Mills came within one vote of gaining approval for the House Committee on Ways and Means to formulate an NHI bill in 1974, consolidating the many proposals before Congress. No one has come that close since. Even though—perhaps because—it would cut across political constituencies, there are some proponents for consolidating all health programs to achieve better continuity and more efficient health care.

Several of those interviewed think that to the extent health needs were covered through NHI, some state rehabilitation funds would be freed. The Health Security Act (Senator Kennedy, Mr. Corman) calls for the most comprehensive benefits, and would provide for more medical necessities for rehabilitation than any of the other NHI bills. Vocational rehabilitation is seen, however, as a separate categorical program.

Nevertheless, rehabilitation agencies would not come under a health service aegis. Although the agency may provide some medical service, if it is incidental to and not the main purpose of the agency, then it seems likely to remain apart from medical or health controls.

While NHI proposals generally do not explicitly include rehabilitation, they do consistently view workers' compensation as a separate program. The Medicare program (Title XVIII) also distinctly avoids duplicating workers' compensation. Operationally though, both pay for health services. Separating clearly job-related disabilities from the balance is far more complex than it first sounds. For example, there are a variety of occupations where certain toxins and diseases are common, but still in substantial dispute. The effect of cumulative job stress on physical and mental health is also under current debate. It is also well known that the extent of disability varies, independent of the specific injury. Thus, the interface between workers' compensation, health insurance, and related health services can be of direct consequence to the rehabilitation field.

CURRENT MAJOR NATIONAL HEALTH INSURANCE PROPOSALS

It does not seem productive to review all NHI proposals. A succession of such bills have been introduced since the 91st Congress. At this point, it appears that if and/or when NHI is adopted, it will not be a complete version of any single present bill. More likely, it will be an amalgamation of those components upon which agreement can be achieved and which are in line with the views of the administration.

Attempting to forecast the short- and long-term cost of NHI is a major dilemma. Congress is daily faced with the progressive rise in cost of Medicare and Medicaid far beyond expected levels.

The Health Security Act (Senator Kennedy, Mr. Corman) has the most sponsors to date, appears the most comprehensive in scope, and is the most ambitious. It has been years in development by the Committee for National Health Insurance (CNHI), popularly called the "Committee of 100," which has formulated the plan under the aegis of the AFL-CIO. It would create a federal administration within the Department of Health, Education and Welfare, which as part of the Social Security System would derive its funding 50 percent from general revenue and 50 percent from payroll and income tax. Coverage would be universal and without deductible or co-payment requirements. No private health insurance organizations would be used under the plan. There would be incentives toward organized arrangements for patient care. Medicare would be terminated and Medicaid in states with remnants left would be supplemental to Health Security. Similarly, CHAMPUS (see later section) would provide only those benefits not provided under Health Security. Coordination of Veterans Administration health care programs is a future possibility, but workers' compensation is excluded. Nearly the entire range of health care services, including catastrophic coverage, would be included.

Of specific interest to Vocational Rehabilitation programs is Section 403: "Funds made available under the Vocational Rehabilitation Act or under Title V of the Social Security Act (Maternal and Child Health) shall not be used, after the effective date of Health Security benefits, to pay for personal health services available under Title I of this Act, but they may . . . be used (a) to pay for institutional services which are either more extensive or intensive . . . or (b) to pay for special medical or other procedures peculiar to Vocational Rehabilitation . . . " (explanation added). Section 27(a)(7), dealing with other professional and supporting services, includes in accord with regulations " . . . rehabilitation services furnished by a freestanding rehabilitation center with which the Board has an agreement. . . . "

A polar opposite in terms of coverage is the *Catastrophic Health Insurance and Medical Assistance Reform Act* (Senators Long and Ribicoff, and Mr. Waggoner). It includes a medical assistance plan to federalize Medicaid and a choice of a federally administered plan or an approved private plan. Financing would be derived from a 1 percent payroll tax—general revenue for public assistance—and encouragement is intended for persons to secure improved basic health insurance to meet the deductible, the first 60 days in hospital, and $2,000 of medical expenses per family. This plan has considerable political appeal in some quarters. It could eliminate the threat of personal economic disaster due to large expenses for health care. It is also seen as improving Medicaid, costing the least, and being an incremental step toward eventual NHI. Its critics say that it would aggravate the inflation of health care costs by removing economic restraint upon high-technology procedures without improving the general level of health care. In any event, since benefits would be payable without regard to coverage of services under other public or private plans, it would complement restorative services and probably save the use of some Vocational Rehabilitation funds.

The *National Health Care Act* (Senator McIntyre and Mr. Burleson) is supported by the Health Insurance Association of America. This bill seeks to strengthen health planning and the development of ambulatory health care centers, and its benefits would be phased in over an eight-year period. Apart from a state plan for the poor, the two private plans (employee and individual) would be open to voluntary purchase with tax incentives. Funding is on a premium basis, with a $100 deductible and an annual limit of cost sharing for a family of $1,000. The plan includes incentives for training professional personnel on location in areas of need. It creates a state insurance pool and would coordinate malpractice and liability insurance. Medicare would continue, and a state plan would be available for the needy which could be selected in place of Medicaid. Vocational Rehabilitation clients insured under this plan would be entitled to full plan benefits which could be supplemented by restorative services.

Among the other major proposals before Congress is the *National Health Care Services Reorganization and Financing Act* (Mr. Ullman) sponsored by the American Hospital Association. It would abolish Medicare, establish new minimum federal standards for Medicaid, and limit assistance in other programs, such as child and maternal health, to noncovered benefits. Catastrophic coverage is a plan feature. The American Medical Association and the U.S. Chamber of Commerce have endorsed other plans. None appear to have an adverse impact upon Vocational Rehabilitation, however.

For historical reasons, because it is still considered by many to be a workable compromise and because it almost passed the House Committee on Ways and Means in 1974, the *Comprehensive Health Insurance Plan (CHIP)* endorsed by the Nixon administration should not be overlooked. It would have introduced a three-part program, each providing the same benefits: a private employee-employer plan; a state-assisted plan for low-income persons; and an expanded Medicare plan. For the private components, there were substantial co-payment requirements and a deductible. The plan had an antiduplication clause and would not pay for services under workers' compensation. Other federal programs for special groups would have continued to operate.

An interesting, and incremental, approach is the *National Health Insurance for Mothers and Children Act* (Senator Javits, Mr. Scheuer). It would provide comprehensive benefits to children and adolescents through age seventeen and a full range of maternity-related benefits to pregnant women. It would not pay for services covered under other government health programs. Children's preventive care services would be without charge, as well as covered services to the poor. Funding would be derived from a .1 percent Social Security tax increase collected from wage earners, employers, and the self-employed. This plan would continuously cover only the young, that segment of the population known to use fewer health services than adults or the aged, and for whom preventive services and early intervention could have the most impact.

The *Consumer Choice Health Plan*, drafted by economics professor Alain Enthoven of Stanford, proposes a regulated competition in the private sector. Modeled after the Federal Employees Health Benefits Program, it would provide competing alternatives and informed choice, with incentives for economy. A tax credit would replace the current deductibles for health insurance, and Medicaid beneficiaries would receive vouchers for qualified health benefits plans. There would be open enrollment, community rating, maximum out-of-pocket costs, a health plan identification/credit card, and continuity of benefits. Given flexibility in benefits, the extent of the tax credit could be phased in. The objective would be the transformation of the health care delivery system into competing organized systems. This proposal was submitted to HEW Secretary Joseph Califano in fall 1977. Enthoven comments that in reality, the alternative to a consumer choice system is a provider-dominated system—or, I would add, a government service.

THE CANADIAN EXPERIENCE

Our northern neighbor, with a territory larger than that of the United States but a population one-tenth the size, has many cultural, government, and other parallels to this country. Canada is a federation of ten provinces in which federal/"state" programs are common. Canada has had a national health insurance program in operation for more than fifteen years. A review of the Canadian experience could be instructive and add perspective to the considerations raised here. Arrangements were made to meet with several current and former officers of the Department of National Health and Welfare in Ottawa. Noteworthy from the start is that Canada's laws set a federal basis for agreements with the provinces, each of which administers its own health service program.

In 1957, Canada adopted the Hospital Insurance and Diagnostic Services Act. The provinces were to be granted overall 50 percent net costs for active treatment without time limit and with no ceiling on costs. The formula for payment to the individual provinces was designed to recognize regional disparity, and a higher percentage was recovered by the less expensive provinces than by the high-cost provinces. Then in 1961, the Medical Care Insurance Act was passed, again on a 50 percent matching basis with the provinces, for comprehensive and universal medical care. Provincial plans had to meet federal minimum standards, and not less than 95 percent of the population had to be enrolled. Professional service rates are essentially annually negotiated fee schedules. Physicians increasingly are salaried, particularly in certain provinces, such as Saskatchewan and Quebec, where their administration has developed health centers in areas of need. Salaried medicine is generally considered very well paid, however.

In any event, the pattern of federal standard setting, provincial (public) administration, and private service delivery (hospitals and practitioners) with rate controls is nationally established. In the early years, several provinces such as Ontario collected premiums to cover part of the cost of health services. Finding that inefficient, however, there has been an increasing proportion paid from general revenue and other more easily applied taxes which are less expensive to collect.

Before adoption of the Medical Care Insurance Act (Medicare), the Canada Assistance Plan (CAP) was passed in 1961. CAP also provides 50 percent federal matching and is very broad in its scope. It includes rehabilitation services. It continues categorical allowances, including unemployment insurance, but it specifically excludes workers' compensation and other third-party liabilities. Mental hospitalization was excluded from the Hospital Insurance Act, but CAP provides 50 percent matching for residential/welfare care, so many people have been transferred to Board Homes. Clients undergoing rehabilitation in psychiatric hospitals have been categorized under welfare, and transferred to the CAP. Similarly, the mentally retarded have been assigned to welfare. It appears to some that the caliber of services available to both chronic mentally disabled groups has declined, but no categorized studies have been conducted to confirm or refute this view.

The Canadian federal government has tried for five years to put a ceiling on Medicare and to renegotiate health insurance. Fully 28 percent of the federal budget now goes to health, or about 5 percent of the GNP, compared to 8.7 percent in the United States in 1976. The Federal-Provincial Fiscal Arrangements and Established Programs Financing Act (1977) combines federal dollars for postsecondary education, Medicare, and hospital insurance and establishes a per capita ceiling subject to cost of living adjustments. The previous legislation, with the exception of fiscal authorizations, continues. The provinces will receive a fixed amount, block grant, per capita plus $20 per capita for special programs such as nursing and home care. This is expected to lead to the conversion of some hospital and mental hospital beds to nursing home beds.

The programs must be universally available, and user charges cannot interfere with consumer access. The deterrent concept of co-insurance and deductible has essentially been dropped. Only Alberta and British Columbia still have user charges. There is concern that establishing a ceiling will lead to expanded provincial introduction of deterrents. The federal government, however, will now match on the basis of gross costs. In summary, the net effect of this Act is to peg the costs of health care. All nonhealth expenses will be transferred to welfare. Provinces able to save funds from their block grants may allocate these resources elsewhere.

The Vocational Rehabilitation of Disabled Persons Act (1960) has enabled provision of assessment, restorative services and counseling, and employment placement. But it serves only those who are potentially employable. Children and the elderly who are handicapped and need certain equipment cannot obtain it under this Act. Federal matching assistance to the provinces is at a 50 percent level. Workers' compensation is excluded.

The Social Services Act was submitted to Parliament in June 1977, with passage not yet completed in December 1977. It would codify the Canada Assistance Plan and has major implications for rehabilitation services. Priorities will be rehabilitation services for the disabled and support or independent living services for the aged and handicapped. It is separate from income support legislation. It is entirely a 50 percent matching program without limit; hence there will be provincial incentive to shift rehabilitative services to this Act, when adopted. It allows wide provincial latitude for contracting to nonprofit agencies, such as crisis centers, but physician and nursing services are not included. All restorative services normally sharable as health services would be excluded from rehabilitation costs. It is planned to transfer prosthetics services to the provinces to increase support for such local industry under this Act. The Act seeks to promote self-reliance, including the development of transportation services, subject to a user charge, much like public transportation. This 1977 legislation has now been withdrawn and replaced by "block-funding" legislation, which does have per capita ceilings but purports to give the provinces more flexibility.

The public funding for rehabilitation in Canada is derived from general revenues: that is, income and corporate taxes. However, grants are widely available to private agencies, and core grants are currently provided to twelve national agencies in the field (e.g., Canada Council of Rehabilitation Workshops, Canadian National Institute for the Blind, Canadian Association for Mental Retardation). The private sector's involvement is consistent with the concept of interdependence and distinguishing rehabilitation from a public welfare program. These core grants of $.62 million are projected to increase to $1 million by 1980. In addition, project grants of $.5 million have been provided to complement government programs and to assist in gap filling, advocacy, and public opinion feedback. This interrelationship is expected to increase, following passage of the Social Services Act.

Along with regulations, the laws are implemented through agreements with the provinces. There are no miminum standards. Provinces are encouraged to meet improved objectives rather than threatened with the "big stick" of regulatory control. Medical rehabilitation is separate from vocational rehabilitation. For the latter, the objective is employment. The quality of rehabilitation programs varies widely among the provinces. Rehabilitation of the alcoholic may be seen as medically oriented in British Columbia and as a social problem in Nova Scotia, and is funded accordingly. In general, there is an effort to normalize the life of the disabled.

Workers' compensation is paid for by the employers and provinces and is without federal involvement. It is also separate from rehabilitation.

Thus, the Canadian trend is to encourage provinces to implement and expand rehabilitation programs, fitting provincial needs rather than federal standards, and to sustain private agency involvement. Workers' compensation is viewed as a separate responsibility which should not encroach upon rehabilitation resources per se. And with expanded universal health care, the health service aspects necessary to rehabilitation have progressively been assumed by health services, enabling rehabilitation programs increasingly to concentrate upon vocational rehabilitation. Moreover, when the new Social Services Act is adopted, the matching funds available to rehabilitation will not have the per capita ceiling placed upon health care.

THE CONNECTICUT EXPERIENCE

As previously noted, the insurance industry is regulated by state law, with the responsible state agency headed by an Insurance Commissioner. There is no legal reason why any state could not adopt and pass a statewide health care act through which it could establish a state health service for direct health care, as distinct from public health or mental health programs or, alternatively, establish minimum standards which any plan/policy must meet and oblige universal coverage. Workers' compensation does this on a state-by-state basis for all job-injured employees.

Some fourteen states have mandated the inclusion of certain mental health benefits in all policies underwritten or delivered in the state. Laws have also been passed requiring the recognition of certain licensed practitioners in all health policies. But the first state approach to legislation of comprehensive health insurance was accomplished in Connecticut. In terms of jurisdictional principle, theirs is a fundamentally different approach. Nonetheless it seems a viable option for any state to establish a model rather than close a gap until NHI arrives. The implications apparently warranted an on-site inquiry with representatives of the insurance industry and the State's Department of Insurance in Hartford.

In 1975 Connecticut passed its Comprehensive Health Care Act No. 75-616, with some "clean-up" amendments the next year. While a few states have passed limited health insurance laws, such as the "catastrophic" health plan of Rhode Island, the Connecticut law was cited as a model for comprehensive, universally available state health insurance. Indeed, it closely follows the COIL Model Bill drafted by the Conference of Insurance Legislators. Group and individual plans must be *available* to all interested parties. A key provision was the creation of a risk reinsurance pool, established by the insurance industry to make coverage available to those who might otherwise be uninsurable. The law became effective in April 1976 but was not operational until October of that year. Has it affected rehabilitation services?

As of June 1977, there were very few subscribers, no group plans had been sold, and fewer than 1,000 individual plans were in effect: 256 by the insurance industry and about 500 by the Blue Cross-Blue Shield Services—this in a state of 3.1 million persons. The Traveler's Insurance Company administers The Health Reinsurance Association (risk-reinsurance pool) for the industry. The plan specifically excludes services for job-related injuries which are covered under workers' compensation. Doctor visits, except for illness and injury, do not meet the deductible; hence preventive care is not included. When first offered, there were also no maternity benefits, as pregnancy is neither an illness nor an injury.

As for rehabilitation, coverage is excluded, not directly but by plan management. There is a coordination, or nonduplication, of benefits provision whereby health and medical services attributable to auto casualty and workers' compensation must be basic. The facility in which the services are rendered must be a medical or hospital setting. This eliminates rehabilitation centers. Services provided by government or in government agencies, whether state hospital or vocational rehabilitation agencies within the state plan, are likewise excluded.

Since the state's Medicaid plan provides more comprehensive coverage than the minimum standards of this Act, there has been no attempt made by the state to buy coverage for this population. Nor would the requirement of a twelve months' wait before prior existing conditions could be covered enable the plan to qualify for federal financial participation: 50 percent matching.

In summary, the Connecticut Comprehensive Health Care Act makes health insurance available for those few persons who do not currently have, or otherwise qualify for, such coverage. But they must also be able to afford the per person deductible cost of $200, $500, or $750 for the low-, middle-, or high-option plans, the 20 percent copayment in excess of the deductible to a limit of $1,000, and the annual premium. Since statutory provision creates a risk-reinsurance association and empowers it to set premiums statewide, it is exempt from antitrust law and can't be challenged with price fixing. Finally, it is structured to cover health services which are attributable only to sickness or injury, and only where these are not otherwise covered by related insurance or a government service.

Many handicapped persons, unless they have access to group health insurance through employment, are not likely to qualify for an individual health policy. The important point is that this Act requires that insurance be *available* to all. While it would not cover sickness or injury problems that are the basis of a handicapped condition for the first year, it would cover all other health problems and, after a year, all health problems. The risk pool amalgamation does, then, close a serious gap in the present health insurance market by making health insurance available to the otherwise uninsurable. Obviously, however, if the insurance industry intends to see the COIL approach become the basis for statewide comprehensive health insurance through the private sector, the legislation will need considerable amendment and a serious effort to sell it.

For those handicapped persons without personal coverage or who do not qualify for Medicaid, the COIL plan could be purchased as part of restorative services. Thus, though its present impact upon the state rehabilitation plan is minimal, the model does have important potential.

CHAMPUS

The Civilian Health and Medical Program of the Uniformed Services (CHAMPUS) is the nation's single largest health plan. Benefits were established by Congress to be as comprehensive as the broadest high-option plan available to federal employees. In all, some 6.31 million persons have this coverage, about 3 percent of the civilian population, 45 percent being the dependents of active duty personnel and 55 percent being retired military personnel and their dependents. Funding for the CHAMPUS is contained in the annual appropriation allocated in statute by Congress for the Department of Defense.

Though the CHAMPUS coverage is extensive, it is second-dollar coverage. Any beneficiary having health insurance by virtue of employment must use those benefits first. Such coverage may, however, be used to meet the deductible and co-payment requirements of the CHAMPUS. Any treatment or care entitlement under workers' compensation must also be drawn upon first. In effect, this program has a history of benefit coordination: that is, nonduplication of benefits, like the "similar benefits" principle followed in the management of VR funds. Regulations also require that where a beneficiary resides within forty miles of a military base health care facility and the health services needed are available, such resources are to be used instead of private health care. All this coordination notwithstanding, this is a major program not only in terms of the number of people covered but also in terms of its cost. A total of $654 million in calendar year 1974 was paid to civilian facilities and civilian health personnel, an average per beneficiary per annum cost of $104.

The extent to which any of the users of health services under the CHAMPUS have also received state VR services is unknown. Given the comprehensive health benefits available, however, the cost to state agencies for restorative services for those involved in a rehabilitation plan should be minimal. In a sense, the CHAMPUS is a national health plan for this segment of our population. It is based upon federal law and the annual budget appropriation by Congress. It could, of course, be readily coordinated into a NHI act.

The CHAMPUS does have a special Program for the Handicapped, adopted in January 1967 for the dependents of active duty personnel. There is a statutory limit of $350 monthly for medically necessary services and supplies, with a scale of co-payment according to pay grade. It is supplemental to the basic CHAMPUS, requires prior authorization, and is restricted to the severely physically handicapped or mentally retarded. Once the diagnosis is established and benefits are authorized, they may continue for an indefinite period subject to annual review. The impetus for establishing this program came from the fact that military personnel, being transient, often did not have access to local services for the handicapped. This special program is quite small, now including some 1,800 persons. The facilities used do not have to be health facilities. Consideration is now being given to developing specific standards for rehabilitation under the Program for the Handicapped.

NATIONAL HEALTH INSURANCE AND REHABILITATION

A Commentary by Joseph LaRocca

National health insurance (NHI) will have maximum impact on the federal-state vocational rehabilitation program, and, if legislated, its extension to include rehabilitation for independent living, provided a number of conditions prevail. Principally they are the following:

- Coverage is universal and broad for all Americans regardless of income.
- Rehabilitation concepts and operational practices are basic elements of the system.
- Specific provision is made for comprehensive physical and mental restorative services—rehabilitation services—and for the duration required in each individual situation, as well as for medical services for the acute care phase of health care.
- Comprehensive rehabilitation services are provided as outpatient as well as inpatient services.

- Accredited rehabilitation facilities are included among the health agencies designated to provide inpatient and outpatient services to the disabled.

In January 1977, there were eighteen proposals before Congress pertaining to some form of national health insurance. No one proposal satisfies all of the conditions, listed above, that would have maximum impact upon the rehabilitation program. Some bills incorporate more rehabilitation elements than others and in varying degrees. As a result, their impact upon rehabilitation would vary. A few proposals offering an opportunity to buy private health insurance at relatively modest cost, but with benefits hedged with co-insurance charges and other limits would, if enacted, have negligible impact upon the rehabilitation program.

The proposals pending in Congress are constantly undergoing change; hence there is no way of making a reasonable assessment of the impact of national health insurance upon rehabilitation until one definitive bill emerges. However, two proposals, the Health Security Act and the Catastrophic Health Insurance and Medical Assistance Reform Act, with widely differing provisions in coverage and benefits, are reviewed below, with qualified assessment of the impact they would have upon the rehabilitation program.

The Health Security Act

This proposal by Representative James C. Corman and Senator Edward M. Kennedy would provide for the establishment of a national health insurance program covering the entire population and offering a broad and comprehensive range of services. For covered services there would be no cutoff dates, no co-insurance, no deductibles, and no waiting periods. The program would be financed by a federal payroll tax on employers and employees, a tax on unearned income and self-employment earnings, and by federal general revenues.

Benefits under this proposal are broad, generous, and virtually free of the restrictions found in other proposals. Benefits would include:

- Physicians' services, including physical checkups.
- General hospital inpatient and outpatient care.
- Psychiatric care in a general or psychiatric hospital—limited to 45 consecutive days of active treatment during a benefit period.

- Skilled nursing home care of 120 days per benefit period.
- Physicians' psychiatric services limited to 20 visits during a benefit period, except when benefits are provided through group practice organizations, hospital outpatient departments, or comprehensive mental health care organizations, in which case there is no limitation.
- Medical appliances and equipment, including eyeglasses, hearing aids, and prosthetic devices.
- Services of free standing ambulatory drug abuse and alcoholism centers, family planning centers, and rehabilitation centers.

In the first year of the program, dental services would be available to children under age fifteen, extended each year to children two years older up to age twenty-five. After seven years, dental care coverage for the rest of the population would be phased in by age or other types of groups.

Free standing rehabilitation centers could qualify as providers of service. Passage of the Health Security Act proposals would profoundly affect rehabilitation programs, as well as other state grant-in-aid programs providing health services or services with health or medical components to disabled people.

First and foremost, federal grants for Medicaid, material and child health, and *vocational rehabilitation* programs would not include funds for the provision of services obtainable under the Health Security Program. In the 1976 fiscal year, state VR agencies spent over $100 million in state and federal funds for physical and mental restoration services and over $75 million for diagnostic and evaluation services, which included some medical and specialty examinations. Assuming that the Health Security program had been in place in the 1976 fiscal year and that the $100 million plus spent for physical and mental restoration services and medical diagnostic services had been available under the Health Security program, then 80 percent, the federal share, of such expenditures would not have been forthcoming to the state VR agencies. Hopefully, federal funds would be provided to the state VR agencies for rehabilitation services of a medical nature that were not provided for under the Health Security program. Additionally, federal funds deductible from the state grants by virtue of the medical rehabilitation services being available under the Health Security program would, we hope, not be deducted. The state agencies would then have added funds with which to serve more clients and to purchase other essential rehabilitation services, such as vocational training, orientation and mobility training, telecommunication and other equipment for clients who are deaf, blind or otherwise severely disabled, and others. These, of course, are budget and policy matters which only the administration and Congress can settle.

The provision in the Health Security Act proposal for the cutoff of federal funds for medical services would *compel* use by the state VR agencies of the Health Security Act. In this regard, it is more stringent than the current provision in the Rehabilitation Act regarding the use of Medicare, Medicaid, and other sources as a similar benefit for physical and mental restorative services. With respect to Medicare, Medicaid, and other medical programs, the Rehabilitation Act and regulations currently provide that the "State Agency will give full consideration to any similar benefit available under any other program to a handicapped individual to meet, in whole or in part, the cost of physical and mental restorative services . . . except where such consideration would significantly delay the provision of such services to an individual." No such proviso appears in the Health Security Bill.

With its extensive mental health benefits, the National Health Security program would offer mental restoration services to clients of the state VR agencies that few, if any, can now provide with their own resources. The dominant disability for persons served by the rehabilitation agencies is mental illness, accounting for over 30 percent of its clientele. Under the National Health Security program, not only might more mental restorative services become available to present clients of the state rehabilitation agencies, but, relieved of the financial responsibility of providing these costly mental health services, the state agencies might be able to serve more persons disabled by psychotic and psychoneurotic disorders. Also, the mental health services provided under the National Health Security program would be an invaluable resource for the state rehabilitation agencies should their programs be expanded to include rehabilitation for independent living. Many people requiring rehabilitation services for independent living are in the upper age groups, and mental problems often accompany their physical infirmities.

The Rehabilitation Act of 1973 made provision, among other things, for postemployment services—services to be provided after clients have been rehabilitated—to assist those who need such services to maintain employment. As the VR program directs its efforts to serving increasing numbers of severely handicapped people, the planning for and provision of postemployment services become more important elements of the state VR agencies' services. Often these are expensive services of a medical nature and, in some instances, essential for life support. State rehabilitation agencies have been concerned with how to provide postemployment services and at the same time maintain intake of new cases with relatively little increase in funds available to them. The national health insurance program proposed under the Corman-Kennedy bill could help in this rehabilitation area.

Under the Corman-Kennedy bill, Medicare would be terminated and the assets and liabilities of both Medicare trust funds would be transferred to the health security fund. A recent study by the Urban Institute found limited utilization by VR counselors of Medicare for the physical and mental restoration services required by recipients of monthly Social Security disability benefits undergoing vocational rehabilitation (Urban Institute, 1976, p. 47). The reason: coverage under Medicare for recipients of disability benefits does not take place until such recipients have been entitled to disability benefits for two consecutive years. Since referral to the VR agency is part of the initial application procedure for disability benefits, Medicare coverage is not available at the time of referral—nor, generally, when the Individualized Written Rehabilitation Program (IWRP) is formulated and initiated. In 1976 the state VR agencies spent almost $15 million trust fund dollars for physical and mental restoration services for recipients of disability benefits undergoing rehabilitation. Presumably, under the Corman-Kennedy bill recipients of disability benefits would qualify immediately for medical and restorative services.

As indicated earlier, the state Medicaid programs would be affected by the proposed Health Security program, which would cover most of the services now provided to the poor by Medicaid. This changeover from Medicaid to the proposed Health Security program would facilitate rehabilitation planning and the provision of service by the state rehabilitation agencies to people in economic need since the rehabilitation agencies would not be faced with the same obstacles and deterrents that now exist with regard to Medicaid usage.

Deterrents to the use of Medicaid are now many and vary from state to state. They are:

- The requirement in some states that the "first dollar" be spent by the VR agency, since the federal matching ratio in the rehabilitation program is more advantageous to the state than in the Medicaid program.
- Cutbacks from time to time in Medicaid services due to funding problems.
- The lack of provision for certain devices essential to rehabilitation (e.g., hearing aids, dentures, repair of prosthetic and orthotic appliances).

- The long delays in the provision of medical services.

According to the Urban Institute study,

> Couselors cited other problems in the use of Medicaid as a similar benefit, problems related to the quality or adequacy of service and the expeditious carrying through of the client's rehabilitation program. Some physicians do not participate in the Medicaid program. These physicians may be the ones who are most knowledgeable about the rehabilitation program, most involved in serving VR clients who are not eligible for Medicaid, and the ones who are most accessible to the client and the counselor. Thus, if required to utilize Medicaid, the selection of the physician by the client and the counselor in the planning and carrying through of the client's rehabilitation program would be severely restricted (Urban Institute, 1976, p. 46).

Counselors also reported that some clients find it demeaning to apply for Medicaid, which they regard as welfare. The Corman-Kennedy bill would establish one program for all people regardless of income. With the means test removed no one need feel demeaned in accepting the services offered.

The Catastrophic Health Insurance and Medical Assistance Reform Act

This proposal by Representative Joe D. Waggoner and Senators Russell B. Long and Abraham A. Ribicoff would establish three programs:

- A catastrophic illness insurance plan providing health benefits for persons in the general population who have incurred unusually large health expenses.
- A medical assistance plan covering the low-income population through a national plan with uniform eligibility standards.
- A program of federal certification of private health insurance to encourage insurance carriers to make available improved basic private health insurance.

The government catastrophic health insurance program would provide benefits to persons who have already incurred long hospital stays or large medical bills. The program, which would cover all of the population, would be administered through the Medicare program and financed by payroll taxes. Employers could voluntarily elect to provide the catastrophic coverage for their employees under a private plan as an alternative to the government-administered program, and a similar option would be available to self-employed persons.

As to the benefits, the program would cover the same services as the Medicare program and, as under Medicare, the services would be provided under separate hospital insurance and medical insurance parts of the program. Hospital insurance would include hospital inpatient care, skilled nursing facility services, and home health services. Medical insurance would include physicians' services, laboratory and X-ray, immunizations, home health services, outpatient physical therapy, medical supplies, and appliances and ambulance service.

The three types of services under hospital insurance would be covered after the individual has received 60 days of inpatient hospital care during a calendar year. Once the deductible is met, the period of eligibility for covered services would continue indefinitely until the individual has been out of both a hospital and skilled nursing facility for a consecutive period of 90 days. If so, the individual would need to meet another 60-day hospital deductible before becoming eligible for benefits again.

Eligibility under the medical insurance part of the program would be on a family basis. The services under medical insurance would be covered for all members of a family after the members together have incurred expenses of $2,000 in a calendar year. Once the deductible is met, the period of eligibility for services would continue indefinitely until the family has incurred expenses of less than $500 in a 90-day period. During the benefit period, all the services under medical insurance would be covered without limitation on the amount of services.

Special provisions would apply to coverage of mental conditions. The hospital insurance part of the proposal would include coverage of inpatient hospital care for mental illness provided in general and mental hospitals. Mental health care services on an outpatient basis would be covered under the medical part of the program. Under a special provision the amount of expenses for outpatient mental illness care which could be credited toward meeting the $2,000 deductible would be limited to a maximum of $500. Once the medical deductible is met, outpatient care would be covered with no limit on the number of visits when provided by a qualified community mental health center. Care by a private psychiatrist would be covered, but limited to a maximum of five visits during a 12-month period, with additional visits covered only if approved in advance by a professional review organization as being necessary to avoid institutional care.

At their option, employers could establish approved private plans as an alternative method of providing coverage for their employees. An approved plan must provide the same catastrophic benefits as the government plan and must meet specified requirements concerning coverage, administration, financing, and other matters. Employees covered under an approved plan would receive the catastrophic benefits under the plan and would not be eligible under the government program.

Self-employed persons could voluntarily establish a private catastrophic plan on a basis similar in many ways to employer plans. Such a plan would cover the self-employed person and the members of his or her family, and persons covered under them would not be eligible for benefits under the government programs.

The second part of the Catastrophic Health Insurance and Medical Assistance Reform Act, the medical assistance plan for low-income and medically indigent persons, would be administered through the Medicare program. It is designed to mesh with the catastrophic plan, as well as other public and private health plans. The program would be financed jointly from federal and state general revenues. The benefits of the program would be available to individuals whose annual family income is below the following amounts without regard to their age, family status, employment, or state of residence:

- Individual, $2,400
- Family of two, $3,600
- Family of three, $4,200
- Family of four, $4,800
- Family of more than four, $4,800 plus $400 for each additional member

Families with incomes higher than the specified amounts could still qualify for benefits under the "spend-down" provision. Under this provision, the family's income for the purpose of eligibility is considered its actual income reduced by the amount of incurred medical expenses the family is legally obligated to pay out-of-pocket: that is, expenses not covered by a private or government plan.

Benefits under this program include:

- Inpatient hospital services (60 days in benefit period).
- Skilled nursing facilities.
- Intermediate care facilities.
- Physicians' services—$3 co-payment for each of first ten outpatient visits per family.

- Laboratory and X-ray.
- Home health services.
- Prenatal and well-baby care.
- Family planning and counseling.
- Periodic examinations for children under age eighteen.
- Outpatient physical therapy.
- Immunizations by regulation.
- Medical supplies and appliances.
- Ambulance services.

The types of mental health services covered under the medical assistance program would be the same services as under the catastrophic program, including inpatient hospital care, partial hospitalization, and outpatient services, subject to the same conditions and limitations, except for the deductible requirements.

The present Medicaid program would be abolished and replaced by the new program. The Medicare program would continue.

The Catastrophic Health Insurance and Medical Assistance Act would affect rehabilitation in several ways. By abolishing the separate state Medicaid programs and setting up a national health insurance program for low-income and medically indigent persons with uniform eligibility requirements and benefits, a number of the rehabilitation problems associated with the use of Medicaid, discussed earlier, would be obviated. On the other hand, the application process in establishing economic need may be time-consuming, interfering with the immediate development and initiation of the individual's rehabilitation program. The process may be demeaning to some people, who would view it as another welfare program rather than a health insurance program.

Some of the services, particularly the mental health services, provided under both the catastrophic health insurance and medical assistance parts of the program, are so limited in time and quantity that it would be very difficult to achieve a rehabilitation goal.

Perhaps the greatest problem with the proposal from a rehabilitation standpoint is that it would seem to encourage continued hospital and nursing home care, since a disabled individual who is out of the hospital or nursing home for 90 days would need to meet another 60-day deductible before becoming eligible for benefits again. While the person is in the hospital, benefits continue indefinitely. On the other hand, rehabilitation seeks to minimize institutionalization and promote independence.

Finally, the proposal seems to focus on acute short-term medical catastrophies and does not give equal emphasis to the severe chronic illnesses and disabilities which are the major concern of the rehabilitation agencies and facilities.

Rehabilitation Recommendations for National Health Insurance Proposals

Various organizations—the American Congress of Rehabilitation Medicine, the American Academy of Physical Medicine and Rehabilitation, the National Easter Seal Society for Crippled Children and Adults, and the Association of Rehabilitation Facilities—have testified before Congress on a number of the bills pertaining to national health insurance. All have urged that NHI proposals clearly provide for comprehensive rehabilitation coverage on both an inpatient and outpatient basis; that a definition of rehabilitation services be included; and that accredited rehabilitation facilities be specifically designated as providers of service. Suggested legislative language to achieve these ends was presented to the Ways and Means Committee by the National Easter Seal Society in its statement on national health insurance, April 15, 1975:

> *Rehabilitation Services*
>
> The term *rehabilitation services* includes any one or more of the following items or services furnished under a medically prescribed plan and related to the achievement of specific outcomes regarding mental and physical functional capacity or the prevention of deterioration in the disabling condition of the patient:
>
> 1. Physician services, including diagnostic and therapeutic services;
> 2. Physical therapy, occupational therapy, and other medically necessary therapies;
> 3. Speech therapy, audiology, and vision services;
> 4. Prosthetic and orthotic devices, including testing, fitting, or training in the use of prosthetic or orthotic devices;
> 5. Social and psychological services;
> 6. Nursing care provided by or under the supervision of a professional nurse;

7. Drugs, biologicals, supplies, appliances, and equipment, including the purchase or rental of equipment;

8. Transportation services necessary for the provision of outpatient rehabilitation services; and

9. Such other services as are medically necessary for the mental and physical restoration of the patient, or the prevention of his deterioration, and are ordinarily furnished by a hospital, SNF, rehabilitation facility, or home health agency.

   Inpatient hospital rehabilitation services are such rehabilitation services as are certified by a physician as required on an inpatient basis for the medical diagnosis or treatment of the patient based on factors such as the need for direct and continual supervision of the patient and the degree of intensity of the service.

Outpatient Rehabilitation Services

The term *outpatient rehabilitation services* means rehabilitation services furnished by a hospital, skilled nursing facility, home health agency, or rehabilitation facility, or by others under an arrangement with, and under the supervision of, such hospital, skilled nursing facility, home health agency, or rehabilitation facility, to an individual as an outpatient who is under the care of a physician,

excluding however—

any item or service if it would not be included under subsection (a) if furnished to an inpatient of a hospital.

Rehabilitation Facility

The term *rehabilitation facility* means an institution (or a distinct part of an institution) which—

i. provides an adequate program of rehabilitation services (one or more of such services) for outpatients and has the facilities and personnel required for such a program or required for the supervision of such a program, in accordance with such requirements as the HEW Secretary may specify;

ii. is accredited by the Commission for Accreditation of Rehabilitation Facilities or another qualified accrediting body;

iii. has policies, established by a group of professional personnel, including one or more physicians (associated with the clinic or rehabilitation facility) to govern the services it provides;

iv. maintains clinical records on all patients;

v. if such facility is situated in a State in which the State or applicable local law provides for the licensing of institutions of this nature, (I) is licensed pursuant to such law, or (II) is approved by the agency or such State or locality responsible for licensing institutions of this nature, as meeting the standards established for such licensing; and

vi. meets such other conditions relating to the health and safety of individuals who are furnished services by a facility on an outpatient basis, as the secretary may find necessary; (p. 61).

As of this time, none of the NHI proposals incorporate all of the recommended rehabilitation provisions. Inclusion of the rehabilitation provisions would reinforce the role of rehabilitation facilities in national health insurance and insure a comprehensive interdisciplinary service to chronically ill and disabled people, essential for their achievement of maximum functional capacity.

Training VR Agency Staff on NHI Coverage and Benefits

Whatever NHI program may be enacted, it will be essential that VR agency staff, particularly the counselors, have full understanding of the coverage and benefits available under that program. This is imperative if there is to be full utilization of the benefits of the health insurance program in the rehabilitation process. The Urban Institute found, in its study of similar benefit usage, that Medicare, Medicaid, and other programs were not fully utilized because, among other reasons, state VR staff had inadequate knowledge about these other programs. Fully 50 percent of the counselors and supervisors participating in the study considered the training they received on similar benefit usage to be inadequate. Moreover, it was felt that, in general, the written materials developed by the state rehabilitation agencies on the utilization of the services offered by the other programs were of limited value. Only a few state agencies had developed a comprehensive manual (Urban Institute, 1976, p. 68).

The vocational rehabilitation process is a planned sequence of services directed to the specific needs of the handicapped individual and designed to bring about his or her optimum employment and/or capacity for independent living. The successful outcome of this process will depend primarily upon each of the needed services being provided in the rehabilitation process when required: that is, when the handicapped person is most receptive psychologically and physiologically to the particular service or services, as well as when the provision of the service or services will have the greatest rehabilitative impact. Under a national health insurance program, the counselors will not have the same time controls over the provision of physical and mental restoration services that they now have in the purchase of these services with vocational rehabilitation funds. Another facet of staff training might be the timely utilization of the benefits available under the NHI program in the development and implementation of the individualized rehabilitation programs.*

RECOMMENDATIONS FOR NATIONAL HEALTH INSURANCE

The principles advanced here are personal recommendations without any official endorsement. They are proposed as a framework for NHI, not only to illustrate some of the potential critical dimensions but, hopefully, to provide a better grasp of the complexity of the entire issue.

Universality

A national health plan must apply to all legal residents, handicapped or otherwise. To assure that it does, it must be automatic, or required. Care for nonresidents should be a personal responsibility or a matter of international agreement.

Phasing

The program should be phased in over a period as long as five years, with the phases forecast in advance, both to facilitate preparation and to minimize dislocation. A sequential implementation should be used to effect a systemic change in health service delivery and in the allocation of health resources. The redirection should be toward optimizing general health in the long run.

The systematic introduction of health education, disability prevention, and health planning should come first and be continuously refined. This should be followed by health enhancement services through, and with the development of, comprehensive ambulatory health care centers and with development geared to community need. Services for acute hospital care are widely available now and should be continued. The next phase should see the decertification of outmoded and unnecessary hospital facilities and, where needed and appropriate, their conversion in whole or part to nursing, convalescent, and residential care centers.

*This ends the commentary by Joseph La Rocca.

Equality

All residents should have equal entitlement to health care regardless of income and without discrimination. The present double standards of quality, all too common between public and private care, would be eliminated. Moreover, prepayment of necessary health care creates an entitlement intended to place providers and facilities at the service of the consumer. The burden of having to pay for services as used would largely be removed, as they would be prepaid, eliminating the need to make personal economic decisions before receiving health services.

Differentiation

It is essential that distinction be made between: (1) active promotion of health and treatment of health disabilities, and (2) continuing care for those no longer able to work or live independently. Health services should be in the private sector, meeting general standards and guidelines. Since all residents will have general entitlement, public services for active treatment should be phased out except for people not in civilian life. A complementary program of long-term and supportive community-based care, encouraging independent living to the extent possible, should be developed under social welfare auspices.

Benefit Coordination

Within plan limits, active restorative health care should be provided to all persons accepted for state rehabilitation services. Any necessary health care beyond the comprehensive entitlements of the NHI plan would be part of the vocational rehabilitation process. A similar nonduplication should be continued for all CHAMPUS beneficiaries and considered for the Veterans Administration (VA) except for certain highly specialized services. In other words, the CHAMPUS and VA health services would only be supplemental to NHI. The main body of health services now provided under their auspices would be subsumed by NHI. The need for automobile medical expense coverage should no longer be necessary.

Because the separation of the health service benefits of workers' compensation programs from cash disability payment could be disruptive and complicate plan administration, it should remain separate from NHI. However, the health care available to job-injured employees should not be less than that under NHI.

Consumer Choice

The consumer must have the option of choice between at least two alternative and competing health care plans and freedom of choice of practitioner and facilities within health plans. The health services must be provided with a guarantee of privileged communication.

Peer Review

The services of all practitioners must be subject to peer review. Since the services rendered, including procedures, drugs, surgery, facilities, appliances, and duration of care, are in some instances under the prescriptive direction of the provider and in most other instances subject to the discretion and judgment of the provider, it appears that if they are to be effective, utilization controls should be directed primarily toward the practitioner. To facilitate this review, an individual provider profile must be maintained on computer for all providers authorized to practice.

Continuity

All basic services must be available on a twenty-four hour basis and an individualized treatment plan formulated upon determination of disability. Individual consumer utilization profiles should be maintained on computer, with spot sampling for potential duplication and fraud.

Mental Health

Since emotional or mental disorder is a primary or concurrent problem for the majority of persons seeking health care and vocational rehabilitation services, it is essential that broad mental health coverage be an integral component of all health care plans. Note should be taken that most NHI proposals would limit services for mental disorder to less than that available for other health problems. Indeed, since the majority of doctor visits are for conditions where emotional distress or mental disorder is a concurrent if not the primary problem, health planning and policy should recognize this lack and consider both psychologists and psychiatrists as primary health care providers rather than backup specialists.

Reimbursement

Hospital and facility per diem and other charges should be based on an annually determined proscriptive rate basis. Similarly, payment for professional services should be annually negotiated. Rates for both hospitals and providers would be determined on a state-by-state basis. Provider fees or salaries would be statewide, with possible incentives for practice in underserved areas. A salaried basis of practice must be available for those practitioners who elect this form of payment, but with waiver of fees. A mechanism should also be available to providers and group practice organizations to submit competitive contract bids for services, including payment on a capitation basis—a rate for each person for whose health care the provider is responsible. All rates and fees should be public knowledge.

Financing

Employee-employer payments would be via payroll deduction to cover the cost of the health plan selected. Self-employed individuals would make quarterly payments, and for those without income or with income below federally determined need levels, funds would be transferred from general revenue to a designated NHI account. To facilitate planning, management, and competition, health care would be financed on a prepaid basis. Employer, employee, or individual payments would be exempt from taxation at any level. According to state option, the health funds collected federally could be transferred directly to the insurers or via the state.

Administration

Necessary laws and regulations would be adopted to assure all major health professions of independent provider status within the scope of their practice, including, but not limited to: physicians, osteopathic physicans, dentists, podiatrists, psychologists, optometrists, nurse practitioners, and social workers. Similar provisions would be adopted federally to facilitate multidisciplinary group practice. Health planning, designation of underserved areas, and oversight of peer review would be a state responsibility. Regulations would provide for federal-state agreements on state plans which substantially exceed the allowable federal minimum program standards.

Provider Status

Each recognized health profession should develop and maintain a national register of its practitioners, based upon explicit standards and definitions. Listing should be based on proficiency and credential review by peers, with areas of specialty competence designated. All practitioners must be licensed, registered, or certified, in keeping with the statutes of the state(s) in which they practice.

Training

The training of needed health personnel should be a component cost of NHI. Those who seek public funding or assistance for their professional training will enter into a return-in-service contract with choice among areas of need. States will annually designate need by community and profession, and contracts will be available according to projected consumer needs for health service.

Research

Since the development of new knowledge and technology is unpredictable, and since the products generally have national application, research funding should be derived from a proportionate share of NHI revenues and allocated federally on a competitive basis. To promote additional research, targeted research, or specialized research centers, suitable appropriations should be made from the general revenue.

REFERENCES

Aday, L. "The Impact of Health Policy on Access to Medical Care." *Milbank Memorial Fund Quarterly* 54, 1976: 215–233.

Alander, R., and Campbell, T. "An Evaluative Study of an Alcohol and Drug Recovery Program: A Case Study of the Oldsmobile Experience." *Human Resource Management* 14, 1975: 14–18.

Alter, J. *Narrowing Our Medical Care Gap.* Jericho, N.Y.: Exposition Press, 1972.

Ayres, J. "Accelerating Skyrocketing Health Care Cost." *New England Journal of Medicine* 296, 1977: 391–393.

Barth, P. "The Effort to Rehabilitate Workers' Compensation." *American Journal of Public Health* 66, 1976: 553–557.

Binner, P., Halpern, J., and Potter, A. "Patients, Programs and Results in a Comprehensive Mental Health Center." *Journal of Consulting and Clinical Psychology* 41, 1973: 148–156.

Bodenheimer, T. "The Hoax of National Health Insurance." *American Journal of Public Health* 62, 1972: 1324–1327.

Burnell, G. M. "Financing Mental Health Care—An Appraisal of Various Models." *Archives of General Psychiatry* 25, 1971: 49–55.

Cailliet, R. "Rehabilitation Medicine: Its Future in National Health Programs." *Archives of Physical Medicine and Rehabilitation* 56, 1975: 97–100.

California. S. B. 110, California Budget Act for 1977–78.

California. *Welfare and Institutions Code.* SS 10651, 10654, 19000, 19018, 19450, 19942, 19946 (West, 1972).

Canada, Department of National Health and Welfare. *Health and Welfare Services in Canada, Research and Statistics Directorate,* 1971.
Cohen, A., and Margolis, B. "Initial Psychological Research Related to the Occupational Safety and Health Act of 1970." *American Psychologist* 28, 1973: 600–606.
Commission on Accreditation of Rehabilitation Facilities. *Standards Manual for Rehabilitation Facilities.* Chicago, Ill.: 1973.
Committee for Economic Development (CED), Research and Policy Committee. *Building a National Health Care System.* New York: 1973.
Conley, R. *The Economics of Mental Retardation.* Baltimore: Johns Hopkins Press, 1973.
Correia, E. *National Health Insurance, Welfare Reform and the Disabled: Issues in Program Reform.* Washington, D.C.: Office of the Assistant Secretary for Planning and Evaluation, Department of Health, Education and Welfare, August 1976.
Cummings, N. "Medicare Reform Testimony to the U.S. Senate." *The Clinical Psychologist* 30, 1976: 21–23.
Davis, K. *National Health Insurance: Benefits, Costs and Consequences.* (Studies in Social Economics) Washington, D.C.: The Brookings Institution, 1975.
Donabedian, A. "Issues in National Health Insurance." *American Journal of Public Health* 66, 1976: 345–350.
Dorken, H. "Psychologist, Is There a Foundation in Your Future?" *Journal of Community Psychology* 2, 1974: 99–103.
———. "CHAMPUS Ten State Claim Experience for Mental Disorder: Fiscal Year 1975." *American Psychologist* 32, 1977: 697–710.
———, et al. *The Professional Psychologist Today: New Developments in Law, Health Insurance and Health Practice.* San Francisco: Jossey-Bass, 1976.
Dwight, J. "Bringing Better Management to Medicaid." *Social and Rehabilitation Record* 2, 1975: 24–26.
Education for All Handicapped Children Act of 1975. Public Law 94-142, November 29, 1975. 89 Stat. 773, 20 USC S1401.
Enthoven, A. "Can We Control the Cost of Health Care?" *The Stanford Magazine,* Fall/Winter 1976: 14–19.
Follette, W., and Cummings, N. "Psychiatric Services and Medical Utilization in a Prepaid Health Plan Setting." *Medical Care* 5, 1967: 25–35.
Follman, J. R., Jr. *Insurance Coverage for Mental Illness.* New York: American Management Association, 1970.
Garfield, S., et al. "Evaluation of an Ambulatory Medical Care Delivery System." *New England Journal of Medicine* 294, 1976: 426–431.
Goldberg, I., Krantz, G., and Locke, B. "Effect of a Short-Term Out-Patient Psychiatric Therapy Benefit on the Utilization of Medical Services in a Prepaid Group Practice Medical Program." *Medical Care,* 8, 1970: 419–428.
Halliday, W. R. "Rehabilitation of Injured Workmen with Psycho-Social Handicaps." In: J. J. Leedy (Ed.), *Compensation in Psychiatric Disability and Rehabilitation.* Springfield, Ill.: Charles C. Thomas, 1971.
Hannings, R., Ash, P., and Simick, D. *Forensic Psychology in Disability Adjudication: A Decade of Experience.* HEW Publication No. 72-10284. Washington, D.C.: U.S. Department of Health, Education and Welfare, Social Security Administration, 1972.
Hatcher, G., Canadian Approaches to Health Policy Decisions—National Health Insurance. *American Journal of Public Health,* 68, 1978, 881–889.
Health Insurance Institute. *Source Book of Health Insurance Data 1974–75.* New York: 1975.
———. *Source Book of Health Insurance Data, 1976–1977.* New York: 1977.
Heck, E. "Professional Psychology and Public Programs: A Critique." *Professional Psychology* 7, 1976: 420–427.

Hewlett-Packard Company v. *Barnes,* 425 F. Supp. 1294 (1977).

Insurance Information Institute. *Insurance Facts 1976.* New York: 1976.

LaVor, M., and Duncan, J. "Vocational Rehabilitation—the New Law and Its Implications for the Future." *Journal of Rehabilitation* 42, 1976: 20–28, 39.

Leonard, Z. "Utilization Control in Medicaid." *Social and Rehabilitation Record* 2, 1974: 29–31.

Lipson, M. "Federal and State Law Developments Which Will Shape and Limit Present and Future Rehabilitation Programs." *Archives of Physical Medicine and Rehabilitation* 57, 1976: 547.

Margolis, R. "National Health Insurance—The Dream Whose Time Has Come?" *New York Times Magazine,* January 9, 1977: 12–13, 32–33, 36, 38, 40–43.

Mathews v. *Eldridge,* 424 US 319, 47 LEd2d 18, 96 S. Ct. 893 (1976).

Mitchell, B., and Schwartz, W. *The Financing of National Health Insurance.* Santa Monica, Calif.: The Rand Corporation, May 1976. R-1711-HEW.

"National Health Insurance: Which Way to Go?" *Consumer Reports* 40, 1975: 118–124.

Pollard, O. "The State-Federal Program: A Point of View." *Journal of Rehabilitation* 42, 1976: 21, 36.

Rehabilitation Act of 1973. Public Law 93-112, September 26, 1973. 87 Stat. 355, 29 USC S701.

Rehabilitation Act Amendments of 1974. Public Law 93-516, December 7, 1974. 88 Stat. 1617, 29 USC S701.

Reynolds, James A. "Carter's Health Expert Fills in the Blanks: Special Report." *Medical Economics,* October 18, 1976: 31, 35, 39–40, 45.

Roemer, M., and Axelrod, S. "A National Health Service and Social Security: Commentary." *American Journal of Public Health* 67, 1977: 462–465.

Scitovsky, A., and McCall, N. "Coinsurance and the Demand for Physician Services: Four Years Later." *Social Security Bulletin* May 1977: 19–27. [HEW Publication No. (SSA77-11700)]

Services and Payment in Medical Assistance Programs. 45 *Code of Federal Regulations* S249.10 (1976).

Spencer, W. "Statement on National Health Insurance Legislation on Behalf of the American Congress of Rehabilitation Medicine and American Academy of Physical Medicine and Rehabilitation to the Committee on Ways and Means, U.S. House of Representatives, April 26, 1974."

U.S. Department of Defense. Civilian Health and Medical Program of the Uniformed Services. *How Other Health Plan Coverage Affects CHAMPUS Payments.* (Fact Sheet 7. 0-219-557.) Washington, D.C.: U.S. Government Printing Office, 1976.

U.S. Department of Health, Education and Welfare. *Proceedings of the Advisory Committee on National Health Insurance Issues, May 20–21, 1977.* Washington, D.C.: U.S. Government Printing Office, 1977.

———. *Towards a Comprehensive Health Policy for the 1970's: A White Paper.* (HEW 0-427-047.) Washington, D.C.: U.S. Government Printing Office, May 1971.

U.S. Department of Health, Education and Welfare, Health Resources Administration. *The Supply of Health Manpower: 1970 Profiles and Projections to 1990.* (HRS 75–38.) Washington, D.C.: U.S. Government Printing Office, December 1974.

U.S. Department of Health, Education and Welfare, Office of Human Development and Social and Rehabilitation Service. "Vocational Rehabilitation Programs, Implementing Provisions." *Federal Register* 40 (228), November 25, 1975: 54696-54731.

U.S. Department of Health, Education and Welfare, Office of Human Development, Office for Handicapped Individuals. "A Summary of Selected Legislation Relating to the Handicapped 1975." In *Programs for the Handicapped.* Washington, D.C.: U.S. Government Printing Office, August 20, 1976.

U.S. Department of Health, Education and Welfare, Office of Human Development, Rehabilitation Services Administration. *Caseload Statistics, State Vocational Rehabilitation Agencies, 1976.* (RSA 77-25078.) Washington, D.C.: 1977.

———. *Distribution of Source of Referral of Cases Closed by State Vocational Rehabilitation Agencies During Fiscal Year 1975.* (Information Memorandum RSA-IM-77-37.) Washington, D.C.: February 11, 1977.

———. *Final Report on Characteristics of Clients Rehabilitated during Fiscal Year 1974.* (Information Memorandum RSA-IM-76-87.) Washington, D.C.: 1976.

———. *Information Memorandum.* (RSA-IM-77-39.) Washington, D.C.: 1977.

———. *Information Memorandum.* (RSA-IM-77-71.) Washington, D.C.: 1977.

———. *Preliminary Report: Comparison of Characteristics of Severely and Non-Severely Disabled Clients Rehabilitated during Fiscal Year 1975.* Memo by Andrew S. Adams, Commissioner. Washington, D.C.: 1975.

———. *Preliminary Report on Clients Rehabilitated during Fiscal Year 1976.* (Information Memorandum RSA-IM-77-21.) Washington, D.C.: 1976.

———. *Preliminary Report: Comparison of Characteristics of Severely and Non-severely Disabled Clients Rehabilitated During Fiscal Years 1975–76.* (Information Memorandum RSA-IM-77-32.) Washington, D.C.: 1976.

———. *State Vocational Rehabilitation Agency Program Data: Fiscal Year 1976.* (OHD 77-25053.) Washington, D.C.: 1977.

———. *A Summary of Selected Legislation Relating to the Handicapped: 1974.* (OHD 75-22002.) Washington, D.C.: 1975.

———. *Vocational Rehabilitation Caseload Distribution: Total, Severe and Non-severe, October 1, 1976 to December 31, 1976.* (Information Memorandum RSA-IM-77-66.) Washington, D.C.: 1977.

U.S. Department of Health, Education and Welfare, Social and Rehabilitation Services. *Statistical History, Federal-State Program of Vocational Rehabilitation. 1920–1969.* (SRS-RSA Pub. No. 134.) Washington, D.C. 1970.

———. *Major Disabling Conditions of Clients of State Vocational Rehabilitation Agencies Rehabilitated and Not Rehabilitated During the Fiscal Year of 1969.* (Statistical Note No. 27.) Washington, D.C.: 1971.

———. *Standards for Rehabilitation Facilities and Sheltered Workshops.* Rev. ed. (SRS 72-25010.) Washington, D.C.: 1971.

———. *The Profile of Mentally Ill Persons Rehabilitated in Fiscal Year 1969.* (Statistical Note No. 23.) Washington, D.C.: 1971.

———. *A Profile of Mentally Retarded Clients Rehabilitated During the Fiscal Year of 1969.* (Statistical Note No. 29.) Washington, D.C. 1971c.

———. *State Data Book, Federal-State Vocational Rehabilitation Program, Fiscal Year 1972.* (SRS 75-25403.) Washington, D.C.: n.d.

———. Rehabilitation Services Administration. *Characteristics of Clients Rehabilitated in Fiscal Years 1968–1972: Federal-State Vocational Rehabilitation Program.* (SRS 74-25079.) Washington, D.C.: n.d.

———. *Selected Characteristics of Clients Closed from Active Caseload Statuses, by Major Disabling Condition, Fiscal Year 1972.* (Statistical Note No. 43. RSA-IM-76-11.) Washington, D.C.: 1975.

U.S. Department of Health, Education and Welfare, Social Security Administration. *The Size and Shape of the Medical Care Dollar.* Chart Book 1975. (SSA 76-11910.) Washington, D.C.: 1976

U.S. Interdepartmental Workers' Compensation Task Force. Policy Group. *Workers' Compensation: Is There a Better Way?* Report submitted to Congress, January 17, 1977.

U.S. National Commission on State Workmen's Compensation Laws. "The Medical Care and Rehabilitation Objective," in *National Commission Report on State Workmen's Compensation Laws.* Washington, D. C.: U.S. Government Printing Office, 1972:77–85.

U.S. Social Security Administration, Office of Research and Statistics. *National Health Insurance Proposals; Provisions of Bills Introduced in the 94th Congress as of February 1976.* (SSA 76-11920.) Washington, D.C.: 1976.

———. *Independent Health Insurance Plans in 1974.* (Research and Statistics Note No. 21.) Washington, D.C.: 1976.

The Urban Institute. *Executive Report on the Performance Standards of the Vocational Rehabilitation Program.* Jerry Turem, Project Director. Washington, D.C.: 1976.

———. *Report of the Similar Benefits Study to the Department of Health, Education, and Welfare.* Jerry Turem, Project Director. Washington, D.C.: 1976.

Wallace, H. "Handicapped Children Under National Health Insurance." *Developmental Medicine and Child Neurology* 18, 1976: 213–228.

Weikel, K., and Leamond, M. "The Decade of Medicaid." *Public Health Reports* 91, 1976: 303–308.

White Paper on Workers' Compensation: A Report on the Need for Reform of State Workers' Compensation. Prepared by U.S. Departments of Labor, Commerce; Health, Education and Welfare; and Housing and Urban Development, May 13, 1974. GPO-875-745. Washington, D.C.: U.S. Government Printing Office, 1974.

3
Rehabilitation Engineering

JAMES B. RESWICK, SC.D.

What is rehabilitation engineering, and what do rehabilitation engineers do? How does their work affect the disabled?

Dr. James Reswick answers these questions in his chapter on rehabilitation engineering. He presents a number of actual situations where rehabilitation engineers of different backgrounds work on the design and testing of devices for meeting the many and varied needs of disabled citizens. The chapter includes a discussion of the barriers to the delivery of rehabilitation engineering services and recommendations on how to overcome these barriers. The educational and professional status of rehabilitation engineers is discussed from the point of view of formal training, continuing education, preceptorships, and certification.

INTRODUCTION

Rehabilitation engineering, an emergent and now nationally recognized profession, may be defined as the application of engineering and other sciences in combination with medicine to improve the quality of life of disabled persons.

We are all aware of the remarkable progress of technology since the beginning of the twentieth century. Our population is mobile at high speed in the air, on land, and on water. We are also aware of the great advances in chemical, surgical, and antibiotic therapy of human disease. Infectious disease can be prevented and often controlled. Many viral diseases have been isolated, and malignancy is beginning to yield to increased understanding of normal and abnormal cell reproduction. Modern X-ray, nuclear medicine devices, and other new instruments for diagnosis have reduced uncertainty. But paradoxically, along with the growth of these technical and medical advances, has been a marked increase in disability of human beings of all ages, resulting from traumatic injury, congenital deformity in the young, and deterioration in the elderly. The human race is now living so long, on the average, that the engineering systems of the body (the pumps, gas exchange systems, filters, fluid flow channels, structures, motors, bearings, information paths, and control centers) begin to degenerate and eventually cause not only disability but often, much later, loss of life.

While technology is responsible for certain injuries and disabilities, it does offer the promise of making the quality of life of disabled people whole and productive, and of making the final years of older people more carefree, meaningful, and free of pain. The application of this technology to overcoming disability is rehabilitation engineering.

The high cost of delivery of health services and its rate of increase are well known. Also expanding is the social awareness in many nations of their responsibility for disabled persons. As individual costs rise, the number of persons who must be cared for also increases, causing a multiplication of costs that are staggering. But while costs are important, it is really the effectiveness/cost ratio of the treatment which is the most important measure. The goal of rehabilitation is to enable people with disabilities to better achieve their own life goals. This is the only valid measure of benefit, but objective measures of change in a disabled person's total life style are difficult to determine. It can, however, be shown that the cost of the rehabilitation systems—their initial cost and subsequent maintenance—are often far cheaper than the cost of chronic long-term hospitalization. From a human point of view, there is no question that the cost/benefit ratio can be greatly increased through enlightened application of technology.

What Is the Magnitude of the Problem?

A recent report (Rehabilitation Services Administration and the Veterans Administration, 1978) conducted jointly by the Rehabilitation Services Administration and the Veterans Administration, presented a table (see Table 1) showing the number of people who had given disabilities by selected types of impairment and age. The numbers shown reflect the U.S. population in 1971. It shows a total of 45,532,000 (all degrees of disability) and 6,579,000 (disability causing limitation in activity). The latter figure, approximately 3 percent of the total U.S. population, can be used as an estimate of those needing rehabilitation engineering services. Categorization by selected types of impairment is probably more useful than categorization by disease categories, since more than one disease may eventuate in the same type of impairment. However, when one considers the broad category of musculo-skeletal disorders (excluding sensory deficits), one finds a surprisingly high degree of incidence. Another recent study (Kelsey et al., 1978) indicates in its summary that:

1. Musculo-skeletal conditions rank first among disease groups in the frequency with which they affect the quality of life of individuals, as indicated by the extent of activity limitation, disability, impairment and handicap. About 20 million people in the United States have musculo-skeletal impairments.

2. Musculo-skeletal conditions rank second to diseases of the circulatory system in total economic cost, and are *first among all disease groups in cost attributable to lost earnings and services from non-fatal illness.* [Emphasis added.] The total annual economic cost attributable to musculo-skeletal conditions has been estimated to be about $20,000,000,000 per year (p. 1).

It is evident, even though the above numbers are probably not exact, that the order of magnitude of the problem is highly significant and the potential for major savings is high. Rehabilitation technology has so much to offer. It can surely improve the quality of life of disabled people and at a cost which, in the end, will be far less than if they were maintained solely by public assistance.

REVIEW OF RECENT LITERATURE

The recent literature in the field of biomedical and clinical engineering is extensive indeed. However, articles on rehabilitation engineering and its implications as a new profession have been very few. A discussion of the nature of rehabilitation engineering as a subclassification in the broad field of biomedical engineering was recently published in *The Bridge* by the National Academy of Engineering (Reswick, 1978). In this article, Reswick suggests that rehabilitation engineering should be defined in terms of the application of science and technology to persons with disabilities, normally after acute care and medical stabilization. This distinction emphasizes the role of the rehabilitation engineer in a chronic care facility and is concerned with the return of the disabled person to the community and work, as distinct from the acute care of patients and the application of science and technology to sophisticated diagnostic instrumentation and patient therapy. A considerable literature does exist concerning rehabilitation engineering research results and the development and application of devices for persons with disabilities. It is not the intent of this review to consider the technology per se, but rather to refer to a limited number of articles and reports that are concerned with rehabilitation engineering as a profession, its

TABLE 1

Number of Disabled People by Selected Types of Impairment and Age (In Thousands)

	1	*2*	*3*	*4*	*5*	*6*	*7*	*8*
	Total	*Under 17*	*17–44*	*Under 45*	*45–64*	*65 & Older*	*65–74*	*75 & Older*
U.S. population, 1971	202,360	66,544	74,703	141,247	41,764	19,349	12,044	7,305
Blind and visually handicapped (all degrees of disability)	9,596	623	2,385	3,008	2,630	3,958	—	—
Blind and visually handicapped (causing limitation in activity)	495	—	—	54	99	342	—	—
Hearing impairments (all degrees of disability)	14,491	863	3,167	4,030	4,765	5,695	2,783	2,912
Hearing impairments (causing limitation in activity)	573	93	155	248	147	176	76	100
Speech difficulty (all degrees of disability)	1,934	995	505	1,500	268	165	—	—
Speech difficulty (causing limitation in activity)	188	57	29	86	54	46	—	—
Paralysis (all degrees of disability)	1,392	158	342	500	446	446	—	—
Paralysis (causing limitation in activity)	861	100	198	298	285	277	—	—

Absence of major extremity	274	—	—	70	127	77	—	—
Impairment of back or spine (all degrees of disability)	8,018	210	3,662	2,872	2,847	1,298	824	474
Impairment of back and spine (causing limitation in activity)	1,976	55	857	912	776	288	189	99
Impairment of upper extremity and shoulder, except paralysis or absence (all degrees of disability)	2,440	120	886	1,006	855	578	—	—
Impairment of upper extremity and shoulder, except paralysis or absence (causing limitation in activity)	485	26	220	246	186	52	—	—
Impairment of lower extremity and hip, except paralysis or absence (all degrees of disability)	7,387	1,281	2,544	3,825	2,017	1,544	853	691
Impairment of lower extremity and hip except paralysis or absence (causing limitation in activity)	1,727	141	481	622	560	543	237	306

Source: *Rehabilitation Engineering—A Plan for Continued Progress II*, Rehabilitation Services Administration, HEW, and the Veterans Administration, Washington, D.C., 1978.

Notes: Column 1 yields two totals: 45,532,000 disabled (all degrees of disability) and 6,579,000 disabled (causing limitation in activity). This latter figure, approximately 3% of the total population, can be used as an estimate of those needing rehabilitation engineering services.

All data in this table were synthesized from the National Center for Health Statistics series on disability—Series 10, Number 99, Tables 1, 2, 4, 5, 7, 9, 10, 11, and 13.

The total listed in column 1 may not equal the sum of items in columns 4, 5, and 6 due to rounding effects.

potential to overcome the handicaps of persons with disabilities, and the barriers to effective delivery of services.

Probably the most informative overview of the present state-of-the-art in rehabilitation engineering is *Rehabilitation Engineering—A Plan for Continued Progress II* (Rehabilitation Services Administration, HEW, and the Veterans Administration, 1978). This document reports on thirteen state-of-the-art workshops in rehabilitation engineering that were held primarily in 1976 and 1977 under the auspices of the Rehabilitation Services Administration and the Veterans Administration. These workshops included:

1. The Role of Engineering in Spinal Cord Injury
2. Mobility for Spinal Cord Impaired People
3. Functional Electrical Stimulation—Application in Neural Prostheses
4. Personal Licensed Vehicles for the Disabled
5. Rehabilitation Engineering Education
6. Locomotion and the Clinical Analysis of Gait
7. Delivery of Rehabilitation Engineering Services in the State of California
8. Environmental Barriers and the Physically Disabled
9. Total Joint Replacement
10. Sensory Deficits and Sensory Aids
11. The Effects of Pressure on Human Tissue
12. External Prosthetics and Orthotics
13. Summary Meeting, National Academy of Sciences

In addition to descriptions of the state of the art, these workshops also produced prioritized lists of areas where future research and development would be most productive. The volume's overview section gives a summary of statistics of persons with disabilities, along with documentation of the sources of data.

In 1975, the National Academy of Sciences-National Research Council organized an ad hoc committee on National Needs for the Rehabilitation of the Physically Handicapped. This committee was to examine what needs to be done to improve the utilization of science and technology in restoring physically handicapped individuals to more active roles in society. The report of the committee appeared in two volumes (*Science and Technology in the Service of the Physically Handicapped,* Vol. I and Vol. II, 1976), the first consisting of the committee's report and the second contained six papers on social science and policy in areas essential to the evaluation of the needs of people with disabilities but not represented by the committee membership. Volume I deals with the nation's needs regarding the application of science and technology to aid both the sensorally and the physically handicapped, and then makes specific recommendations to meet these needs with an emphasis on the role the NAS/NRC might play. The papers contained in Volume II deal with cost-benefit analyses, public policy toward disability, the benefits and costs of federal/state vocational rehabilitation programs, social issues in rehabilitation, public expectations, consumer perspectives and critical issues facing the health care system, and significant contributions.

One of the recommendations contained in *Rehabilitation Engineering—A Plan for Continued Progress* (National Academy of Sciences, 1971) was the formation of a network of national Rehabilitation Engineering Centers. The first such centers were Rancho Los Amigos Hospital, Downey, California, and Moss Rehabilitation Institute, Philadelphia, Pennsylvania, in 1971, under grants from the Rehabilitation Services Administration, then part of SRS-HEW. Since then, the number of U.S. centers has grown to fifteen, with three in other countries. Leclair and Reswick (1977) give an overview of some of these centers in *American Rehabilitation.* They present the objectives of the centers and give examples of products which have been developed there as the result of their core research and development efforts.

The delivery of rehabilitation engineering services throughout the nation, providing disabled persons with equipment which already exists, is severely impeded by a number of barriers. Recognizing the need to define and understand these barriers, the Department of Rehabilitation of the State of California, in collaboration with the Veterans Administration, the Rehabilitation Services Administration, and the Rehabilitation Engineering Center at Rancho Los Amigos Hospital, brought together a number of persons concerned with service delivery at a 1977 workshop. They subsequently held a series of mini-workshops throughout the state, at which local participants reviewed and added to the findings from the first workshop. The report of this workshop, *Development of a Model Rehabilitation Engineering Delivery System in California—A Beginning* (California State Department of Rehabilitation, 1977) is one of the most complete and succinct statements of the problems faced by all those who help disabled people to take advantage of the many technical devices that now exist. This report is discussed in more detail later.

As a result of the workshops, improved information exchange was identified as a key factor in an effective rehabilitation engineering service delivery system. Realizing that judicious use of information retrieval and processing offered a significant potential for enhancing service delivery, the Technology Utilization Office at NASA's Ames Research Center funded an initial study on information needs concerning rehabilitation engineering and its products. This study, *Suggested Approach for Establishing a Rehabilitation Engineering Information Service for the State of California* (Christy et al., 1977) was undertaken by SRI International's Technology Application Team as part of its mission to transfer NASA experience and technology to the public sector.

To develop the initial model for an information service, the SRI Team first undertook an information needs profile of selected segments in rehabilitation. These profiles provided the basis for the second major portion of the study, which identified existing information models and systems both from within the world of rehabilitation and from other sources.

A California Rehab-engineering Information Service (CRIS) was proposed to support the provision of rehabilitation services to handicapped individuals through the use of technology and information. CRIS consists of three separate organizations that gather and disseminate information:

1. A Rehab-engineering Information Center to prepare catalogs of assistive devices and systems and repair and service directories; provide equipment design and consultation; operate mobile training units; staff a telephone call-in service; and process consumer feedback on devices and services.
2. An independent, nonprofit evaluation center and clearinghouse to assemble testing results and develop criteria for a cost/benefit analysis of technical devices and rehabilitation engineering services.
3. A Rehab-Technology Applications Unit to link user and designer needs with a data base and research expertise.

The purpose of this study was not to make final recommendations concerning an information service for CRIS but rather to provide an orientation and basis for further discussions among NASA, the California State Department of Rehabilitation, and the rehabilitation community.

The National Science Foundation has recently been active in supporting research studies on the needs of persons with disabilities and the potential of science and technology to meet these needs. Two reports that contain significant statements and which, incidentally, have excellent bibliographies should be mentioned. The first, *The Application of Technological Developments to Physically Disabled People,* was published by the Urban Institute in Washington, D.C. (La Rocca and Turem, 1978). It reviews the disabled population in the United States in terms of number and functional limitations as well as income and employment. It deals with technological developments, particularly communications systems, and discusses the impact of public policy on the use of technologies for handicapped people. It then deals with the problems of development, manufacturing, and marketing facing manufacturers and the problems of funding the development of technologies. Of particular interest is the section on technologies in housing, employment, and transportation that aid handicapped people. A second report, *Human Rehabilitation Techniques—A Technology Assessment,* was prepared by the Texas Technological University under an NSF grant (Texas Tech. University, 1978). It is organized around eleven broad issues ranging from problems presented by unstandardized definitions within rehabilitation to the distinction between rehabilitation and maintenance. Particularly significant is the chapter on representative disabilities, wherein a variety of disease categories are dealt with in terms of their definitions and degrees of resultant disability. The chapter "Disability as Life Function Impairment or Limitation" distinguishes between life function needs and multiple disabilities, showing that a classification by disability and function is more appropriate than by disease category. The chapters on human rehabilitation in relation to society and policy-related consequences are interesting in that they are built around generalized economic models of the nation and the potential impact of growth projections.

The questions of production and marketing of rehabilitation engineering devices are discussed in many of the references cited. In particular, the problem is dealt with explicitly by R. K. Jurgen in his article "Devices for the Disabled: A Production Dilemma" (1976):

> Although numerous innovative devices to aid the handicapped are constantly being developed, many do not progress beyond the prototype stage. As a result, the disabled are being denied the benefits of technological advances that could make them more self-sufficient and employable.

> The problem is complex. Industrial firms, used to the commercial marketplace, are often reluctant to manufacture a rehabilitation device for which there may be no clearly defined market, or a known small market, or a market made up of customers who often cannot afford to pay for the product. Those companies that have entered the rehabilitation-device manufacturing field have often had to develop unique marketing strategies based, if possible, on government and institutional funding in combination with their own financial resources and, more often than not, with a strong feeling of social consciousness (p. 45).

Some of the most relevant material in the field of rehabilitation engineering and problems facing the delivery of services has been developed during congressional hearings. Of particular relevance are the oversight hearings before the Select Subcommittee on Education of the Committee on Education and Labor, held during the 93rd Congress on November 30 and December 1, 1974. Part III of the published document from these hearings contains a number of verbal transcripts and prepared statements by professionals from the field, dealing with the need for enhanced research and development and the problems which face manufacturers of rehabilitation engineering devices. Similarly, the hearings before the Committee on Science and Technology, U.S. House of Representatives, during the 94th Congress on September 22–23, 1976, deal with the same problems and include a number of examples of successful rehabilitation engineering device applications.

These 1976 hearings led Olin E. Teague, Chairman of the Committee on Science and Technology, to appoint a Panel on Research Programs to Aid the Handicapped. The panel was authorized "to conduct a study of the problems of the handicapped and how research or the application of present scientific and technological achievements should be put forth in programs to ameliorate or resolve the problems of the handicapped" (Panel on Research Programs to Aid the Handicapped report, 1977, p. iv). Panel findings generally confirmed needs as stated in previous references—need for research, consumer participation, increased investment in research and demonstration, improved communications about and distribution of rehabilitation engineering services, and others. However, a particularly critical need recognized by the panel was for coordination of research and demonstration and delivery of services within the federal government. This led to its major recommendation: the creation of a National Council for Research and the Handicapped. Most of the report deals with the recommended structure and function of the proposed organization.

But the concept did not catch hold, and Congressman Teague appointed a second Panel on Research Programs to Aid the Handicapped which reported to the Committee on Science and Technology in March 1978 (Panel Report, 1978). This second panel report contains the first panel report as an appendix. After examining and approving the methods, findings, and recommendations of the first panel, the second panel concentrated on a recommendation that "The U.S. Government should establish and fund an entity with authority, responsibility and accountability for coordinating, supporting, and guiding research and development programs for the benefit of handicapped persons" (Panel Report, 1978, pp. 2–3).

The panel developed a list of program responsibilities and then concerned itself mainly with possible locations for a host agency. It proposed, after studying a number of models, that NASA host the new entity and that it be guided by a twelve- to eighteen-member Science and Technology Board for Handicapped Persons, appointed by the President of the United States.

Apparently neither the recommendation of the second panel nor that of the first panel will be realized, at least exactly as made. At the time of this writing, a conference committee of the House and Senate is considering a third proposal that has been written into both the Senate and House versions of the 1978 Amendments to the Rehabilitation Act of 1973. This is for the creation of a National Institute for Rehabilitation Research, the form and structure of which is a central issue for discussion in the conference committee.

It is not unreasonable that this brief literature review end on the above note, for most of the references are concerned with the unmet needs of persons with disabilities and the potential of rehabilitation engineering to meet their needs. That the efforts of so many responsible and concerned persons have resulted in congressional recognition of the problems and potentially significant legislative action is encouraging indeed.

BARRIERS TO THE EFFECTIVE DELIVERY OF REHABILITATION ENGINEERING SERVICES

As stated earlier, in 1977 the California State Department of Rehabilitation, with support from the Veterans Administration and the Rehabilitation Services Administration, convened a workshop on rehabilitation engineering. The purpose was to define barriers to delivery of effective rehabilitation engineering services and to generate recommendations to overcome these barriers. Among the participants were representatives of the following groups:

1. Consumers—disabled persons who need the devices.
2. Ombudsmen—physicians and other allied health professionals who diagnose the patient's needs and prescribe the devices.
3. Agencies—federal, state, and local, which have the health, social, and vocational responsibility for disabled persons.
4. Suppliers—manufacturers and institutions which make the equipment available to consumers.
5. Authorizers and providers—health agencies (e.g., Medi-Cal, Medicare) and insurance companies which must authorize purchase of equipment and provide payment.
6. Inventors—rehabilitation engineers and others who design and develop equipment to meet the needs of people with disabilities.
7. Educators—university and college professionals who train rehabilitation engineers and rehabilitation technicians to develop, manufacture, and maintain equipment.
8. Legislators—politicians and staff personnel at federal, state, and local levels who pass and administer legislation concerning the rehabilitation of disabled persons.

It is interesting to note the nature of the differing groups, all of which have important roles to play in helping disabled persons. Together they comprise a system that is very complex and cannot be improved without an understanding of the system as a whole—the interrelationships of the groups and how they function.

The report of the Pomona Workshop, *Development of a Model Rehabilitation Engineering Delivery System in California—A Beginning* (1977), summarizes the barriers as seen by members of the above-listed groups. The following list is adapted from that report (comments relate primarily to the State of California but are applicable in other states):

1. Lack of effective information dissemination and communication.
    a. Consumer (disabled person) lacks information about *what* is available, the *quality* and *effectiveness* of devices, *where* and *how* they may be obtained, and *how* to get reimbursement for devices.
    b. Counselors, physicians, therapists, advisors, and others lack information on devices and their appropriateness for particular patients.

c. Developers and suppliers lack sufficient market data.
d. Designers lack awareness of existing equipment and may end up "reinventing the wheel" because they do not know about some technology or device which is already available in the United States or in other countries.
e. Designers lack information on the real needs of consumers. Too often, they do not understand the needs of the disabled person and spend their time trying to invent and develop devices which are not needed.
f. Providers lack information on cost/effectiveness of devices so that they can justify payments. An expensive device may really be cheaper in the long run.

2. A hodgepodge of agencies, with overlapping functions in some cases and gaps in others, deal with the disabled person. Naive consumers have a difficult time becoming educated about the sources of support for them and how to reach for them. It is almost impossible to allocate costs among a number of agencies, such as Medicare, Medi-Cal, CHAMPUS, CCRS, Blue Cross, and the Department of Vocational Rehabilitation. Agencies have different goals; for example, Medi-Cal is concerned with *medical* care, while the state departments of VR are concerned with *vocational* effectiveness. Many times a single device solves both kinds of problems. Often neither agency can pay full costs, but they might share if the mechanisms existed.

3. There is a general lack of funds for:

   a. Research on needs of the disabled.
   b. Research and development of devices.
   c. Initial support for establishment of rehabilitation engineering.
   d. Evaluation of new and existing equipment.
   e. Support to manufacturers for start-up costs when the market is limited and needs to be developed.
   f. Research on cost-effectiveness of existing delivery systems and potential new systems.

4. There is a major lack in the availability of rehabilitation engineering services. Only a few scattered, relatively small enterprises for retrofit and maintenance exist.

5. There is a great need for product evaluation. Even if manufacturers' catalogs are available, there is a great need to be able to differentiate between devices and to have good information on

reliability, ability of the device to meet the patient's need, maintenance, and other factors.

6. There is a need to improve the ability of providers to approve and pay for devices. Payment schedules at present are completely unrealistic. The system is incapable of updating itself in terms of new technology, products, and costs. The Schedule of Maximum Allowances (SMA) of Medi-Cal is out of date. Determination of eligibility for Medicare/Medi-Cal is difficult. Medi-Cal looks for the least expensive way to solve a problem (even if it may be more expensive in the long run). The "scope of benefits" limits Medicare/Medi-Cal, which cannot reimburse for "new" items. Budget is sufficient to cover only approved items. There is a lack of guidelines for purchasing innovative devices.

7. Problems of suppliers-manufacturers: It is difficult to get new devices to the marketplace and often unprofitable for private industry. The cost of providing rehabilitation engineering services is high. A low-volume market, product liability, device legislation, and the cost of selling goods and services all inhibit new developments. Lack of market data dampens industry enthusiasm. The high cost of development is difficult to recoup in limited market.

8. Educational Problems

   a. Curriculum not defined for rehabilitation technician or rehabilitation engineer.
   b. Lack of coordination within the allied health education of the educational institutions in California.
   c. No provision for teaching users (e.g., nurses, social workers, technicians, physicians).
   d. Lack of good text material (e.g., books, tapes, TV, audiovisual materials).
   e. Standard biomedical engineering curricula not appropriate.
   f. Need for means to expose students from all disciplines to multidisciplinary curriculum and practice.
   g. Need for a variety of exposures—controls, electrical, mechanical, architectural, construction—at the hands-on level.
   h. Motivating students a problem because of the poor rehabilitation engineering fit into the hospital and agency hierarchy they are likely to go into. In other words, rehabilitation engineers, instead of being accountable to the medical director, are more likely to report to the plant engineer. They have to be part of the *clinical* team.

i. No licensing and certification. The rehabilitation engineer should have a clinical responsibility and be part of the patient care team.
j. Guidance counselors in high schools at the appropriate time —probably not now—need to steer students into rehabilitation engineering. Guidance counselors at this time are unaware of this field.
k. No journal for the exchange of information for many purposes—certainly for the educator's.
l. Lack of communication between educators and other professionals—between educators and users and consumers.

9. Transportation for disabled people for delivery of services is inadequate. Difficult for patients to receive devices and to continue follow-up.

With all of the problems listed above, it is remarkable that so many of the rehabilitation engineering needs of disabled people are being met today. In fact, there now exist a wide range of devices in successful use. As suggested by the above list, the main problems center on information and delivery of services. There appears to be one overriding need which, if addressed, would go a long way toward solving many of the problems listed above. This is the need for an *effective evaluation system* for rehabilitation engineering devices.

Evaluation is where the buck stops. Evaluation should tell us whether a device really meets the needs of disabled persons. Everyone concerned with disabled people—and especially they themselves—need and seek information. But information without relevance and value to the recipient is useless. In fact, it is often damaging and counterproductive. The importance of an effective evaluation system—which does not now exist in the United States—is discussed in further detail later.

HOW DOES THE REHABILITATION ENGINEER SERVE PEOPLE WITH DISABILITIES?

To explain the role of the rehabilitation engineer, brief activity portraits of persons engaged in this type of work are presented below. While not totally comprehensive, the activities of the engineers who are described do represent a major portion of the field; each one illustrates a different role, work environment, and set of issues. The composite is intended as an overview of the field of rehabilitation engineering—its functions and certain of its problems.

The Rehabilitation Engineer as a Member of the Patient Care Team

Bruce B. is a recent graduate of a biomedical engineering program of a large university. He joined a research group in a rehabilitation engineering center while still a student and completed his master's thesis on research done as part of the group's research activity in functional electrical stimulation. This preceptorship provided him with experience in a clinical environment and created in him a strong motivation to continue his professional career in rehabilitation engineering. As a result of his demonstrated competence and interest, he became a full-time engineer in the research group and, after several years, assumed leadership responsibilities.

Working closely with physicians and allied health professionals concerned with the rehabilitation of stroke patients, Bruce was able to present a number of new concepts for stroke therapy based on his knowledge of feasible technology and his increasing awareness of the goals of stroke therapy. At the same time, the medical and allied health professionals proposed modes of treatment which required technology that Bruce could test for feasibility and actually design. From this milieu of interaction and exchange of ideas emerged a number of new devices and methods of stroke therapy based on the application of functional electrical stimulation and biofeedback. These are now proving their effectiveness for a large number of stroke patients in a major rehabilitation center. Neither Bruce nor any of the other health professionals responsible for patient care can claim to be the sole innovator of these successful ideas. Rather, they have resulted from a truly interactive team effort that took place in the clinical environment while patients were being treated.

The Rehabilitation Engineer as a Member of the Vocational Rehabilitation Team

Clyde S. is supervisor of a model shop in a large rehabilitation center. Clyde is an all-around craftsman who works with metals, plastics, textiles, and the like. He is also skilled in basic electrical circuits and controls. He did not graduate from an engineering school but developed his natural talents in a series of different work settings. As one might expect, he keeps his own home in top condition, repairing appliances, doing his own plumbing and electrical work, and minor maintenance work on his car. He typifies, as do so many other Americans, the "Yankee spirit of innovation" and "do-it-yourself" capability. He is satisfied only when his products work safely and reliably and exhibit the kind of aesthetic qualities that result from the skills of a craftsman.

Clyde is a rehabilitation engineer not because of his training and skills but rather because he applies these skills to the problems of disabled people. In the large rehabilitation hospital where Clyde works, a new program has been developed to provide rehabilitation engineering services to clients who are referred by counselors of the State Department of Rehabilitation. Typically, a client is seen by a team of which Clyde is a member and which includes the client and family, the counselor, and appropriate occupational and other therapists, as well as social and sometimes psychological counselors. In the team meeting, the client's problems are reviewed, the potential for vocational and avocational activities is assessed, and the applications of technology which will help the client are defined. These may include special wheelchair modifications and controls, functional lap-board systems, modifications in the home, special driving controls with associated training, modification of an on-the-job work station, or, in the case of severely disabled clients, highly sophisticated computer-controlled environmental communications systems. Wherever possible, Clyde will recommend commercially available equipment that, in his judgment, best meets the client's needs. In most cases, he will design and build special adaptive devices that match the client's unique limitations to the control of the equipment. Clyde's effectiveness depends not only on his own technical skills but also on his ability to relate effectively as a team member who understands, with the help of therapists and others, the overall goals of the client and how physical and other limitations may be taken into account in the design of equipment. One of Clyde's major problems is to get the other team members, especially the authorizer of payments, to understand that his time, the time of his technicians, and the materials he uses can culminate in much higher than expected costs for a one-of-a-kind device. It is usually difficult for the nontechnical person to relate the very low cost of a highly developed mass-produced device to the development cost of a special device that ends up looking much like it.

The Rehabilitation Engineer in Research and Development

Carol F. was a physics major in college. Her graduate work required her to become familiar with both the hardware of modern computer systems and their software and programing. Several years in industry gave her practical experience with the specification of computer components and their application to real problems. She joined a research group in a rehabilitation engineering center that is concerned with the analysis of human functioning, using a wide variety of physical measurement techniques along with the computer analysis of data. Measurements are made on persons disabled by disease such as cerebral palsy, stroke, multiple sclerosis, polio, and arthritis; on patients who have been traumatically injured; and on amputees. Such measurements include energy consumption analysis, EMG, accelerometry, goniometry, events of floor contact by the foot during gait, and stress measurements on orthotic and prosthetic devices. From such measurements, when compared with those typical of normal function, surgeons are better able to plan their surgical interventions. Objective comparisons between pretreatment and posttreatment may be made.

Carol is a member of a team that includes medical and other allied health personnel as well as other technical support persons. She assists in the development of evaluation protocols for various categories of patient disability; and plans and engineers the acquisition and development of devices to perform measurements at high speed and telemeter results to a computer center. In particular, she assists the medical professionals in designing data formats and processing techniques to produce significant parameters which are true measures of human performance and which are useful to physicians in their decision making. She plans the continuing growth of a computer facility, taking advantage of the increasing capability of modern technology. Her work requires her to understand the details of electrical circuits and the operation of transducers, and she is personally able to troubleshoot a system and make it work. The job is not easy because, in addition to solving demanding technical problems, she must remember the needs of the patient, who may be severely disabled and possibly confused (as is sometimes true with brain trauma). In the end, the data produced by the complex system must be truly meaningful to the physician. As a member of a team dealing with patients in a clinical environment, which necessarily results in a constant communication and interaction with the patients and the professionals who care for them, Carol is able to apply her skills to produce meaningful results.

The Rehabilitation Engineer in Industry and Private Delivery Systems

Harry F. is a graduate electronics engineer. For some years, he has been employed by a large manufacturer whose success is derived from the international distribution of heart-pacing devices. This firm is actively expanding into other areas in rehabilitation. Harry is a "new idea" man. He travels a great deal, making contacts at national meetings and responding to interest expressed by physicians with innovations of their own who need technical and manufacturing support. Harry manages a group of prototype engineers and technicians who are able to put together highly sophisticated devices for implant in the human body. He maintains active liaison between the groups in clinical settings and his firm. In addition to engineering skills, he must be aware of and responsible for his company's compliance with increasingly demanding regulations of federal and state governments relating to new medical devices. He must also be aware of the costs of development, manufacture, and distribution to ensure that the final product can be marketed profitably in our free-enterprise system. New products require extensive and careful evaluation. Harry therefore finds himself concerned with developing effective evaluation protocols and coordinating evaluations in multiple centers where new devices are used with human beings for the first time.

For example, Harry has been deeply involved in the development and evaluation of a new implant stimulator to overcome the disability of drop foot in stroke patients; a similar implantable stimulator for correcting the curvature of the spine due to scoliosis; and an implantable electric stimulator that reduces chronic pain by electrically stimulating the spinal cord of a patient. Harry's success depends on his close interaction with those responsible for patient care. During early evaluations, he may find himself observing and assisting in the operating room, where he can become aware, firsthand, of the problems facing the surgeon during an implant procedure and provide the surgeon with technical assistance. Of course, the surgeon is primarily responsible for any device used in a patient, but to a large degree, Harry must share this responsibility. His technical expertise and that of his company are an indispensable part of a particular treatment program.

Scott D. is president of a small company that delivers rehabilitation engineering services directly to disabled people. His firm specializes in converting standard automotive vans to be used by those who use wheelchairs. He designs, builds, and attaches electric lift devices to provide access to the rear of the van, adds numerous electric controls for opening and closing doors, and modifies the driving controls to enable paraplegics to drive with only their hands. Scott provides a vitally needed service, but he operates under many constraints. He ensures, to the best of his ability, that his conversions are reliable and safe. He must often modify a given approach to meet the unique needs of a particular client. Much of his work is handcrafted, which is expensive in both time and materials. He must raise capital to launch his business, and he is responsible for meeting payrolls and debt service as well as completing the myriad forms and reports required of a small business. To keep his costs within reason, he must operate efficiently and yet be sure that his work is of the highest quality. His largest problem is that of product liability. A single failure resulting in an expensive lawsuit and settlement could bankrupt him at any time. The cost of liability insurance is so high that he literally cannot afford to protect himself and still provide his services at a reasonable level. His only recourse is to do the best job he can, keep his attachable assets relatively low, and hope for the best.

The Prosthetist/Orthotist Rehabilitation Engineer

Mike Q. is a certified prosthetist/orthotist. He is a graduate of a baccalaureate program and represents the increasing number of young men and women who enter the field as college graduates. While orthotics and prosthetics is a worldwide profession, increasingly its practitioners are being required to broaden their knowledge and practice to become skilled in the application of new materials and electronic devices. Mike is not only skilled in conventional bracing and casting techniques but is, for example, able to apply and maintain externally powered and electrically controlled prostheses, environmental control systems, and communication devices.

Mike brings to rehabilitation engineering a kind of training and experience that others must often acquire. As a certified orthotist/prosthetist, he was trained to work in a patient care team and to assist the physician in orthopedic care of patients. As a businessman, he is familiar with the process of third-party billing and payment, an area in which most rehabilitation engineers are naive.

Mike leads a research group that has pioneered the application of vacuum-formed polymer materials in the design of lightweight and cosmetically pleasing prostheses. His research also deals with new fracture-bracing devices that permit better control of pressure on the tissues, and he is concerned with the mechanics of novel traction techniques. Thus, while he does not hold an engineering degree, he does, through his practice and training gained in a rehabilitation engineering setting, function as a rehabilitation engineer.

DISCUSSION

The Unique Qualities of the Rehabilitation Engineer

From the preceding descriptions, we can see that a number of common factors characterize the rehabilitation engineer. These factors arise more from what a rehabilitation engineer *does* than from his or her formal education and training. Most are, in fact, graduates of engineering and/or biomedical engineering programs. While no formal rehabilitation engineering education programs now exist, it is certain that they will soon become part of the curriculum in a number of universities. But whether rehabilitation engineers have engineering degrees or enter the practice of rehabilitation engineering through other paths they will exhibit the following characteristics:

1. Rehabilitation engineers must, first of all, be a competent professional in a field of specialization (e.g., mechanical, electrical, systems, chemical, materials engineering, orthotics/prosthetics). This is necessary for two reasons.
    a. They must be able to practice professional engineering in a competent way.
    b. They must be recognized by peers as competent professionals if they are to gain the respect necessary to collaborate on a peer basis with the health professional.
2. Rehabilitation engineers should have natural propensities for working with health professionals as a member of a patient care team and sharing responsibility with other team members. This characteristic, perhaps more than any other, distinguishes rehabilitation engineers from other biomedical engineers who, for the most part, are individually concerned with research and the development, use, and maintenance of hospital systems and devices that focus on acute diagnosis and care.
3. Rehabilitation engineers practice a profession which assumes the highest ethical norms of both the engineering and health professions. They must share responsibility for patient care with the health professional and must therefore understand and practice the highest professional ethics.

4. Rehabilitation engineers must often relate closely to the commercialization of devices. They must understand the special problems inherent in marketing medical devices and be prepared to counsel industry before a manufacturing project is undertaken. Further, they should be prepared to assist an industry in the production and distribution of devices.
5. Above all, rehabilitation engineers are patient- or client-oriented. Whether in the development of a new device or therapy mode, or in the actual delivery of a rehabilitation engineering service, the goal is to improve the quality of life of the disabled person.

Evaluation of Rehabilitation Engineering Devices

Probably the major barrier to effective delivery of rehabilitation engineering services in our country today is the lack of a comprehensive evaluation system. The problem is often referred to as one of "information transfer" or bridging the gap between research and prototype development and commercial distribution. The fact is that while information transfer is critically important, the information itself must be based on effective evaluation of devices in clinical and home environments. The central problem with commercializing rehabilitation engineering devices lies in marketing and distribution, which comes back again to effective evaluation. Evaluation is the only way in which the true market potential of a new device can be determined and its criteria for use ascertained.

Evaluation is far more difficult and costly than is often assumed. To be effective, a *program* for each device to be evaluated must be undertaken, with a central management function that evolves protocol and criteria for evaluation; monitors the actual evaluation in a number of clinical and/or home settings; stimulates proper data taking; and finally, correlates field reports into an informative and comprehensive document. When one considers the many thousands of devices, each of which should go through this process, one can see that from a national point of view, the problem is immense.

Consider, for example, wheelchair cushions. There are more than 100 different wheelchair cushions marketed commercially in the United States today. These range from simple foam pads that may be custom-fitted to patients, through gel and visco-elastic polymer-filled cushions, to externally powered and controlled alternating pressure pads. To evaluate these cushions, it would be necessary to define patient populations with specific indications (stroke, polio, paraplegic, quadriplegic, cerebral palsy, etc.) in order to form statistically significant control groups and to devise protocols and instrumentation for objective data taking. Multiply this by the wide variety of cushions, and one comes up with a study costing hundreds of thousands of dollars and involving a large number of people in many places.

The wheelchair cushion is only one of hundreds of devices and may be among the most straightforward to evaluate objectively, yet this has never been done. The consumer has only manufacturers' catalogs to rely on and, in most cases, is provided a cushion which is in vogue at the time in the center where he or she is a patient. The health professional who prescribes the cushion and the provider who pays for it are equally in the dark. The manufacturer of a new cushion has no way of learning if this unique design is valid and will be able to sustain itself in the marketplace. The same remarks may be made over and over again with respect to countless other rehabilitation engineering devices.

A proper evaluation thus involves (1) procuring a sufficient number of devices to be statistically significant, (2) a substantial number of worker hours in arranging the evaluation, as well as the worker hours involved in the actual evaluation, and (3) to be effective, substantial workshop and/or travel costs. Thus, the evaluation cost of a single item can be very substantial. Of course, much evaluation data can be obtained on a less formal program basis from simpler devices, especially those which have already achieved some market acceptance. But the problem can be attacked only through a large-scale effort. While aware, to a great extent, of the need for evaluation, the federal agencies have been largely unable to come to grips with the magnitude of the problem. Only the Veterans Administration has maintained a moderate evaluation program with respect to devices suitable for veterans, and while their efforts have produced much useful information and have been of considerable assistance to manufacturers in launching their products, the overall problem remains. What is needed is a "consumers union" for rehabilitation engineering devices.

The author visualizes a central facility of substantial size capable of both coordinating evaluation in centers throughout the country and having an in-house testing and evaluation function. It would soon become a center of information and should have a number of dissemination modes (e.g., a direct "800" telephone, computer network, frequent evaluation bulletins, comprehensive reports, and other innovative uses of communications systems). It would be a place to which consumers, providers, authorizers, manufacturers, and government agencies at all levels could turn for immediate answers and continuing information updates. Such an evaluation center will be costly to create and to run. A system of fees could reduce operation costs, once established, but a major allocation of funds, probably federal, would be required to bring it into being. The potential for cost saving in the yearly costs of delivery of health services and the benefits to consumers far outweigh the substantial costs of initiation. Will our nation provide this desperately needed facility?

CONCLUSION

In the foregoing sections, the author has attempted to define rehabilitation engineering, both in terms of its emergence as a new profession and by examples of what a rehabilitation engineer does. There is a great unmet need for rehabilitation engineering services among the population of disabled persons. Research and development must be continued and expanded, but the need to bring the devices and techniques that now exist to disabled persons is even more important. Barriers that inhibit the delivery of these services are many and complex; most of them are part of our social and political system and therefore beyond the control of the rehabilitation engineer and other professionals who care for persons with disabilities. Research leading to an understanding of the total system is badly needed. Only a total approach that identifies and strengthens the weakest links in the delivery-of-services chain will be effective in meeting all of the needs. Among the weakest links are (1) the lack of information, particularly information based on good evaluations, (2) the lack of an evaluation system to produce this information, and (3) the disarray in the system of authorizations and payments. These problems inhibit the ability of all persons in the delivery system to do their jobs effectively. It seems clear that steps must be taken at all levels —local, state, and national—to initiate actions to define these problems and overcome them.

This chapter has been mainly concerned with rehabilitation engineering, complex systems of service delivery, and the like. These somewhat cold terms should not divert us from the people to whom all of this is directed. They are human beings who simply have physical or sensory disabilities which the majority of people do not. Whether or not the disability produces a handicap must be determined in terms of the limitation imposed on creativity, effectiveness, and personal happiness. It is in this sense that the goal of rehabilitation engineering is to minimize handicaps. This point was never better stated than by Her Excellency, Mrs. Jehan El Sadat, wife of the President of Egypt, in her opening address at the Rehabilitation Engineering Conference, Wafa Wa Amal, held in Egypt in June, 1975:

> You represent a procession of peace, love and good will, a procession illuminated by the offering of this experience, its science and its incomparable potentials enhanced by noble sentiments for the sake of Man's happiness. For the sake of making him feel that he does not live isolated from the love, tenderness and care of his brothers in humanity (pp. 1–3).

It is this thought which underlies the logo that is gaining world acceptance as the symbol of rehabilitation engineering. The right hands of the physician and the engineer are seen holding together the parts of a broken Ankh—the ancient Egyptian symbol of humankind that includes both body and soul.

REHABILITATION ENGINEERING

REFERENCES

Christy, L., Kelton-Fogg, G., Lizak, R., and Vahlkamp, C. *Suggested Approach for Establishing a Rehabilitation Engineering Information Service for the State of California.* SRI International, Menlo Park, Calif., September 1977.

Development of a Model Rehabilitation Engineering Delivery System in California—A Beginning. Report of Kellogg-West Workshop, January 16–18, 1977, and subsequent "mini-workshops" held throughout the State of California. California State Department of Rehabilitation, Sacramento, Calif., 95814.

Hearings before the Committee on Science and Technology, U.S. House of Representatives, 94th Congress, September 22–23, 1976.

Human Rehabilitation Techniques—A Technology Assessment. Final Report to National Science Foundation, Grants ERP-75-10594 and ERP-75-10594-A01, Texas Tech. University, 1978.

Jurgen, R. K. "Devices for the Disabled: A Production Dilemma." *Spectrum* September 1976, 45.

Kelsey, J., Pastides, H., Bisbee Jr., G. *Musculo-Skeletal Disorders: Their Frequency of Occurrence and Their Impact on the Population of the United States.* Prodist Press: N.Y., 1978.

La Rocca, J., and Turem, J. "The Application of Technological Developments to Physically Disabled People." The Urban Institute Report to the National Science Foundation, Grant No. PRA-76-82314, May 1978.

Leclair, R. R., and Reswick, J. B. "Looking at Engineering Centers." *American Rehabilitation* 2, 1976–1977: 20–23.

Oversight Hearings before the Select Subcommittee on Education of the Committee on Education and Labor, House of Representatives, 93rd Congress, Part 3, November 30 and December 1, 1974.

Panel on Research Programs to Aid the Handicapped. *Report to the Committee on Science and Technology,* U.S. House of Representatives, 95th Congress, First Session, Serial A, April 1977.

Panel on Research Programs to Aid the Handicapped. *Report* to the Committee on Science and Technology, U.S. House of Representatives, 95th Congress, Second Session, Serial V, March 1978.

Rehabilitation Engineering—A Plan for Continued Progress. Report of the Committee on Prosthetics Research and Development, National Academy of Sciences, Washington, D.C. 1971.

Rehabilitation Engineering—A Plan for Continued Progress II. Rehabilitation Services Administration, HEW, and the Veterans Administration, Washington, D.C., 1978.

Reswick, J. B. "Some Thoughts Relative to the Rehabilitation Engineer." *The Bridge* 8, 1978, 7–9.

Science and Technology in the Service of the Physically Handicapped, Vol. I and Vol. II. Report of the Committee on National Needs for the Rehabilitation of the Physically Handicapped, National Academy of Sciences, Washington, D.C., 1976.

4
Sheltered Industrial Employment*

CAROLYN L. VASH, PH.D.

The U.S. citizen with a disability is enjoying a newfound status of being legally protected from discrimination in employment. This is a dramatic change from centuries ago when the cripple *was an openly castigated social pariah, or only a decade or so ago when the* invalid *was an object of pity and protection. The Rehabilitation Act of 1973 offers legal protection to disabled persons with respect to employment under federal contracts and program participation under federal grants. The act ushered in a new era of mainstream employment for workers with disabilities; the emphasis changed from* whether *to* how *and* when.

These developments are traced in "Sheltered Industrial Employment," *a state-of-the-art review of worldwide experience and conceptualizations regarding accommodated or sheltered employment in both the segregated and mainstream worlds of work for workers with disabilities which constitute vocational handicaps. The review also provides information for vocational rehabilitation administrators and planners to use in future planning of implementation strategies for sheltered employment projects in the public and private sectors in the United States.*

This chapter describes work opportunities for people with such severe disabilities and vocation handicaps that they cannot fit into a vacant position as easily as the average person - some kind of accommodation *or* shelter *is needed. Whatever words we choose, many aspects of jobs are now being modified to meet the needs of workers or potential workers rather than forcing them to make all the adjustments.*

The chapter is organized into five major sections which include definitions and legal and philosophical issues; information on sheltered workshops and

*This chapter is based on a monograph of the same title that appeared as one of a series called "Emerging Issues in Rehabilitation," published by the Institute for Research Utilization (Washington, D.C. 1977), with funding support by the Rehabilitation Services Administration. The author wishes to thank the following individuals who contributed to the preparation of the earlier monograph: Mr. Henry Redkey, Mr. Dean Phillips, Mr. Al Frederickson, Ms. Saralea Altman, Mr. Tom Burns, Mr. Robert Melody, Mr. Wyn Cochran, Mr. Dwight Guilfoil, Mr. Wesley Geigel, Mr. Charles Richman, Dr. Frank Gentile, Dr. Thomas Backer, Ms. Susan Stoddard, Dr. Herbert Dorken, Dr. Elizabeth Pan, Dr. Frederic Schlamp, Ms. Judith Senkovitch, and Ms. Charlene Howlett.

mainstream employment; and a description of American industry's experience preparing disabled persons for work in mainstream settings.

The final section presents considerations for the future and some ideas, conclusions, and suggestions for how past experience might be used in planning future action. Appended to the paper is a selected bibliography.

INTRODUCTION

Shelter is a word we have traditionally used in talking about ways in which a job situation is altered to conform to the needs of the worker who has a disability. Lately, however, there is growing discussion about such phenomena as the four-day work week, flex-time, job sharing, job-site child care facilities, and so forth. These are also ways in which a job situation can be altered to conform to the needs of the worker, but not because the worker has a disability. Often it is because the worker has parental obligations. In these cases, we do not speak of shelter; we generally use the word *accommodation.* Whatever words we choose, we are assuredly in an era in which many aspects of jobs are being modified to meet the needs of workers or potential workers, rather than forcing them to make all of the adjustments. Providing accommodations needed by disabled workers is only one part of this trend. Another way of clarifying the distinction is this: *Accommodation* is something an employer provides to enable a worker to perform up to standards. *Shelter* is something the employer provides for selected employees who are unable to meet the standards. Accordingly, the term *shelter* will here be used solely in cases where some degree of reduced production or inappropriate work behavior is tolerated.

Figure 1 illustrates the conceptual framework of this topic. It presents an ascending scale of increasing integration into the mainstream world of work, coupled with decreasing accommodation or shelter. Some additional terms used in Figure 1 require definition.

1. The term *industry* reflects the general sense, so familiar in rehabilitation, of work that exists anywhere other than a workshop with a prime purpose of providing services to client-workers, not the production of goods. It also means employment in the real world of work, including all types of business and professional pursuits, not just the narrow meaning of industry as manufacture and processing.

2. The term *mainstream* is borrowed from education, where it has become very familiar over the past five years. It is used here with respect to employment in a similar way and refers to employ-

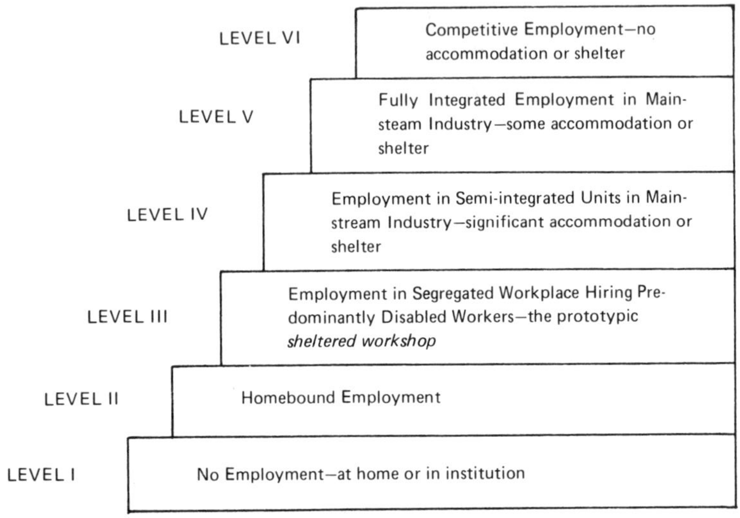

FIGURE 1

ment, again in the real world of work, rather than in a separate track. As in education, it is not an all-or-nothing proposition; there are degrees of mainstreaming.

3. The opposite of mainstream employment is *segregated employment* in a separate, specialized, sheltered workshop where most of one's co-workers are also disabled.

4. A step up from segregated employment is what is here called *semi-integrated employment.* The blind-operated vending stands in public buildings offer a familiar example of this in the United States. The blind and otherwise disabled workers in these concessions come to work in the same plant as nondisabled workers, allowing for some familiarizing contact and socialization between them, even though they are not integrated into the same work force.

5. Finally, there is employment for disabled workers that is fully integrated into a mainstream work operation. *Fully integrated employment* comes close to what is typically referred to as *competitive industrial employment,* but where accommodations have been made to permit the disabled worker to perform adequately. Occasionally, even a little shelter may be offered.

Scope and Purpose

This chapter has two objectives. One is to provide a state-of-the-art review of worldwide experience and conceptualizations regarding accommodated or sheltered employment in both the mainstream and segregated worlds of work for workers with disabilities. The other is to provide an information base for future planning of implementation strategies for accommodated or sheltered mainstream projects in the public and private sectors in the United States.

The primary focus of the chapter will be upon levels 4 and 5—those characterized as semi-integrated and fully integrated employment with elements of accommodation or shelter. However, because segregated employment is often a critical factor in disabled workers' movement into mainstream employment, some attention will also be given to Level 3, segregated employment. As much as possible, this will be limited to work that is truly employment—a way of earning a living—not a vehicle for work evaluation, work adjustment, or other rehabilitation services.

Legal Background

The U.S. citizen with a disability is enjoying a new status of being legally protected from discrimination in employment. This is a dramatic change from centuries ago, when the "cripple" was an openly castigated social pariah, or only a decade or so ago, when the "invalid" was an object of pity and protection. The term *invalid* seems laughable in relation to the militancy reflected in acronyms such as the BADD Action Coalition and HASSLE—two political action organizations of people with disabilities.

The Rehabilitation Act of 1973 contains two sections which offer legal protection to disabled persons with respect to employment under federal contracts (Section 503) and program participation under Federal grants (Section 504). Following a month-long, loosely coordinated seige of simultaneous, nationwide demonstrations by disabled leaders in the consumer movement—many of whom were very severely disabled, very militant, very eloquent, and very effective—the long-delayed regulations governing Section 504 were signed by the HEW Secretary in April 1977. This ushered in a new era with respect to mainstream employment for workers with disabilities. The emphasis moved from "whether" to "how" and "when," although "when" may be as much a problem as with architectural barrier legislation.

Federal laws of this nature have very limited direct applicability. Their primary value is as enabling legislation, serving as a springboard for states to develop similar laws with greater opportunity for enforcement. In the case of nondiscrimination in employment, many states were ahead of the federal government in passing laws which ensured that job applicants or workers with disabilities would be protected from unfair employment practices.

A January 1977 survey (Wheatley, 1977) conducted by the Civil Rights Office of the California State Deparment of Rehabilitation reveals that fifteen states have laws which protect both physically and mentally disabled people and eleven states have laws which protect physically disabled people only. Eighteen states reported having no laws protecting either group, and seven states did not respond. The fifteen states which protect both the physically and mentally disabled are Illinois, Indiana, Iowa, Maine, Michigan, Minnesota, Montana, Nebraska, New Mexico, New York, Ohio, Oregon, Texas, Washington, and Wisconsin. The eleven states which protect only the physically disabled are California, Connecticut, Hawaii, Kansas, Kentucky, Nevada, New Jersey, Rhode Island, Vermont, and Virginia, as well as Florida, which reported no laws but has a constitutional statement that "No person shall be deprived of any right because of . . . physical handicap."

Philosophical Perspectives

Historically, the advent of "Aid to the Totally and Permanently Disabled" welfare programs heralded an awakening to the fact that just because an individual lacks the usual and expected abilities to use his or her body or mind, this does not automatically mean lifelong institutionalization.

The concept that a totally paralyzed person needing respiratory assistance could go home and manage a household, if given the necessary equipment and service supports, was bold and beautiful—in its time. It helped to create the very environment that has now caused it to become obsolete. The original concepts of "totally" and "permanently" disabled no longer make sense in a world where the director of a large state agency with an annual budget nearing $100 million has permanent paralysis of 98 percent of his muscles and must spend fourteen out of every twenty-four hours in a tank respirator.

Many of the work disincentives built into the current welfare program for people with disabilities are carryovers from the older thinking: that if a person is "totally" and "permanently" disabled, work is simply not an issue to be reckoned with. Now we know that it is, and the brave new social legislation which so recently opened up new worlds of independence and freedom has become old and interfering with respect to disabled people moving from the welfare system to the employment system for their income.

Wage Versus Welfare

Delong (1975) asks whether the individual who cannot fit into a normal work situation should be treated as a social welfare case or be considered a potential contributing member of the work force; one who can realize his potential if he can find employment in a situation suited to his capabilities.

Black (1965) looks at the issue in a somewhat different way. He questions whether the need to work involves a basic human right wherein society must provide the opportunity for work to the handicapped and asks who society is in this instance (industry, government, sheltered workshops). He asks whether the business community's greater charity is providing work to some proportion of the "higher risk" employees or contributing charitable dollars to the partial support of a sheltered workshop that takes such employment off its hands.

It would be nice to think that such questions were dredged from the historical archives, but the dates indicate that they were not. These are only two of many examples that might have been selected. The current literature is full of them.

Nelson (1971) cites Jacobus Ten Broek's scathing critique of sheltered workshops which concludes that there is no place for them in vocational rehabilitation, at least for the blind. He calls the use of work as a beneficial process for training or rehabilitation a "dubious duality" and asserts that if the blind cannot find work in competitive industry, they should be given adequate sums to enable them to manage their own affairs. They should not work in workshops just for the sake of working. If they work, they should always be paid an adequate wage for an adequate standard of living. This view highlights not only the wage-versus-welfare issue but shows its relationship to the underlying issue of the work ethic itself. Ten Broek obviously did not hold to an "occupational identification at any cost" philosophy, as many people still seem to do.

Some Alternatives

Nelson (1971) also discusses some alternatives to workshops which might circumvent Ten Broek's and others' criticisms. He suggests that industry might be paid to take handicapped persons into their regular programs and enable them to become acceptable employees. This is now happening on a broad scale for poor people, generally, through the Comprehensive Employment and Training Act (CETA). In many areas of the country, rehabilitation agencies and consumer advocate groups are pressing hard to ensure that CETA moneys are used for disabled poor people.

Another alternative cited by Nelson is that industry could be paid to set up social programs to accomplish what workshops now do. Still other alternatives are that nonprofit agencies buy and take over industrial firms or that handicapped persons organize companies and operate businesses for themselves. He points out that these proposals are close to the regular work process and do not appear to be seeking charitable help. Examples of each of these alternatives will be presented in the ensuing sections, along with many other approaches which have been taken or conceived of to make work opportunities for disabled people closer to the mainstream world of work.

SEGREGATED EMPLOYMENT

Although the literature abounds with material relating to sheltered workshops, where a high proportion of the jobs available for seriously disabled workers are, very little of this voluminous material relates to the jobs which exist in those workshops. That aspect is almost hidden, while articles discuss exciting new trends in rehabilitation services. Work evaluation techniques, work adjustment methods, and work experience outcomes—all these have professional respectability. If the workshop can claim to do job skill training, respectability skyrockets. Placement, of course, is the *summum bonum* of life.

Placement in this context means forcing the person to leave your employ and go to work for another industry—variously referred to as "open," "regular," "competitive," "ordinary," or "mainstream." In a burst of honesty, the writer may confess that not all clients are placed elsewhere because they are *very* severely disabled. Other writers charge that they place only so-so workers in open industry and keep and exploit the best. Whatever the truth on that issue, the more deeply one delves into the topic of the-workshop-as-job-resource, the clearer Ten Broek's "dubious duality" concept becomes. Although the workshops are a major employer of disabled people—at least from the disabled person's point of view—it is all too often a discredited function in the eyes of the workshop staff.

This section will report the worldwide literature and interviews with key experts on the subject of segregated industrial employment for disabled workers who require some degree of accommodation or even shelter in their work situation. Descriptions of workshops will be very selective, due to the voluminous nature of partially and/or tangentially related material. Those selected offer potentially the largest job market or have elements considered to have potential as models for future planning.

United States Experience

Goodwill Industries

Goodwill Industries is probably the best-known opportunity for employment for people with disabilities in the United States. In fact, Goodwill and the Salvation Army may be the only rehabilitation phenomena in the country which have achieved the status of being "household words." The Salvation Army, however, is best known for its relief work throughout the world, whereas Goodwill is better known as "the place where you go to get a job if no one else will hire you."

Dean Phillips, President of Goodwill Industries of America, indicates that Goodwill began as a joint effort to provide inexpensive clothing for the poor and a sheltered workplace for physically disabled people. Goodwills have continued to offer such work opportunities since 1902. They began to add vocational training, the first rehabilitation service, during World War II.

Historically, the primary source of work for the disabled workers and income for the Goodwill installation has been the salvage operation: the refurbishment of donated goods for resale. Today, however, Goodwills are moving increasingly into industrial subcontracts as a source of work and into rehabilitation services as a source of revenue. Many factors have contributed to this trend. Products are no longer produced for repairability in this era of the handy, dandy, disposable everything. The flea market and garage sale manias, which are proving to be long-lived, have further undercut the potential of salvage operations. Vocational training, plus work evaluation and work adjustment, all of which are consumed voraciously by the state Vocational Rehabilitation agencies, have become prized sources of involvement and income for workshops, and Goodwills are no exception.

Phillips indicates a personal belief that whatever Goodwills do with respect to services, they must continue as a sheltered place to work. This is because, according to the Greenleigh study (1969), for many people it's the only game in town.

Abilities, Inc.

Abilities, Inc., in Long Island, New York, is also a nonprofit organization. Vice-President Frank Gentile (1975) describes it as a demonstration industrial and clerical work center which could serve as a model for any modern industrial and business complex. All workers are either disabled, retarded, or aged, and they work a full forty-hour week up to industrial standards. The worker receives the minimum wage or higher, commensurate with experience, plus all the usual fringe benefits. These include life insurance, medical insurance, and a pension plan, all at no extra cost.

Gentile (1977) indicates that they have considered putting *satellites*—their term for *enclave* and perhaps a better one—into regular industry but have not yet done so. In a sense, they have reversed this process. They have a bank branch on the company premises where they train people to be bank computer operators. The Indianapolis Goodwill-Western Electric program is similar in concept to this one.

Abilities Inc. lent key staff members to help form a Florida organization to provide training and employment for disabled and aged workers. Their basic policies were: to create a normal, competitive, industrial setting; to secure contracts by competitive bids; to pay prevailing wages; to use modern industrial equipment and production techniques; to give physical examinations *after* the decision to hire had been made; and to emphasize the demonstration motive of the project for others. Locascio considers this demonstration highly successful and cites the fact that the new organization survived a recession as evidence.

The Paraplegics Manufacturing Company, Inc.

The Paraplegics Manufacturing Company, Inc. (PAMCO), in Bensenville, Illinois, offers a unique example of a for-profit industry created by disabled veterans especially for the purpose of providing employment opportunities for people with disabilities. PAMCO's public relations brochures indicate, "Since the company's founding in 1951, PAMCO has specialized in contract manufacture of electrical, electronic and mechanical assemblies." They describe themselves as specialists in wiring, soldering, assembly, testing, and packaging.

PAMCO's inception was similar to that of the Invalid's Cooperatives in Poland (described below). That is, it was begun by seventy paraplegic veterans who pledged a purchase of stock and mortgaged their homes and cars to raise the needed $25,000. The European literature reveals that the Invalid's Cooperatives were begun by thirty assertive disabled veterans who needed to create a solution to their own problems.

PAMCO has celebrated its twenty-fifth anniversary and appears to be doing well. It is a unique model which both the professional and official communities have largely ignored. Perhaps the consumer community will learn from it and attempt to emulate it elsewhere. (See "Business by the Disabled, for the Disabled," below.)

PAMCO currently employs about 100 people, most of whom are disabled. However, Dwight Guilfoil, President of PAMCO, indicates in a personal communication that increasing opportunities for disabled people to find employment in regular industry are making it difficult to find sufficient disabled employees. Since it is a for-profit corporation, it will undoubtedly have to hire nondisabled workers to take up the slack. Perhaps in the future, PAMCO will be included in the "mainstream" rather than the "segregated" section of a chapter such as this one!

Business by the Disabled, for the Disabled

"Business by the disabled, for the disabled" is a term that could have been invented twenty-five years ago by the founders of PAMCO, and maybe it was. However, it was introduced recently by leaders in the consumer movement as an important component in their independent living programs. The forerunner of these programs, the Center for Independent Living in Berkeley, California, has such an operation in its wheelchair and van repair shop. The center performs a needed service for disabled people in the community and, at the same time, earns enough money from the endeavor to support several other needed but nonremunerative program components.

The independent living programs, which are appearing all over the country, are very aware that they cannot exist forever on startup grants and that they must find revenue generators they can control and count on. Their own versions of business by the disabled, for the disabled will probably be one of the answers for a number of these programs.

The Javits-Wagner-O'Day Act

The Javits-Wagner-O'Day (JWOD) Act is of inestimable importance to any nonprofit workshop providing employment opportunities to disabled workers. The original Wagner-O'Day Act, passed in 1938, was designed to make mandatory the purchase, by all government agencies, of certain items from qualified agencies for the blind. A central agency, the National Industries for the Blind (NIB), was established to represent the workshops, allocate orders and give technical assistance. The Committee for Purchase from the Blind, composed of officials from the major procuring and operational departments of the federal government, was given the legal authority to execute the responsibilities of the act. It selects the items and publishes them in catalog form. It also establishes a fair market price for the items, which can be changed as market conditions change.

In 1971 the act was extended to include sighted, severely handicapped people. The legislation was sponsored by Senator Jacob K. Javits and others.

Just as NIB was established to help implement the 1938 act, the National Industries for the Severely Handicapped (NISH) was established to help implement the new provisions of the 1971 act. Like NIB,

NISH researches commodities and services from federal government purchasing sources and tries to match them to workshop resources. If a workshop wants to develop an item, NIB or NISH asks the committee to assign it to them. The committee then seeks clearance from those with priority under the act.

NISH Executive Director Harry Clements (1977) provides a progress report on this new organization, which came into being in 1974. In it, he observes that the legitimacy of the procedures and the adequacy of the committee and its staff have been challenged in two recent court cases and two administrative appeals to Congress' General Accounting Office, brought by private companies concerned with certain products being processed in the program. However, all four decisions supported the committee and have reportedly strengthened the evenhanded but often slow-paced program.

The purchase of Modglin-Maid by the National Industries for the Blind reflects an entirely different approach to several problems. Rusalem and Ricterman (1971) describe the process by which NIB took over the failing industrial plant in the late 1960s. In the course of fulfilling its function vis-à-vis the JWOD Act, NIB came to see the need for an experimental laboratory-type workshop. They purchased "both the goodwill and assets" of Modglin-Maid Corporation, a plastics business, for this purpose.

Blind persons were given preference in hiring, equipment was modified, existing staff was retrained, and rehabilitation staff was brought in. Cooperative arrangements with other workshops were established wherein Modglin-Maid manufactured components of products produced at other NIB workshops. The venture was considered highly successful, and the authors conclude that with proper planning and administrative controls it is realistic to consider purchasing an ongoing industrial enterprise and converting it into a workshop. They warn that the technical assistance available from an organization such as NIB is critical.

Experience Abroad

England

England's Department of Employment published "Sheltered Employment for Disabled People: A Consultative Document" in 1973. In a historical note, they point out that sheltered employment began as a voluntary effort, with health and welfare the aim and charity the means. This pattern was redrawn along employment lines as a result of wartime needs in World War II and progress in medical science. In 1941, the Tomlinson Committee suggested that sheltered workships produce articles required for war or other public purposes. The most important recommendation was that the central government should set up a company to build and run the workshops. In 1944, the Disabled Persons' Employment Act was passed to implement this recommendation through a company known as Remploy, Ltd.

Remploy is a nonprofit company, and its government subsidy goes toward the cost of employing severely disabled workers, not price reductions. At the time of the 1973 report, there were eighty-five such factories and the total number of severely disabled workers had reached 8,000.

Most Remploy establishments were built soon after World War II. They tend to be largely factories employing 100 or more people. Recently, local authority developments have concentrated on providing smaller (30- to 40-worker) workshops in less predominantly industrial areas. Most sheltered work is manual, although there are some clerical and supervisory opportunities. Remploy manufactures branded products for the national market but is turning increasingly to subcontract work, which requires a minimum of capital and work engineering for the facility and a minimum of skill on the part of the worker. Some workshops produce and sell goods on their own account, ranging from traditional goods in local markets to national markets of branded goods, such as Remploy furniture. In the latter case, a large organization is required to bear the risks and sustain the overhead involved in a national marketing operation.

The Remploy wage structure is based on a minimum standard for all trades, settled by negotiation between management and a consortium of trade unions. Merit and proficiency payments are included. There is also a travel-to-work scheme to help with excessive fares.

Since Remploy is a national company, the annual difference between its expenditures on wages, materials, and overhead and its income from sales is met in full by the government, as is the capital cost of new buildings and equipment.

The 1973 report indicates that operating costs are disturbingly high in relation to wages paid and that "A situation where a man could be paid more for staying at home than for going to work must give grounds for concern." The Department of Employment's research and planning team carried out a detailed financial and economic analysis from 1968 to 1970. The analysis looked at Remploy and a sample of twenty other workshops. The basic questions were: How does the cost in public funds of providing sheltered employment compare with the cost of providing the alternative social benefits to which the individual would be entitled if unemployed? and How did the real resources consumed in the provision of sheltered workshop employment compare with the real resources produced?

The Department of Employment believes that the analysis showed clearly that the cost in public funds was greater than the cost of the alternative social benefits; that the net economic input was greater than the net output; and that performance of the blind workshops was appreciably lower than that of the sighted workshops. The report concluded that sheltered employment is justified on social, not economic, grounds. The problems mentioned are the same ones we talk about here: the economy of small-scale production; the overhead per unit labor equaling that of ordinary industry while the output is less; management and marketing skills lacking; inability to dismiss or lay off when open industry would; need for continuous flow of suitable work; and reluctance to take risks. The report claims the single most important factor is marketing. It also recommends the development of more enclaves to improve the cost-effectiveness of sheltered employment. Many of the commercial problems of sheltered employment arise from segregation and would not arise in enclaves where marketing facilities, management expertise, and suitable work are readily available.

The Netherlands

The Netherlands' Social Employment Act became effective January 1, 1969. It superseded legislation which had for twenty years regulated Social Employment in the Netherlands, during which time it had seen enormous growth. "Social Employment" refers to government-provided jobs for men and women who would like to work and have the skills but are excluded from open industry because of a disability or for certain other reasons. The government has created adapted employment for them, which is aimed at maintaining, recovering, or developing work capacity. Social Employment can be found in about 180 special industries in the Netherlands. Every effort is made to find work to suit the worker, instead of a worker to suit a job. Implementation is entrusted to local authorities, who must find or create suitable work.

The activities are carried out in working projects with sound management frameworks. Although the worker is employed by the government, the contract is not similar to that of a civil servant. People are employed only after a selection procedure, during which they may be placed in one of two categories: (A) workers who are evidently able to do productive work, and (B) those for whom there is less certainty. When it is certain that the person placed in category B belongs in category A, he or she is given a permanent contract. If it is certain that placement in category A is impossible, then the temporary employment contract is terminated and other activity is found for the person.

For persons employed, the act provides legal status with rights, obligations, and an appeal system for grievances. The level of wages is such that the worker should be able to earn a living for self and family. The wage levels depend on both the amount and quality of work performed. There are different wage groups for manual and clerical work, and "The devotion given to the work and the attitudes toward the environment are also important." Wage scales are geared to the prevailing wage in government and open industry, and sometimes a Social Employment wage is received in addition to a Social Benefit. According to the Incapacity for Work Insurance Act, the pension is reduced to an amount which, together with the wage, equals 90 percent of the worker's former wage.

With respect to financing, there is a subsidy system by which the central government assists the municipal authorities. Since the average production of the worker in Social Employment is lower than in open industry special provisions have to be made on their behalf.

Dolnick (1970) observes that most social workshops in the Netherlands cannot be identified by their appearance or name. They are well designed for industrial purposes and are decorated with original art. The workers are usually members of trade unions and earn at least 95 percent of the minimum wage for the types of work done. They may earn up to a 20 percent bonus for good performance.

Reubens (1970) points out that the Dutch believe the subsidies are offset by the savings to government from reduced claims on other benefits. The Dutch define Social Employment as a substitute for institutional or home care and indicate that fewer personnel are needed in the work setting than in custodial or home care.

The Netherlands has a highly unified organization, since all created jobs are administered by a single agency in the Ministry of Social Affairs in Public Health. Henry Redkey (1977) points out that while the Social Employment activities are carried out by the municipal authorities, funding is almost 100 percent national, and the central government employs a number of monitors who keep very close watch on possible abuses. He further indicates that it costs the nation about $8,000 per year to keep a person in a Social Employment workshop, compared to only $5,000 to keep the same person at home. He considers $3,000 an accurate estimate of what it costs to keep a disabled person working at a normal wage and off the welfare programs. Others disagree sharply, saying that many of the social service costs, for which other citizens are also eligible, are included in the cost of running the work operation.

Sweden

Sweden is characterized by Redkey (1975) as a "cradle-to-grave welfare state." The Swedes hold that every disabled person should have a chance to work. Sweden's workshops are models of industrial layout, with the best equipment of modern design. Labor unions negotiate contracts and standard wages are paid, some on piecework and some on an hourly basis. Again, there is little enthusiasm for quota laws. A program of job subsidy exists whereby the government pays 40 percent of the workers' wages, but the Swedish people are very dissatisfied with its potential for abuse. All sheltered employment and vocational rehabilitation in Sweden are administered by the National Labor Board.

Work evaluation, work adjustment, and the other things done in transitional workshops are not done in Swedish workshops. They take place in Regional Evaluation Centers, which are magnificently equipped and staffed by experts. This leaves the workshop free to concentrate on equipment, efficiency, management-labor relations, and good wages.

Denmark

Denmark is also described by Redkey (1975) as a "cradle-to-grave welfare state," but whereas he sees Sweden as taking a "labor market approach" to rehabilitation, he sees Denmark as taking a "social services approach." All disabled people receive a pension, which is granted on three levels according to severity. Workshops are primarily operated by voluntary agencies, with the exception of a newly organized government program for mentally retarded people. Redkey feels that the work ethic is very strong in Denmark, and that the pension does not deter from a desire to work in the shops.

The Communist Countries

Hampton (1970) toured workshops in Prague, Budapest, Sophia, Moscow, Warsaw, and East Berlin in 1970. He introduces his topic by admitting, "I had for a long time wondered many things about how workshops are operated in countries where the state runs everything" (p. 22).

Hampton describes a small workshop in Budapest which, like most, was established with local government funds. Two four-hour shifts are used as an accommodation. He indicates that the workshop must maintain a high percentage of handicapped workers and staff members in order to keep its tax privilege. Although the nature of this tax relief is not described, it apparently serves as an important ongoing subsidy.

Hampton characterizes Prague as having one of the largest workshops in Europe—1,600 workshop slots plus a large homebound program. Moscow also has a large facility with 1,000 slots. He observed that throughout his trip, he noticed that the profit motive was automatically built in. Nobody said to him, "We doing rehabilitation can't make a profit." Profit is considered by Hampton a necessary part of the total production in order to meet the needs of handicapped people.

Finding this hard to comprehend, in view of the English and Dutch contentions that sheltered employment costs more than paying the same individual to stay home, I asked Redkey to help interpret the apparent conflict. In personal correspondence, Redkey indicates that in Poland, at least, the subsidies are substantial and come not only from tax waivers but from less obvious sources.

Redkey is sure that the rehabilitation aspects of the workshop programs are funded from outside sources. The biggest difference, in his opinion, is that in the socialist system, production is state planned and allocated to shops for the disabled, just as with other industries. Even more important, prices are set by the state. With production and prices both on an administered basis, the profit margin can be whatever is desired. Another factor is their excellent equipment, compared with the pathetically outdated equipment in most shops.

Hampton notes that the blind seemed to have preferential legislation in all countries visited, but that the "deaf union" is quite strong in a few countries, especially Bulgaria. Their "Silent Industries" have work stations for more than 800 deaf and hearing-impaired workers. His final observation is, "I got the feeling that in these countries workshops are not looked down on as ours often are either by the general public or by individuals within the workshop, who seemed to take great pride . . ." (p. 25).

Poland. Poland may have the most sophisticated segregated employment program in the world. According to Trampczynski (1973), Poland's first Cooperative Societies of the Disabled were established by ex-servicemen after World War I. They were created to ensure that the disabled got an adequate supply of food at prices they could afford. Although they did not intend to engage in rehabilitation, the cooperatives were an indication of solidarity among the disabled.

In 1949 a single central organization was created. Poland's planned economy, with its emphasis on providing work for all, has opened up a vast field for action for the collective resourcefulness of the disabled. At the time of Trampczynski's report, there were 421 cooperatives employing 224,000 individuals, 171,000 of whom were disabled. The cooperatives of the blind belong to a special union of their own.

The economic activities of the cooperatives have to be conducted in accord with the principles binding other cooperatives in state enterprises. They do enjoy certain tax reliefs and privileges to compensate for the higher outlays involved in the employment of severely disabled people. About one-fifth of all those working in the socialized sector of the Polish economy are employed by the cooperatives of the disabled.

The primary function of the cooperatives is to carry on business operations based on the labor supplied by the members. The most common form of business carried on by the cooperatives is production, followed by services and small-scale retail trade.

There are two components to remuneration: direct payment for the work done and a share in profits, if any. Output standards are established to achieve a rational distribution of production tasks and sensible use of working time. Some employees, however, are paid on time rates, in an effort to reduce the incentive to raise output at the cost of excessive effort or stress. Trampczynski asserts that if wages were paid strictly according to the results of the work, they would not be sufficient to secure adequate living standards.

Dolnick (1972) believes that the Polish homebound component has much to offer as a U.S. model, citing not only their experience but also their sense of responsibility for this population which the United States tends to forget. Poland's 42,000 homebound workers make up about 25 percent of the total cooperatives for the disabled work force. None of the reports related interviews with homebound workers to learn if they agree that home is the best, or only, place for them to work.

China. China has had the Redflag Rubber and Hardware Factory since 1958, when it began as the Experimental Factory for the Blind. It now engages persons with varied types and degrees of disability. It is administered by the Civil Affairs Bureau of Peking Municipality. It produces rubber balls, shoe soles, stoppers, locks, and other national market items.

A 1976 article in *Rehabilitation World* indicates that production equipment is designed for the convenience and safety of disabled workers and that workers with different afflictions cooperate on work tasks. The People's Bus Company sends a special bus to take them to and from work. A workers' union organizes recreational activities, and child care facilities are available, with children of disabled workers receiving top priority. There are living quarters for fifty disabled workers and their families a few blocks from the factory. The article stresses that disabled workers are encouraged to take on leadership and creative roles. In strong contrast to the United States, all workers engage in political study as part of their workday.

MAINSTREAM EMPLOYMENT

This section presents American experience with semi-integrated and fully integrated mainstream employment, followed by European and other foreign experience. As will be seen, Europe reports more and more innovative work at the semi-integrated level, and the United States reports greater advances at the fully integrated level. Australia, the only other continent from which relevant reports were obtained, offers one of the most progressive programs of all.

The reason the above classification system arises at all is that employers are generally reluctant to hire workers with disabilities as part of their primary work force. Therefore, segregated and semi-integrated opportunities are created for them.

Why don't employers want to hire disabled workers? Greenleigh Associates (1969), in comparing their interviews of rehabilitation agency personnel with those of employers, found an interesting discrepancy. The agency personnel believed that employers rejected disabled workers out of concern for insurance payments and personal reactions to their disabilities. In fact, the employers simply did not expect to find the same quantity and quality of task performance among disabled workers as among nondisabled workers.

With respect to opportunities in the public sector, the Greenleigh report makes a damning statement:

> General observations made during the field research suggested that job opportunities for the handicapped were even more circumscribed in the public than in the private sector. . . . These requirements appear to be based on outdated assumptions about the capacities of the handicapped, and also on the belief that there are some widespread aversions to the handicapped. . . . Some states have not adopted any alternatives to the civil service examinations for those for whom such examinations might impose an insurmountable obstacle.

The report then cites some exceptions. Maryland, for example, like the federal government, permits the VR agency to certify mentally retarded people for certain positions, obviating the need for a qualifying examination. Another state allows visually handicapped dictaphone typists to be given civil service tests with verbal instructions. However, the benefit of this is mitigated by the fact that a lower salary scale is used for the visually handicapped clerk-typists.

Greenleigh Associates asserts that much more should be done to develop a labor market for the disabled in the public agencies. They point out that this will require a compilation and analysis of the applicable statutes and practices, followed by a concerted campaign to amend public policies. These statements were made in 1969. In 1977, following the signing of the regulations governing the implementation of Section 504 of the 1973 Rehabilitation Act, perhaps this is on the verge of gradually coming about.

United States Experience

Semi-integrated Employment

One type of employment which might be labeled semi-integrated is the integration of people with different types of disabilities or disabled workers with other hard-to-employ workers, such as older or socioeconomically disadvantaged people or those whose work skills have become obsolete because of technological advances. Apparently in Europe there is even greater segregation of disability types in both service and work settings than in the United States. That, however, is not the concern of this section. A step toward integrating disabled workers into the mainstream world of work is the focus here.

Business enterprise programs. Probably the best-known example of a semiintegrated employment venture in the United States is the Business Enterprise Program (BEP), made possible through the Randolph-Sheppard Act of 1936, otherwise known as the vending stand program for the blind. This program is semiintegrated in that while the blind worker is not integrated into the same work force as the other workers in the building, she or he at least comes to work at the same plant, and an opportunity is created for contact between sighted and nonsighted individuals. Once that is present, familiarization and socialization can follow. Then the myths and stereotypes can be broken down.

Because of his long experience with the Blind Enterprise Program, I asked Robert Melody, Chief, Business Development Services, California Department of Rehabilitation, what he considers its most salient features with respect to semi-integrated employment. Melody believes the program proves that many blind people can be highly successful. Some operators of the larger food service operations in California are making more money than the VR director in their state. Melody also feels that this should be an encouragement for operators to move outside of the program. However, he noted that when a state senator proposed this in California in 1969, he was booed down by a group of organized blind people. They apparently didn't want to move out of these protected settings and into the competitive world of independent business, however capable they might be.

On the issue of integration into mainstream employment, Melody thinks this was never the intent of the BEP. The new amendments may actually lead to more segregation and more incentives to stay in the program than to graduate and move on and out. Moreover, a 1974 task force comprised largely of blind people who are advocates for the blind was vehemently opposed to diversification of the BEP, fearing it would "weaken the program." It would appear that the BEP will remain on the border between segregation and semi-integration for the foreseeable future.

Business development section. Similar in intent to the BEP for the blind is the Business Development Section (BDS) of the California State Department of Rehabilitation, under the direction of Robert Melody. The mission of this newly created section is to develop self-employment opportunities for severely disabled individuals.

The section's first major accomplishment is to have established three retail shops in the Los Angeles County Hall of Administration shopping mall. Here, clients can operate one of these businesses for three years, learning and saving toward a business of their own in the private sector. One business is a floral shop, one is a drycleaning drop station, and one is a services center for paying utility bills, copying documents, purchasing bus tickets, postal services, and a theater ticket agency. Melody believes that just fifteen to twenty stations throughout the state are needed because of their transitional character.

The section also provides consultation to counselors, does feasibility studies and market research, and locates sources of funding. It also provides followup for up to 1½ years after "closed, rehabilitated, employed." One of the biggest needs, Melody says, is for counselors to learn how to develop a loan package. The Small Business Administration has "Handicapped Assistance Loans" which require 20 percent equity before they will lend the other 80 percent. He indicates that in the past, the SBA has systematically turned down counselors' loan packages because they were not adequately prepared.

Enclaves. An *enclave* is a specified part of a work site, usually a factory, which is set aside for workers with disabilities. Jobs and work sites may be modified as needed, and special hiring, firing, and supervisory practices may be maintained. Attempts to locate experience with enclaves in the United States were not very successful. They are being tried in several countries in Europe, however. These European efforts will be described in more detail below.

Apparently one enclave did exist at Hughes Aircraft in California from the time of World War II until the late 1950s, when its progenitor, Justin Johnson, died. Disabled workers were needed in the aircraft industry during the war because the abled-bodied men were off fighting. By the late fifties, this was no longer true, and without the guidance of a committed individual, the program did not survive. It was designed to be transitional—a point of entry from which enclave workers would eventually move into the regular factory, thus creating a vacancy for another disabled worker in the enclave.

A model closely resembling the enclave approach is *group place-*

ment, which has been used primarily with patients with mental-emotional disabilities. The only known examples, such as Fountain House in New York City, are transitional in nature, with the intent of helping the emotionally disabled worker to develop or redevelop appropriate work habits and skills. They are clearly rehabilitation service programs, not just employment opportunities, however.

The *work crew* is a final approach which might be labeled semi-integration. This is being tried in many places both in the United States and abroad, usually for severely retarded people, in the janitorial and grounds-keeping areas.

The Exceptional Children's Foundation in Los Angeles is one of many organizations serving retarded people who are training house-cleaning crews. Hansen (1969) describes a project in Folsom, California, where six trainable retarded youth worked as a cleanup crew at the Folsom Dam recreational area. The work is primarily lawn work, ditch cleaning, weed pulling, brush removal, and general gardening. The tools and equipment are purchased jointly by the State Department of Rehabilitation and the local school district. From the experience, Hansen concludes that these youth can do work under highly supervised conditions, and that a healthy competition is engendered. He believes the crew idea could profitably be explored in the American economy because of the increasing usage of recreation areas and the tremendous need for cleanup.

Fully Integrated Employment

Unquestionably, the most important issues associated with accommodated, mainstream employment are affirmative action programs for workers with disabilities and the inclusion of disabled people as a protected population under fair employment practice laws. Sections 503 and 504 of the 1973 Rehabilitation Act and the various states' positions on protecting physically and/or mentally disabled people from unfair employment practices were described in the introduction.

In addition, Section 501 of the 1973 Rehabilitation Act requires that all agencies of the executive branch of the federal government submit annual affirmative action plans for the hiring, placement, and advancement of handicapped individuals to the U.S. Civil Service Commission.

The U.S. Civil Service Commission. The U.S. Civil Service Commission must annually report on progress to Congress. The second such annual report (1975) indicates that historically, particular emphasis was placed on utilizing disabled persons as a manpower resource in the early 1940s, during World War II. In 1957, a system was established wherein coordinators were designated in all federal installations with appointing authority to ensure that counseling and placement assistance was offered to disabled applicants. In the 1960s, the Office of Selective Placement Programs was established, and its ten regional and sixty-five area offices now work with federal and other public and private agencies concerned with employment of disabled persons.

Accommodation and/or shelter can take many forms in mainstream employment and can occur at many steps along the path of getting, doing, and keeping a job. One of the earliest and greatest barriers to getting a job for many people with disabilities is the examination process, especially in civil service. If you can't take the written examination, you can't even be considered a candidate for the job, unless someone is willing to make accommodations in the examination procedure or waive it altogether. In 1964, the latter step was taken when special appointing authorities were established outside of the ordinary competitive structure. This reflected recognition of the fact that some severely physically and mentally disabled people can perform well in specific jobs even though they cannot compete well in the usual selection process.

Here are some of the specific accomplishments reported on with respect to competitive examining procedures:

- The test for blind competitors is available in large print, Braille, and on tape.
- The use of an abacus or arithmetic-type slate is granted.
- The test for deaf competitors emphasizes clarity of expression.
- The use of interpreters in clarifying instructions is encouraged.
- Test content inappropriate to blind or deaf individuals is deleted.

One of the solid achievements reported by various federal agencies was mobility barrier identification and, in some cases, removal. Most other "achievements" involved bureaucratic tasks such as establishing liaisons and reporting systems. The 1975 report singled out one serious problem area: the allotment of resources to do the job, including appropriate staff. Too many selective placement coordinators have little interest in the program, and their status is considered "other duties as assigned."

Earlier, of course, the federal program wherein written examinations were waived for mentally retarded applicants for certain job classes had proved to be a highly successful and well-utilized opportunity. An area which still needs work is written examination procedures for people with upper extremity impairments or dyslexia and who simply cannot record their answers intelligibly.

A Wisconsin project. A Wisconsin project described by Lobes (1975) sought to place nearly 100 mentally retarded or restored individuals with that state's civil service system and to answer several research questions. It was called Project Skill, and its primary concern was: Is competitive employment more attainable when training and work adjustment are part of an employer's system?

Wisconsin reports that the first difficult task was demythologizing and destereotyping disabled people in order to get job slot commitments. Only three out of twelve departments with appropriate positions agreed to participate. The report indicates that it is too early to say whether the project is a success.

California. A California policy reflects a less formal approach which focuses upon more severely disabled people, primarily those with physical limitations. An administrative directive issued by the Director of the Department of Rehabilitation in 1975 stated, in essence, that the department would provide whatever equipment and services were needed for an employee to perform the job function, including those required by employees with various handicaps. That might include Braille writers, Optaicons, special wheelchairs, transportation equipment, drivers, readers, attendants, and interpreters. The equipment remains the property of the state and is to be used only on state business. The employee provides his or her own transportation to and from work and assistive devices which are not solely work related (e.g., prosthesis, wheelchairs, glasses). The department also makes whatever alterations are needed in the work environment, including mobility barrier removal and work site modifications.

All of these adjustments constitute accommodations, not shelter. That is, they allow the worker with a disability to meet performance standards; they do not relax the standards. The department has many severely disabled staff members, ranging from those at the clerk-typist level to the Director. A number of these might be still on Supplemental Security Income at an annual cost of $15,000 or more if they were not working for an organization which is willing to provide the supports necessary to permit them to work. It is hard to imagine that the accommodation costs could so overbalance the value of the work performed that the cost of such a work slot could exceed that of maintaining the person on $15,000 per year welfare, as the above-reported English and Dutch experiences might suggest.

Welfare tax credit. The welfare tax credit is a potentially promising phenomenon that has been little explored in rehabilitation. Wyn Cochran, labor and industrial relations specialist with the California Department of Rehabilitation, has had a great deal of experience in applying the Work INcentives (WIN) tax credit program to disabled clients who are also WIN eligible. He indicates that on the welfare tax credit, such as the WIN tax credit, if the employer hires a WIN registrant or a WIN eligible person and retains that person for 180 days of employment, or if he or she is fired for cause, then the employer is forgiven up to 20 percent of the individual's wages for the first twelve months of employment from the taxes the employer owes. Cochran indicates that there has been no follow-up on the effects or effectiveness of this program and no selling of the concept. He believes a similar tax credit for SSI recipients and other disabled persons should be tried, but to work, it must be advertised.

Industrial injuries. So far, the focus has been upon *getting* disabled workers into mainstream employment. The issue of *keeping* them there is equally important, since so many disabling conditions occur after the person becomes occupationally established.

A state of California report (1970) presented the results of a statistical study of 3,635 workers injured in California during a six-month period. Only those with a permanent residual disability which prevented them from returning to their old jobs were studied. A key finding was that more than half the workers were returning to their original employer in new or modified positions, indicating that both insurance carriers and employers engage in significant voluntary rehabilitation efforts.

Most of these involved fairly minor injuries. I attempted to locate a sizable sampling of cases involving severe disabilities resulting from industrial injuries, followed by significantly accommodated reemployment by the same firm. The search was almost totally unsuccessful. Here is an example from the tiny sampling I found: Mammoth Mountain Ski Corporation has a paraplegic safety director, a former patroller who was caught in an avalanche. They have provided him with a van and modified his home, and he lives there year-round as an overseer. My informant tells me that the insurance carrier has not publicized this case. The resort has cost them so much that they have canceled its policy.

Special wage certification. For people who cannot produce up to a given standard, even on low-level jobs and regardless of the accommodations made, there currently exists a mechanism for paying less than the minimum wage. Special minimum wage certification may be applied for by employers in regular industry, just as it can be by sheltered workshops. The process is very seldom used, however, for two major reasons. First, great fears are expressed by many rehabilitation people that the mechanism will be abused and workers with disabilities will be exploited for the opportunity to pay them less. This seems a needless fear in view of the other reason: few employers have wanted to use it. The employer is forced to submit the application for the certification.

The rehabilitation worker cannot assume this burden. As a result, both worker and employer simply refuse to become involved.

Experience Abroad

Semi-integrated Employment

The European approach which has captured the most attention from the United States is the enclave. Unlike the one which existed at Hughes Aircraft in the 1940s and 1950s, those in Denmark and Great Britain tend not to be transitional. Employment, not transition to an ordinary work setting, is the goal.

England. One of the early efforts began in 1960 in the city of Leeds. A dozen people liable to epileptic seizures worked under the supervision of a foreman trained to deal with any seizures that might occur. They performed the full range of tasks associated with the care of public parks and gardens. The Department of Employment subsidized the arrangement. Similar schemes had spread to at least seven other communities at the time of writing in 1973.

In 1963, the Industrial Therapy Organization (ITO) began making arrangements for ten ex-mental hospital patients to work with local firms. Before allocation to an enclave, workers try out in ITO workshops and may return if work in the enclave ends. The ITO acts as the employer in every respect. The firms measure and pay the ITO for the work performed. From this, the ITO deducts the cost of nursing supervision and administration. That sum is reimbursed under the Department of Employment's scheme of grants.

The 1973 report analyzes the problems associated with direct subsidy in employment. It states unequivocally that these objections do not apply to the enclaves, in which workers are employed by an independent workshop which, in turn, is paid by the firm for all the work done. The report states that the enclave system is a logical extension of the subcontract work used in workshops. Moreover, the open-air enclave is considered particularly conducive to rehabilitation, and the per capita costs are much less than in sheltered factories. It is also pointed out that enclaves could be established within easy travel distance of most severely disabled people. Local authority open-air enclaves appear to be spreading, and whereas the scope for factory enclaves is greater, less progress has been made.

The British recognize that essentially all sheltered work opportunities in England are manual work. In an effort to correct this, they plan to pursue the Swedish model of archives work for severely disabled people for whom clerical/administrative tasks are appropriate. The Swedish archivist projects will be described below.

An article in *Lancet* (early 1975) indicates that the British Department of Employment has now accepted that groups working under supervision in open industry are superior to sheltered workshops in the management and re-training of the disabled. The author describes such a program for former mental patients and claims that year by year, the cost per place in sheltered groups has been consistently much lower than in the sheltered workshops. He further points out that in sheltered groups, all costs other than psychiatric supervision and administration costs are carried by industry.

Sweden. Sweden's archivist program has captured the interest of many writers. It is a mechanism for providing employment for disabled people with high-level skills, and approximately 12,000 people are currently so employed. Redkey (1975) believes this type of program could be readily adapted to the United States. The Swedish government pays the full cost of these white-collar projects if they are initiated by branches of the central government. If initiated by the municipalities, one-third of the costs are subsidized, except in extraordinary cases of areas with high and persistent unemployment and a diminishing number of inhabitants.

To paraphrase Reubens (1970):

> The archives work evolved from Special Public Works jobs for unemployed professional and technical workers. These opportunities were later opened up to workers with disabilities, refugees with little knowledge of the Swedish language, and musicians. Both the Swedish and Dutch have a great concern for artists, compared with the lack of concern found in the U.S. The archive works are limited to the public and non-profit sectors, although private enterprise could conceivably be tapped for contracts. Some typical sites for archives work are: museums, government offices, schools and universities, hospitals, libraries and laboratories. . . . In Sweden and elsewhere it may be anticipated that handicapped white collar and professional workers will constitute an increasing proportion of all on created jobs for the handicapped (pp. 262–263).

Denmark. In Denmark, while enclave workers have separate space, they are on the factory payroll. In both Denmark and Sweden, there may also be a state subsidy. Redkey (1975) indicates that in the Danish enclaves there is no standard method for determining wages and prices. Everything is left to negotiation. He also observes that efforts to integrate mentally retarded workers in this fashion have not enjoyed the success experienced with other disability groups.

The Netherlands. In the Netherlands, under the Social Employment program, the employment office has the task of keeping a lookout for opportunities in open industry in its efforts to find or create suitable work. Included among the 44,000 workers covered by the Social Employment Act are 4,300 white-collar workers and 8,000 workers in open-air projects (Dolnick, 1970). It is not clear what proportion of these are disabled to a degree we would consider substantial.

Israel. The Israelis have found that the work crew approach can be successful for mentally retarded people. One project there (*SRS Abstracts,* 1970) attempted to motivate severely retarded Israeli adolescents and young adults through the technique of group work. Employment was found in groves, parks, and agricultural areas still using manual labor for four groups of ten young people. Some of the findings were that all groups showed increasing productivity, friction with employers or other workers was minimal, and the prospects for expansion to urban parks looked good.

Fully Integrated Employment

Australia. Australia offers a most innovative and far-reaching example of fully integrated, accommodated employment in Centre Industries in Sydney. It was established in 1961 to provide real, not token, employment for cerebral palsied workers in competition with able-bodied workers in open industry. Jonas (1976) claims that no favors or preferences are given the more than 250 severely handicapped trainees who work alongside 600 able-bodied workers, use the same machines and are paid the same piece work rates.

The factory is a prime manufacturer of telecommunications equipment. It has not only been successfully self-supporting but has contributed significantly to the support of the Spastic Centre for Children. Centre Industries receives no preferential contracts from the government, and subsidization is limited to building expansion and some costs of training and transportation.

Jonas has attempted to replicate the model in Kansas, apparently with some success. Center Industries in Wichita does subcontract work in a variety of areas, including Kansas state license plates, and has adjacent housing facilities and vans for transporting workers to and from the job. The ratio of disabled to nondisabled workers almost reverses the Sydney Centre, however; 65 percent are disabled in Wichita, compared with 30 percent in Sydney. Thus, the American version might fit better under the semi-integrated employment classification.

Jonas points out that the biggest difference is that in Sydney, the disabled workers are already considered to be in open industry; thus, there is no point in stressing placement. In Wichita, the hope and expectation is for graduation from what is considered a sheltered work environment to ordinary industry.

Thus, we see the usual American stress on services in conjunction with created work opportunities. A more faithful replication of the Sydney model, the creation of work opportunities in an integrated environment, is still to be tried in this country.

European countries. European countries generally place very little stress on moving disabled workers out of the segregated or semi-integrated settings created for them and into the mainstream world of work. Dolnick (1970) indicates, for example, that in the Netherlands no particular effort is made to provide placement services into industry. The initiative is left up to each worker. However, the Netherlands, like England, Sweden, and other European countries, has a quota system wherein all industrial firms employing more than twenty-five persons must hire at least 2 percent disabled workers. There is essentially universal agreement among all writers and all countries which have a quota system. *It doesn't work.* It is seldom adhered to, and lack of adherence is seldom followed by negative sanctions. When a fine is levied, it is simply paid and tolerated as a cost of doing business. Quota systems have not brought more disabled workers into mainstream jobs.

It seems that the less sophisticated the segregated and semi-integrated work facilities and job opportunities, the greater the stress upon placement in mainstream industry. This makes sense. When you "solve the problem" in one way, there is less pressure to solve it in others. Generally, European countries have much more sophisticated programs at the segregated and semi-integrated levels than we do, with the Communist countries ahead on segregated solutions and non-Communist countries ahead on semi-integrated solutions. The United States, lagging behind in both areas, places its emphasis on ultimate competitive mainstream employment.

Sweden, however, is one European country with an open industry placement emphasis which has caught worldwide attention. The Swedish Adjustment Team is described by Redkey (1975) as a promising new concept. Each firm has a team comprising an employer representative, an employment office representative, and a representative of the workers' council at that plant. Their job is to find jobs in industry for disabled workers. Redkey indicates that they are in operation at 4,000 plants in Sweden and rely more on good communication and education than legal sanctions. He points out that there is a last resort if this method fails. The government can require an employer to hire only from among those referred by the employment office if a good faith effort is not shown.

Sweden has had pioneering experience with respect to wage subsidies, and many observers conclude that it may be best not to try it. Redkey (1977) puts the problem very simply. The scheme is plagued with possibilities for abuse and the necessity of monitoring and investigating disability.

REFLECTIONS ON THE FUTURE

It has been my observation that it is rare to hear a consumer bring up the issue of sheltered workshops during planning and consumer input conferences. It is usually workshop staff who attend these meetings as consumer advocates who raise the topic and stress that there are urgent needs.

Once the topic is open, the consumers may have some things to say, possibly critical, and may agree that some needs exist which should be met. When the topic can be changed without discourtesy to sincerely concerned workshop people, it usually is—and to something of less peripheral concern to the consumers. Supplemental Security Income disincentives and architectural barriers are very likely topics. If the new topic is employment, it will almost surely be mainstream, not segregated. The rehabilitation services which go on in workshops go largely unrecognized as such.

Nonetheless, there appears to be good consensus among both American and European writers that there will always be a group of disabled workers whose handicaps to job functioning are so severe that they cannot exceed 30 percent productivity by ordinary standards. I don't know just how this relates to the old management truism that the average worker is about 45 percent productive. In any event, there is a "low group" which definitely needs shelter, not just accommodation. Whether they also need segregation is another matter.

Recapitulation of Some of the Major Issues

Unionization

Unionization of workshop workers seems to be taken for granted on the European Continent. Here, however, the topic has power to strike fear into the hearts of workshop administrators. They reason that if the clients average productivity is significantly less than the prevailing wage and yet they are forced to pay it, then it will only be a matter of time before their workshop becomes the *former* only-game-in-town for a number of severely disabled people. Moreover, programs which employ other high-risk employees, such as ex-public offenders, will simply stop doing so if they are forced to pay them the same as they would pay a standard-risk employee. The goose may not be laying golden eggs now, but even the tarnished silver ones would disappear.

Greenleigh Associates (1975) points out that a problem inherent in any proposal to simulate realistic industrial operations in sheltered workshops involves potential conflict with organized labor. Except for a few JWOD-related skirmishes, labor is not particularly interested in the low-level types of work and small total capacity of most sheltered workshops. However, if they are upgraded in some of the ways proposed, then they would be competing for work which might otherwise provide jobs for the regular labor force. Thus, they predict, wages will probably have to be subsidized to competitive rather than minimum wage levels.

Marketing

Marketing is also a very important aspect, with considerable implications for the future. Malone (1976) believes attention to marketing is essential to the workshops' survival, and that those who choose not to become marketing oriented will find work increasingly hard to get. He sees deinstitutionalization trends as requiring workshops to both expand and change direction from being transitional to providing extended employment. He stresses the need for executive directors to assume the role of marketing manager and to look beyond the usual industrial subcontracts to NISH, state use, supermarket industry prime manufacturing, direct mail prime manufacturing, and industrial new product manufacturing.

European Countries

A recapitulation of what we have to learn from European countries is provided by Redkey (1975).

- *Denmark:* Subsidizing people who are disabled does not necessarily destroy incentive to work; subsidy of sheltered workshops is an absolute must; enclave projects are worth more study.
- *Sweden:* Regional evaluation has everything to recommend it; archives programs could be readily adapted to the United States; we should face up to the costs of sheltered work in a program that pays normal wages.
- *Poland:* We should do the following: separate services from extended employment so that the latter can concentrate on production; consider the cooperative form of organization for our extended employment shops; make our workshops better

equipped; consider making shops for those who cannot work in normal industry the focal point for health, social, and recreational service delivery; assign sheltered work a respectable role in the national life; consider tax waivers as a form of subsidy.

- *West Germany:* Quota systems don't work; the size of sheltered workshops is important to efficiency; chain operation of workshops might increase their efficiency.
- *The Netherlands:* Social employment is a simple but expensive method; open-air projects are an excellent way to employ disabled workers and get needed work done; we should consider using groups of sheltered employees to do contract construction for public and private industry.

There is no one point I disagree with, but I believe the timing may be particularly right for trying the cooperative approach here. War ravishment, and the solidarity that shared tragedy can bring, stimulated the growth of the Polish cooperatives many years ago. In the United States today, the rapidly growing solidarity among disabled people may be ready to support such a movement here. The viability of PAMCO suggests that a group of disabled people looking after their own economic self-interest can both establish and maintain a for-profit as well as a nonprofit enterprise.

Government Control of Workshops

Government control of workshops is an issue which looms large in the foreign literature, particularly the subissue of centralized control. The Netherlands has it; England wants it. Bertram Black (1965) states unequivocally that workshops in the United States should not and will not be government controlled, and that as long as the products made and services rendered are those normally prepared in the private business sector, that is where the sheltered workshop will be in our society.

Redkey (1975), on the other hand, sees flexibility in administration with several options, such as operation by private organizations, state operation, singly or as a chain, or cooperatives. Government monitoring he sees as essential, as is true for any business. I agree, and would like to see each of these approaches tested and their advantages and disadvantages documented.

Mainstream Employment

In these days of monitored affirmative action plans for disabled workers, it is not likely that myths such as "They will make the other employees uncomfortable" will survive much longer. Who will pretend to care if the alternative is losing federal contracts or wasting time in getting hassled about it? However, if union problems are created because a disabled worker is seen as getting equal pay for unequal work, that is a different issue.

If the issue is a cut in profit margin, the employer will surely try to find a way to avoid "hiring the handicapped." As has been pointed out, employers say they are concerned about getting a worker who will produce a quality product on time. They fear they will not get this from a disabled employee. Therefore, this is a major issue which must be dealt with in job development.

Job Development

Job development, or what passes for such, would usually more accurately be called "job solicitation" (Greenleigh Associates, 1975). Job development is not just a matter of asking an employer to place a disabled worker in a given vacant position. It involves a creative process of simultaneous discovery and development resulting in a modified or new position which (1) takes care of a work need of the employer and (2) can be done by a specific disabled worker or is uniquely fitted to a particular group of disabled workers, such as people who are deaf or lack upper extremity function. Thus, job development is a mixture of job solicitation, job modification, and job creation.

Rehabilitation people going into businesses and industries and proffering "expert" advice on job redesign and related phenomena, motivated by a desire to make a place for a client and not particularly by a desire to help the employer, need to be very careful not to oversell themselves. The result has been to turn off employers to others coming later who might have had solid knowledge of work flow processes which could benefit the employer as well as make a place for a client. A team of experts is probably needed, since it is unlikely to find the diverse kinds of expertise needed in one person.

The Rehabilitation Engineer

The rehabilitation engineer can be an important member of a job-development team. A magnificent example of the potential of this field is the "talking calculator," which has opened up a host of mathematical occupations to blind people which were never before possible. This is a crucial area of job accommodation possibilities which will allow severely disabled people to work and meet performance standards comparable to those of workers without disabilities.

Accommodations

Accommodations of other types which need to be explored and exploited for disabled workers are job sharing and flex-time. It may be that such provisions would not be needed for the lifetime of the disabled person's career with a given firm. They may be needed only at the beginning, while the individual works out the special arrangements for transportation, attendant care, and any other life support systems which might be needed. If we accept the fact that these arrangements take some trial-and-error adjustments, and therefore time, and don't slam the gate on the individual because he or she does not, and probably cannot, have them worked out in advance, it is certain that many severely disabled people who have not been able to get into an employment situation would be able to do so.

Irrelevant Training

Irrelevant training is one of the saddest phenomena on the rehabilitation scene. The number of disabled people who are trained for employment through the state-federal VR system, only to find that there are no jobs available in their area, is far too high. It is fashionable to blame the rehabilitation counselors for this and part of the responsibility does reside there.

But the problem is more imbedded in the system than a lack of job and labor market information on the part of individual counselors. No one in the entire Vocational Rehabilitation organization knows what jobs exist where. Moreover, no one in the vocational schools and colleges that deliver the training knows either. They rely on faulty statistics from the state service-delivery arm of the U.S. Employment Service. It turns out that they don't know either. Their projections of supply and demand occupations are based on the job order information that comes into the state employment agencies from a tiny subset of employers who use them for filling jobs. Estimates range as low as 5 percent. People in vocational rehabilitation have long admitted and lamented that counselors know a great deal about clients but next to nothing about the world of work. A U.S. Department of Labor report (1967) indicates that the same is true for Employment Service interviewers.

Finding there is no job following training is one part of the problem. Another part is finding that although a job area seemed feasible, it is not, and no accommodations can make it so. Neither client, counselor, nor supervisor was aware that there were critical aspects of a particular job that a person lacking dexterity, visual acuity, or other abilities simply would not be able to do. What is needed in such a case is job analysis.

The outcomes of this kind of error in rehabilitation planning are often (1) an unemployed client or (2) a client who must work in an unnecessarily sheltered setting when, if he or she had been trained in an appropriate area, no shelter would be required. The counselor is more directly responsible for this type of error, but again, the system supports are lacking. We must take corrective steps so that needed job analyses are done; so that severely disabled people, who have often lost many years already to hospitalization, don't lose more years because, "Oops! I never thought of that!"

Incentives and Disincentives to Employers

Phillips (1977) insists that employers don't need incentives; they just need to be given reasonable assurance that they're not going to lose their shirts if they hire workers with disabilities. In other words, he stresses the removal of disincentives.

One of the most important disincentives is liability for second injuries. Many states have no second-injury laws, and the states that do generally consider theirs inadequate. In California, for example, if the total disability is judged to be 70 percent or greater, the employer is not adversely affected. If it is less than that, however, the employer may be liable for the costs of a disability which the individual had prior to coming to work for that firm. The laws governing second injuries need to be improved to eliminate this kind of disincentive to employers.

With respect to incentives, European countries which have tried direct wage subsidies to disabled workers in open employment seem to have had considerable problems with that approach. However, there is no evidence that the tax relief approach has been problematical. This country has tried the welfare recipient tax credit and the WIN tax credit with modest success. They are also modest credits, however. Perhaps if they offered more significant tax relief and were publicized more, the response to them would be less lackadaisical. Perhaps analogous programs for Supplemental Security Income recipients or any other substantially disabled persons could be successful if these changes were made.

Innovations

The *Dictionary of Occupational Titles* divides the world of work into three types of employment: jobs that deal with people, data, and things. One of the inherent limitations of segregated, sheltered workshops is that almost all of the available jobs are "thing" jobs, regardless of the predilections of the worker. People who are making subminimum wages on assembly and benchwork tasks might be able to make very respectable salaries in a suitable field. For example, whereas my annual income has exceeded $30,000 for several years, when I was time-studied on the assembly of convention badges at a workshop I directed some time ago, I was worth exactly 19.5 cents per hour. There are very few opportunities for "data" and "people" jobs in most workshops today.

Other avenues must be found for workers who need shelter but would enjoy and be more proficient at the other kinds of jobs.

In an extensive series of interviews with facility and VR agency people, Redkey (1976) found that essentially all concerned saw a need for employment. He relates discussions on the idea of an intermediate employment agency which could maintain high management standards, be well equipped, maintain good labor relations, pay prevailing wages, subsidize wages from federal funds when necessary, and emphasize employment, leaving rehabilitation to other agencies. He believes this would put a premium on workers managing their own lives by paying adequate wages and dropping Supplemental Security Income payments. Whether or not this is the perfect model is not the issue. What strikes me as positive and important is that here is someone who is willing to put forward a model to be subjected to others' critical scrutiny and tested empirically.

Phillips has reported a promising new cooperative type of venture. GIA is now setting up an arrangement with NIB to sell blind-made products at Goodwill stores. He agrees that Goodwill stores might also have boutiques and galleries of wares made by the participants at the various independent living programs for the severely disabled. He believes the development of proprietary products for workshops is generally desirable. NISH shops are making laundry bags, picture frames, file boxes, and other products for the government; he sees no reason why they couldn't produce more to sell to the public. NIB shops are currently selling items to the public that don't meet government specifications.

Enclaves

According to Phillips, Goodwill Industries of America has submitted a proposal to the Department of Labor for a CETA-funded Projects with Industry which entails transitional enclaves. He expresses the opinion that one result of the Section 504 regulations of the 1973 Rehabilitation Act will be the establishment of enclave units in mainstream industry which can pay piece rates to disabled workers. Regular industry cannot do this if other workers are being paid an hourly rate.

The Fountain House group placement model is a highly successful transitional enclave approach. John Beard, administrator of Fountain House, indicates in a personal communication that the model has been imported by a large number of facilities working with mentally disabled people and one program serving people with epilepsy. Surely this basic model can and should be replicated in many sites for many different disability populations.

Finance Consultants

Finance consultants are needed. In response to Redkey's caution about language and politicoeconomic barriers to understanding, I believe we should send a cadre of American economists and business/industrial experts, who also know the Polish language, to visit the Cooperatives of the Disabled in Poland, now that the rehabilitation experts have had a chance to determine whether the approach is generally consonant with American philosophy. We also need to bring Polish consultants here for part of the preparatory work in establishing a demonstration of how a cooperative might work in the United States. Hopefully, this will also lead to an understanding of why countries such as Poland are reporting profits from their workshops while countries like England report that sheltered employment costs the government more than maintaining the person on welfare.

Proposed National Center for the Handicapped

The proposed National Center for the Handicapped might serve as an information clearinghouse on what has been tried and whether/why it succeeded or failed. It might also take the initiative for demonstrations of the workability of enclaves, cooperatives, and other approaches in the United States. Proposed by Goodwill Industries of America as a result of their 1976 feasibility study conducted for the Rehabilitation Services Administration, the primary thrust of the Center would be to train leaders for the full range of rehabilitation organizations.

A significant research and development component is also proposed, and a third component would be an experimental workshop where ideas and procedures developed in the other two components might be tried out. Phillips expects the research and demonstration component to prove to Congress that rehabilitation saves money: that it is an investment, not a cost. Specifically, he disagrees with Redkey's conclusion that sheltered slots cost more money than they save. He speculates that in Europe, the institutional programs cost less than here, and since there is no emphasis on placement, the sheltered slots actually have big and costly service components, compared with the institutions. These conflicting views form the nucleus of what could be an exciting set of social experiments and demonstrations.

Military Service

Military service was the topic of one of the most stimulating conversations of the entire research period for this chapter. The fact that disabled people are unabashedly discriminated against with respect to participating in the federally funded military services has long irritated me. Consumer groups are not clamoring for their right to be inducted, for both obvious and not-so-obvious reasons. Some disabled people, specifically young men during wartime, feel that being 4-F is one of the few benefits of disability. Most, however, don't realize the many benefits they are giving up by maintaining this protected status.

I recall an abortive attempt to discuss this as a serious issue with a recruiting officer on a local TV program some years ago. He nearly exploded, and the moderator changed the subject quickly since I had obviously lost my reason by suggesting that severely disabled people may have not only a responsibility but an inalienable right to serve their country. Recalling this, with some trepidation, I asked Phillips what he thought about the issue. For a moment he was silent; then he cocked his head to one side and began to speak:

> Well, you kind of got me there. I just hadn't thought of it. Why, of course, disabled people should have the opportunities military service provides! The Marine Corps is the only branch that requires everyone to be combat ready at all times, so disabled people ought to be inductible into every other branch. The opportunities for trade training and the many benefits of veteran's status should certainly be available to disabled citizens. The Peace Corps and VISTA are alternatives, but they don't offer anything comparable to the fringe benefits of military service . . . complete health care for self and family, lodging, meals for self, cheap, convenient supplies for self and family, experience and salary—plus the whole host of benefits that accrue to the veteran, whether from peace or wartime.

Most military occupational specialities have civilian counterparts, and most civilian jobs can be done by someone with some kind of disability. If a paraplegic, say, can do a clerical job in the civilian sector, there is no reason why she or he cannot do it in the military sector. If one can, one ought to have the opportunity to do it and reap the benefits, like anyone else. Phillips is currently attempting to arrange a meeting with Vice President Walter Mondale on this issue.

Synthesis

In the opinion of this writer, two major philosophical questions underlie all of the foregoing considerations. One was asked directly by Riscalla (1974) in the title of her article, "Could Workshops Become Obsolete?" The second has been asked or implied by nearly every writer reviewed: "Which is the better way—welfare or wages?" The two questions are independent of one another.

When Redkey acknowledges that the English analysts may be right

—that it does cost more to keep disabled persons in sheltered employment than it would to support them at home—he is doing something much different than surface appearances might suggest. I believe he is saying, "I don't care whether it saves money or costs money; what's right is right!" He is convinced that providing opportunities for valued work is right for disabled people. If it actually proves to save rather than cost money, then that is a nice bonus. But the financial costs should not be a deciding factor in whether we do it. X-ray machines cost money, too, but we don't decide to forgo them because of that fact.

The inevitability of employers trying to avoid "hiring the handicapped" because of possible costs was alluded to earlier. However, that is only true given the system we now have. Suppose we had a different system? Imagine one in which the employer simply understands that he has some employees who can perform only if accommodations, which have costs attached to them, are made. It is also clear that these costs must either be covered by a government (tax) subsidy or passed on to the customer in increased prices for goods or services, just as for all of the other costs encountered.

In Civil Service employment, this approach should be relatively easy to implement because either way, tax moneys will be used. They can be used to pay welfare to people who are doing no work in exchange for it, or they can be used to pay for the job accommodations needed by severely disabled people so that they *can* work in exchange for a salary which is, hopefully at least, somewhat larger than their welfare grant would have been. Outside of the Civil Service employment system, one encounters the problems of assigning "pass-through" costs in the competitive enterprise sector. The concept will not be easy to implement there. However, it is not necessarily impossible.

One thing is certain. The planning needed to implement this or any other workable system *must* encompass our entire national economic system or it is doomed to worse than failure. It will be laughable. It is time to show that the lives and work efforts of disabled citizens are important enough to be integrated into our overall national planning effort.

My final suggestions are that a cost analysis of the California Department of Rehabilitation policy to provide whatever supports are needed by disabled employees be conducted and the results widely disseminated; that the concept be explored and implemented on a demonstration basis in various locations throughout all levels of Civil Service; and that an appropriation be pursued to initiate planning to extend the concept into the private employment sector, with a view toward letting the consumer price traffic bear what it will bear before government subsidies to employers and/or disabled workers are created.

REFERENCES

Abilities, Inc., of Florida [Clearwater]. *Employment of the Physically Handicapped in a Competitive Industrial Environment.* RD-00493-001. 1966.

Big Bend Community College. *Columbia Basin Jobs Project.* Moses Lake, Washington: June 1976.

Black, Bertram J. "The Workshop in a Changing World: The Three Faces of a Sheltered Workshop," *Rehabilitation Literature* 26(8), August 1965: 230–235, 243.

Brickey, Michael. "Normalization and Behavior Modification in the Sheltered Workshop," *Journal of Rehabilitation* 40(6), November–December 1974: 41, 44–46.

Brubeck, Thomas. "They Come to Work," *Social and Rehabilitation Record* (8), 1974: 18–22.

California, Department of Rehabilitation. *Special Assistance to Handicapped Employees.* Sacramento: September 1975.

California, Department of Rehabilitation. *Report of the California Conference on Handicapped Individuals.* Los Angeles: November 1976.

California, Division of Industrial Accidents—Workmen's Compensation Appeals Board. *Industrial-Vocational Rehabilitation Study: Report on the Rehabilitation of Injured Workmen.* Sacramento: July 1970.

Clements, Harry R. "NISH Finds Its Niche," *Journal of Rehabilitation* 43(3), May–June 1977: 15–25.

DeLong, Vaughn R. "Some Thoughts on Sheltered Employment," *Rehabilitation World* 1(2), October 1975: 7–9.

Department of Employment (England). *Sheltered Employment for Disabled People: A Consultative Document.* Department of Employment, Disabled Persons Branch, DPS; 168 Regent St., London, W1R 5TB, England, 1977.

DeSimone, Anthony. "Industry's Commitment to VR," *Social and Rehabilitation Record* 1(5), 1974: 23–27.

Dolnick, Michael. *Sheltered Workshop Programs in the Netherlands and England.* Washington, D.C.: U.S. Department of Health, Education and Welfare, Rehabilitation Services Administration, September 1970.

———. *Trip Report: Poland.* [Unpublished report.] Washington, D.C.: U.S. Department of Health, Education and Welfare, Rehabilitation Services Administration, March 1972.

Early, Donal F. "Sheltered Groups in Open Industry: A New Approach to Training and to Employment," *Lancet* 1, June 21, 1975: 1370–1373.

"Factory for the Handicapped," *Rehabilitation World* 2(1), Winter 1976: 20–21.

Ferguson, Robert G. "Evaluating Vocational Aptitudes and Characteristics of Mentally Retarded Young Adults in an Industrial-Agricultural Workshop," *American Journal of Mental Deficiency* 62(5), 1958: 787–791.

Futro, Aleksander. *Invalids' Cooperatives in Poland.* Union of Invalids' Cooperative. Warsaw: 1970.

Gentile, Frank D. *A Model Sheltered Workshop.* Final report to U.S. Department of Health, Education and Welfare, Rehabilitation Services Administration on Independent Living Workshop-Seminar, Berkeley, California: October 1975.

———. Personal communication, 1977.

Gersuny, Carl, and Lefton, Mark. "Service and Servitude in the Sheltered Workshop," *Social Work* 51, July 1970: 74–81.

Gozali, Joav, and Killian, John J. "Projects with Industry, New Role for the Rehabilitation Counselor," *Journal of Rehabilitation* 38(2), March–April 1972: 28–29.

Greenleigh Associates. *A Study to Develop a Model for Employment Services for the Handicapped.* Final report to U.S. Department of Labor, Manpower Administration, August 1969.

———. *The Role of Sheltered Workshops in the Rehabilitation of the Severely Disabled,* VIII. Final report to U.S. Department of Health, Education and Welfare, Rehabilitation Services Administration, May 1975, 279–280, 313–328.

Hampton, R. C. "A Visit to Workshops in Communist Countries," *Rehabilitation Record* 11(5), September–October 1970: 22–25.

Hansen, Carl E. "The Work Crew Approach to Job Placement for the Severely Retarded," *Journal of Rehabilitation* 35(3), 1969: 26–27.

Humphrey, Hubert H. "Senate Bill 506," *Congressional Record* 123(16), January 26, 1977.

Israel Association for Rehabilitation of Mentally Handicapped Children. *"The Use of a Group Approach in the Rehabilitation of Severely Retarded Adolescents in Agriculture in Israel." SRS Abstracts* 3, October 1970: 1183.

Jonas, John F. "Australian Employment Concept Flourishes in Kansas," *Rehabilitation World* 2(3), Autumn 1976: 13–15, 17.

Lobes, Carol, et al. *Project Skill: Demonstration Project on Employment of Handicapped Persons in State Civil Service Positions, First Year Report.* State Bureau of Human Resources Services, Madison, Wisconsin: April 1975. Prepared for Manpower Administration, U.S. Department of Labor. (NTIS, PB-241–238.)

Los Angeles, Mayor's Office of Human Resources. [*A Proposal for*] *On-the-Job Training Program for the Disabled.* William Elkins, Exec. Dir. Submitted to U.S. Department of Health, Education and Welfare, Rehabilitation Services Administration, June 1976.

Malone, Edward A., Jr. "The Marketing Concept: A Survival Plan for Workshops for Severely Handicapped People," *Journal of Rehabilitation* 42(4), July–August 1976: 14–17.

McLelland, Shelton W. "Sheltered Employment in Great Britain and Asia," *Rehabilitation World* 1(2), October 1975: 10–13, 30–31.

Ministry of Social Affairs, The Hague, Holland. *Social Employment in the Netherlands: A Brief Survey of the Social Employment Act.* January 1969.

Nelson, Nathan. *Workshops for the Handicapped in the U.S.: An Historical and Developmental Perspective.* New York: Charles Thomas, 1971.

92d Congress, S. 557. *Public Law 92–98,* June 23, 1971.

Nunn, Harold D. "The Abilities, Incorporated Experience," *Journal of Rehabilitation* 43(3), May–June 1977: 24.

Phillips, Dean. Personal communication, 1977.

Redkey, Henry. "Sheltered Workshops Abroad: What We Might Learn About Sheltered Employment," *Rehabilitation World* 1(2), October 1975: 2–6.

———. *A Way of Looking at Sheltered Workshops for the 1970's.* Rehabilitation Lectures Series. Menomonie, Wisconsin, University of Wisconsin, Stout, Vocational Rehabilitation Institute, December 1975.

———. *An Evaluation of the Work of the Northwest Association of Rehabilitation Facilities.* [Unpublished report.] Office of Rehabilitation Services, Federal HEW Region X, November 1976.

———. Personal communication, 1977.

Reubens, Beatrice G. *The Hard to Employ: European Programs.* New York: Columbia University Press, 1970.

Riscalla, Louise. "Could Workshops Become Obsolete?" *Journal of Rehabilitation* 40(6), November–December 1974: 17–18, 36.

Rusalem, Herbert, and Richterman, Harold. "From Faltering Industrial Plant to Experimental Workshop Laboratory," *Rehabilitation Record* 12(4), July–August 1971: 20–23.

Samuel, Allen T., and Evans, George M.E. *The Wagner-O'Day Act: A Manual for Agencies for the Handicapped.* Printed for the International Association of Rehabilitation Facilities by Goodwill Industries of America under DHEW Grant No. 44-P-1516713-01, 1972.

Santa Fe Springs, California. *Work Experience Program: A Joint Project Between the City of Santa Fe Springs and the California State Department of Rehabilitation.* [Undated brochure.]

Trampczynski, Boleslaw. "Co-operatives of the Disabled in Poland," *International Labor Review* 108, 1973: 423–437.

U.S. Civil Service Commission. *Employment of Handicapped Individuals Including Disabled Veterans in the Federal Government.* Report prepared for Senate Committee on Labor and Public Welfare, Senate Committee on Veterans Affairs, House Committee, Washington, D.C.: 1975.

U.S. Department of Health, Education and Welfare, Office of Human Development. "Vending Facility Program for the Blind on Federal and Other Property." *Federal Register* 42(56), March 23, 1977, Part II.

U.S. Department of Health, Education and Welfare, Social and Rehabilitation Service. "Employer Job Sites: A Key Resource in Habilitating the Mentally Retarded," *Research and Demonstration Briefs* 2(4), December 2, 1968.

U.S. Department of Labor. *Sheltered Workshop Report of the Secretary of Labor.* Submitted to Congress September 18, 1967.

Viscardi, Henry, Jr. *The Abilities Story.* New York: Paul S. Erickson, Inc. 1967.

Walker, Robert, et al. "Social Restoration of Hospitalized Psychiatric Patients Through a Program of Special Employment in Industry," *Rehabilitation Literature* 30(10), October 1969: 297–303.

Wheatley, James A. "Other States' Laws Protecting the Disabled in Employment." Report to the Directorate, California Department of Rehabilitation. [Unpublished internal memorandum.] April 1977.

5
Continuing Education in Rehabilitation*

JAMES A. BITTER, ED.D.

This chapter provides an overview of the scope, activities, and current issues in rehabilitation continuing education in the United States. Continuing education is defined here as the postemployment development of rehabilitation personnel. A number of federally supported programs address this postemployment need, including state rehabilitation agency staff development programs, national and regional short-term training, Regional Rehabilitation Continuing Education Programs, Rehabilitation Research and Training Centers, and Rehabilitation Facility Administration training programs.

Rehabilitation continuing education activities are described with respect to their content, training delivery approaches, media development, training needs assessment approaches, and training evaluation. Resources for continuing education materials are identified. Also discussed are some current issues for rehabilitation continuing education, including certification for rehabilitation counselors, approaches for assessment of training needs, measurement of training outcomes, and the need for national and regional long-range planning for training.

Rehabilitation continuing education has existed since the beginning of the state-federal vocational rehabilitation program in 1920. It received a considerable boost, however, when training for rehabilitation personnel was authorized by the Vocational Rehabilitation Act Amendments of 1954 (Public Law 565: 83rd Congress). The 1954 amendments authorized training for physicians, nurses, rehabilitation counselors, physical therapists, occupational therapists, social workers, psychologists, and other specialists. As a result, grants were made to colleges and universities to assist in the development of preservice campus training programs and to provide incentive in the form of traineeships to students.

*Grateful acknowledgment is made to William E. Martin, Jr., doctoral candidate in rehabilitation counseling at the University of Northern Colorado, for his assistance in researching the literature for this chapter.

The act also provided the authority for postemployment training, including short-term training, seminars and workshops, and in-service training programs in state rehabilitation agencies. This was perhaps the formal beginning of what has come to be known as continuing education in rehabilitation.

This chapter provides an overview of the scope, activities, and current issues in rehabilitation continuing education in the United States. In addition to proposing a definition for continuing education, it describes a number of federally supported programs. Major rehabilitation continuing education activities are also reviewed and described in five areas: content, training delivery approaches, media development, training needs assessment, and training evaluation. Current issues discussed include certification, the assessment of training needs, the measurement of training outcomes, and the need for national and regional long-range planning for training.

THE SCOPE OF CONTINUING EDUCATION

Continuing Education Defined

The Regional Rehabilitation Continuing Education Program (RRCEP) directors (1975) define *rehabilitation continuing education* as a "career-oriented process of personal and professional development intended to train newly employed and inexperienced staff and also to ensure that experienced staff maintain professional competence in current rehabilitation practice" (p. 23). For the purpose of this chapter, continuing education is defined simply as the postemployment development of rehabilitation personnel. Such a definition encompasses the efforts of a number of federally supported programs, including state rehabilitation agency staff development programs, national and regional short-term training, Regional Rehabilitation Continuing Education Programs, Rehabilitation Research and Training Centers, and Rehabilitation Facility Administration training programs, and some job-related degree programs.

Publicly Supported Programs

State Rehabilitation Agency Staff Development Programs

Rehabilitation legislation authorizes grants to be made to state rehabilitation agencies for the continuing development of state agency staff. Staff development programs in state agencies are intended to be comprehensive and available to all categories of personnel and to assist in expanding the availability of services for people with disabilities, particularly those with severe handicaps. Such programs must include a determination of training needs, career development plans for all personnel, and an evaluation of training effectiveness.

Short-term training. The public program also funds national and regional short-term training sessions. Like other post-employment training, the purpose of short-term efforts is to improve the professional practice skills of rehabilitation personnel serving disabled clients. Program priorities are identified by the Rehabilitation Services Administration (RSA) of the Department of Health, Education and Welfare (DHEW). Training projects of national scope (i.e., those which transcend regional boundaries) are solicited by RSA. Training projects having regional significance are identified and solicited by regional DHEW Offices of Rehabilitation Services. The program priorities identified for short-term training vary from year to year. However, they generally relate to improved knowledge of disabilities, rehabilitation service delivery methodology, management considerations, and current rehabilitation issues.

Regional Rehabilitation Continuing Education Programs (RRCEP)

RRCEP's were established in 1974 to provide comprehensive and integrated sequences of training for delivery primarily on a multiagency basis. RRCEP's are intended to complement state agency staff development programs and the national and regional short-term training efforts. A principal intent of the RRCEP's is to provide training which is common across state rehabilitation agencies and can be more efficiently done on a multistate basis. The RRCEP directors (1975) identified four broad goals of RRCEP's: (1) to deliver continuing education programing to rehabilitation personnel; (2) to provide assistance in post-employment training program development within rehabilitation agencies; (3) to coordinate continuing education resources and serve as resource centers for a variety of training materials and informational data, and (4) to develop continuing education instructional content for meeting identified personnel training needs.

Rehabilitation Research and Training Centers

The Rehabilitation Research and Training Centers (RTC) were authorized by legislation in 1961. As of 1978, there were nineteen Research and Training Centers. Eleven of these focus on medical rehabilitation, three on vocational rehabilitation, three on mental retardation rehabilitation, and two on deafness rehabilitation. It is anticipated that two additional Research and Training Centers will be established in 1979, one on psychiatric rehabilitation and the other on blindness rehabilitation. The Research and Training Centers have two principal purposes: (1) to conduct research which will produce new knowledge leading to improved rehabilitation methodology and service delivery, and (2) to conduct training programs which promote the utilization of research findings. Though much of this new knowledge can also be disseminated through pre-employment training programs, RTC training generally emphasizes postemployment development of rehabilitation personnel.

Rehabilitation Facility Administration Training Programs

The first facility-oriented training programs began in 1963. In 1978 there were eleven which emphasize management training and five which focus on programming, particularly vocational rehabilitation.

Job-related degree programs. Some universities and colleges have developed degree programs specifically for employed rehabilitation personnel (e.g., the University of San Francisco, DePaul University, Southern Illinois University-Carbondale). In recent years nontraditional degrees have been emerging, offering rehabilitation personnel a greater opportunity to integrate education and the job. Various program delivery options are available. For example, some programs offer rehabilitation personnel the opportunity to attend classes on weekends, supplemented with job application assignments. Others conduct a week of classes every three months, also with independent study and assignments between on-campus sessions.

CONTINUING EDUCATION ACTIVITIES

Content

A study reported by Dickerson and Roberts (1973) indicated that one-third of 345 state rehabilitation agency counselors in three Midwestern states received no in-service training. This may be representative of the state of the art in rehabilitation. However, continuing education is, theoretically, for everyone. The range of content available in postemployment training is all-encompassing. It includes information and concept development, the development of skills and proficiency, and the development of self-awareness for changes in disposition (Miller & Obermann, 1969). Examples of training in these areas taken from an evaluation report of the Regional Rehabilitation Continuing Education Program (Rehabilitation Services Administration, 1977) are the following:

1. *Information and concept development:* legal aspects of placement; providing rehabilitation services to severely disabled clients; sexuality and physical disability; managing time; rehabilitation of the spinal cord injured; the role of the rehabilitation teacher in the vocational evaluation of blind clients; motivation and communication; the psychology of disability; evaluation of mentally retarded people; legal aspects of case documentation.

2. *Skill development and proficiency:* interviewing techniques; training techniques for supervisors; micro-counseling; job analysis; audiovisual utilization; management by objectives; management utilization of the computer; leadership skills for supervisors; behavior modification in rehabilitation facilities; effective use of assessment data; program evaluation and consultation; effective caseload management.

3. *Self-awareness and disposition:* training sessions which focus on learner feelings and attitudes generally overlap with content and skill development purposes. An example is an orientation program for rehabilitation secretaries developed by the RRCEP conducted by the Virginia Department of Vocational Rehabilitation. This program focuses on the secretary's job in a rehabilitation context; provides information about the rehabilitation program and clients; and is designed to create an identity with rehabilitation and a positive attitude toward rehabilitation clients and the service process. Training sessions for supervisors conducted in at least three regions (DHEW Regions II, VI, and VIII) emphasize acceptance of a training or coaching role with subordinates in addition to their traditional managerial responsibilities. Similarly, counselor training related to job placement of severely disabled clients and to case management usually contains strong attitudinal objectives, since many counselors typically resist development in these areas.

There is considerable overlap between the various postemployment training programs in rehabilitation. However, state rehabilitation agency staff development programs concentrate on training needs specific to the agency (e.g., orientation programs for all new staff). National and regional short-term training generally address legislative and programatic priorities, and are often offered only once. RRCEP's conduct training which is considered to be recurring and sequential, and identified as a training need for more than one agency within a geographic region. Research and Training Centers develop new knowledge and communicate it to rehabilitation personnel through training. Rehabilitation Facility Administration training programs concentrate on facility personnel, and degree programs for employed rehabilitation personnel offer a core of knowledge for career mobility.

Training Delivery Approaches

One of the most significant experimental efforts in continuing education for rehabilitation counselors was a project conducted at the University of Iowa between 1966 and 1969 (Miller & Obermann, 1969; Miller & Roberts, 1971a; Miller & Roberts, 1971b). Three studies were conducted in that project. The first involved the development of thirty learning units. Each unit was concerned with one topic and was packaged with a tape-recorded auditory presentation and printed supplements which require counselor responses. The study involved a pretest and posttest control group design with 100 experimental group counselors and 69 control group counselors. Significantly greater gains in knowledge were made by the experimental counselors on a 300-item test.

A second study was designed to test an experimental program for improving counselor skills during initial interviews with clients. However, the collected data turned out to be insufficient for analysis.

The third study involved an experimental training course on rehabilitation facilities. Materials included a manual of readings, tape recordings of interviews with directors of three major rehabilitation facilities and a set of slides depicting the facilities. A one-group pretest and posttest study design engaged 274 counselors in four sessions, with each lasting about 2½ hours and held at two-week intervals. The course was conducted in small groups in local rehabilitation offices. It was found that counselors significantly improved their knowledge of rehabilitation facilities.

The University of Iowa Studies in Continuing Education for Rehabilitation Counselors were significant in the rehabilitation field because they explored alternatives to the more traditional classroom instruction and short-term conference approach to continuing education. Still, most postemployment training in rehabilitation today is of the one-time, two- to five-day variety. A possible disadvantage of the more intensive approaches to the curriculum which involve continuous training lasting several days is that trainees do not have sufficient time to assimilate information. A study by Saxon (1977), however, found that a four-day interpersonal communication training program was as effective as training spread over a six-month period.

There are some variations to the two- to five-day approach. Cornell University (1977), in its rehabilitation management training program, conducts training sessions which involve participants for three days in the classroom, followed by three weeks in their own work settings to assimilate and apply instructional insights and culminating in a second three-day session designed to clarify skills and knowledge. This approach has been utilized by many schools. The Seattle University RRCEP has conducted placement training for rehabilitation counselors in a similar mode. The delivery of training in that program involved multidisciplinary informational sessions followed by single-discipline skill training and finally by in-state multidisciplinary training sessions emphasizing field application. The three training phases were separated by appropriate time intervals (RRCEP Directors, 1975).

A variation of these approaches which space the training has been utilized by the DHEW Region VIII RRCEP at the University of Northern Colorado in two of its training programs: (1) an orientation to rehabilitation for new counselors, and (2) facility management. The obvious advantage of such a format is the opportunity to apply the concepts discussed in the first session and to discuss application experiences in subsequent sessions.

Some universities utilize other nontraditional approaches for delivering continuing education to employed rehabilitation personnel. North Texas State University, for example, conducts institutes for rehabilitation facility managers which involve week-long on-campus sessions followed by a second week at locations with individual states at a later date. Southern Illinois University-Carbondale (SIU-C) and DePaul University deliver concentrated graduate courses at off-campus community sites within their geographic region. The format for the SIU-C program includes four to five weeks of independent study to complete reading assignments, five to six days of concentrated instruction, and ten to eleven weeks for individual student projects or papers. DePaul University offers courses which require meeting two weekends during an academic quarter. Students receive textbooks and a syllabus at the beginning of the quarter, are given three to four weeks for independent study, and then meet for a three-day concentrated weekend in select geographic locations. A second weekend session is held three to four weeks later, with the final four weeks of the quarter devoted to independent study projects. The University of San Francisco (USF) offers a masters degree in rehabilitation administration in a different format. USF students attend six eight-day on-campus sessions over an eighteen-month period. Fourteen subject areas are offered in the curriculum, and students apply what they've learned in the classroom to their job in required follow-through activities or projects. The student is given application guidance by a field coordinator who visits the student at his or her facility between each on-campus term.

McDonald and Lorenz (1977) recently proposed a graduate degree delivery format for rehabilitation facility administrators which captures most of the elements of the above approaches. They suggest:

> [a] 44-hour concentrated block of instruction prefixed and suffixed over a 16-week period as follows: *(a)* one-to-four hour orientation to the course designed to familiarize the students with the area of study, the course objectives, reading assignments, etc; *(b)* independent study for four-to-five weeks designed to familiarize students with the body of knowledge and prepare them for a knowledge-based test; *(c)* a 44-hour concentrated, week-long period of instruction in which two or more instructors teach, discuss and apply the area of study to the course goal(s); and *(d)* a ten-to-twelve week period for the student to develop a project to apply the new learning to the anticipated job situation (p. 21).

Another approach to continuing education is what the Seattle University Rehabilitation Workshop Administration training program calls *vertical training.* Vertical training involves individualized training for the staff of one rehabilitation facility. Participants include staff from various positions and managerial levels. This same concept has been successfully implemented by the University of Colorado Rehabilitation Research and Training Center (RT-10) for training hospital personnel in concepts and programing for cardiac rehabilitation.

RT-10 also conducts community-oriented training efforts. In a cooperative effort between RT-10 and the Department of Physical Education at Colorado State University, cardiac rehabilitation education is provided to physicians, nurses, and paramedic personnel in the community, teaching them to supervise exercise sessions for outpatients with cardiovascular disorders. Advantages to such outreach approaches include cost effectiveness, the opportunity to better identify and meet local needs, improved utilization of local resources, and increased access to local citizens who can be involved (Brammell, 1978).

Internships represent still another continuing education approach for employed rehabilitation workers. The Nebraska Psychiatric Institute at the University of Nebraska College of Medicine began an internship program in 1974 for rehabilitation counselors employed by state rehabilitation agencies. The program's purpose is to enhance counselor understanding of psychiatric problems and clients (Blose & Schill, 1977).

Browning and McGovern (1974) conducted a national survey to determine short-term training methodology in rehabilitation. Based on eighty-six responses from training personnel, they determined that a number of methods for instruction were utilized, including lectures, small group discussions, instructional materials, demonstrations, role playing, case study illustrations, touring facilities, on-job training, simulations, report writing, and national laboratory training techniques. The three methods which were considered to be best were small group discussions, simulations, and on-job training.

Competency-based instruction has been debated as an educational strategy in rehabilitation education. Those who favor it believe it aids the development of performance skills, selection of instructional methodology, and evaluation (Anthony, Dell Orto, Lasky, Power, Shrey, & Spaniol, 1977; Steger, 1977). Those opposing the competency-based approach think it is conceptually narrow and distorts objectivity and evaluation (Diamonti & Murphy, 1977).

Telecommunications as a training delivery method has received considerable attention recently. Telecommunications provide a mechanism for delivering programing—for example, films, videotapes, slides, and audiotapes. In addition to involving more of the senses of learners, a study by Sadlick and Penta (1975) suggests that videotapes can positively affect attitudes toward handicapped persons.

In a project conducted by the METREK Division of MITRE Corporation (1977), it was found that considerable software was available (such as films and videotapes) which could be delivered by telecommunication systems, and that this form of communication was probably underutilized in rehabilitation continuing education. A project survey found that rehabilitation agencies were not taking full advantage of the telecommunications systems that they already had. The project also concluded that there was no single clearinghouse which facilitates awareness of training programs and materials developed by state rehabilitation agencies or other training resources.

The Denver Research Institute at the University of Denver is engaged in several studies related to telecommunications in rehabilitation. Denver Research Institute staff of a National Institute of Education planning project are presently investigating the potential applications of satellite-delivered continuing education services for persons working with aged individuals, parajudicial personnel, library staffs, and vocational rehabilitation staffs. The intent is to design systems and methods for selecting course material for satellite delivery. In addition, a Rehabilitation Services Administration project was funded to identify telecommunication systems which either are or have the potential to be cost beneficial in delivering rehabilitation staff training and training materials.

Media Development

Perhaps the largest developers of postemployment media training materials are the Rehabilitation Research and Training Centers. More than 550 media titles are described in a 1975 edition of the *Audio-Visual*

Aids Directory of the Rehabilitation Research and Training Centers (Rehabilitation Services Administration, 1975). The directory includes audiotapes, discs, films, slides, overhead transparencies, filmstrips, and videotapes.

Some Regional Rehabilitation Continuing Education Programs have also developed media materials and instructional packages. For example, the Region V program located at Multi-Resource Centers in Minneapolis has developed a number of instructional packages and audiovisual materials (e.g., Sexuality and Physical Disability, Medical Aspects of Disability, Case Management, and Program Evaluation). Similarly, the Region III RCEP conducted by the Virginia Department of Vocational Rehabilitation has developed the four-part orientation to rehabilitation for rehabilitation secretaries mentioned above. The package includes slide-tape presentations, exercises, and other materials which are intended to be utilized by an instructor.

The Materials Development Center located at the University of Wisconsin-Stout was established in 1969 to acquire, reproduce, and develop materials, including training materials, related to rehabilitation facility personnel. It is funded by a Research and Demonstration Grant from the Rehabilitation Services Administration.

Directories of materials are emerging. The Region II RCEP at the State University of New York in Buffalo publishes a training resources directory which includes reviews of various training materials: books, films, slide-tapes, and manuals. The material is not only described and evaluated, but its potential training utilization is also identified. In addition, the Region II RCEP maintains a library of such materials for loan, principally within Region II.

A catalog of audiovisual materials related to rehabilitation was compiled by the Alabama Rehabilitation Media Service, located at Auburn University in Alabama, from more than 200 other audiovisual catalogs. The catalog includes very brief descriptions of media materials and their sources.

Another resource for rehabilitation materials is the Information Clearinghouse located at Oklahoma State University in Stillwater. The Clearinghouse collects and distributes many materials, particularly papers, articles, and other manuscripts, upon request. As a service, the Clearinghouse periodically distributes an information memorandum of recently acquired materials.

More recently, on the basis of a feasibility study and recommendations by a Rehabilitation Services Administration project to The George Washington University (Pan & Senkevitch, 1975; Pan, Senkevitch, & Fern, 1975), the RSA established a national rehabilitation information center at Catholic University of America in Washington, D.C. Services include supplying copies of research reports and audiovisual materials which were prepared with RSA funding, journal articles, conference proceedings and other manuscripts, preparing bibliographies for specific requests, and locating answers to factual questions.

Another training materials development concept (and continuing education approach) which has existed since 1947 is currently called the Institute on Rehabilitation Issues (IRI). The IRI began as the "Guidance, Training, and Placement Workshops" and became known as the Institute on Rehabilitation Services in 1962; the current name was adopted in 1973. The purpose of the institute is to bring together personnel from state and federal rehabilitation agencies, voluntary agencies, universities and colleges, and select Research and Training Centers to develop training resource documents on selected issues. Topics are suggested by RSA, with input from state rehabilitation agencies. A Planning Committee then determines the particular topics, usually three each year, which are assigned to prime study groups made up of about twelve persons representing various perspectives in rehabilitation. The study groups prepare documents which are presented and critiqued in an annual workshop. Approximately 200 persons attend the annual workshop, following which the material is revised, printed, and distributed for use as a training resource by rehabilitation agencies and training programs.

Two IRI documents are directly related to continuing education and offer methodological guidance to training personnel. One is entitled *Training Methods in Vocational Rehabilitation* (Fourth Institute on Rehabilitation Services, 1966); the second is called *Guidelines for Staff Development* (Eighth Institute on Rehabilitation Services, 1970). Another similar and excellent document is one developed by the Rehabilitation Administration and Management Programs (1977) at the University of Oklahoma. It is entitled *Staff Development Manual.*

Training Needs Assessment

Bitter (1978a) defines a training need as "the difference between desired individual performance and present performance. It is a training need only if present performance can be enhanced with the acquisition of knowledge and/or skills" (p. 3).

Many methods are used in rehabilitation to identify training needs. Fargher (1977) described a number of approaches which could be potential training-need assessment techniques: organizational analysis, job analysis, personnel analysis, career planning, interviewing, operational analysis, analysis of records, nominal group process (a structured process for group decision making), task forces, and committees.

Various training-need assessment approaches have been implemented and reported in rehabilitation. Clark (1977) describes a competency-based approach for determining training needs. The approach involves identifying desirable or required competencies, present levels of performance, priorities, and employee and supervisor commitment to learning.

The Region VII Rehabilitation Continuing Education Program, located at the University of Missouri-Columbia, tested a personal interview approach with 104 rehabilitation personnel in thirteen facilities from one state, Missouri. The procedure involved coordination and commitment by the facility executive directors, the state rehabilitation agency facility specialist, and the president of the Missouri Association of Rehabilitation Facilities. Two-day site visits were established by telephone, and a confirmation letter with instructions and printed questionnaires were sent prior to the interviews. In addition to learning of specific content needs, the interview survey revealed that facility personnel preferred specific information, experientally based educational training, and small group approaches with practical exercises. Training which did not have direct application to the job, was too advanced or too elementary, and involved heterogeneous groups was thought to be ineffective (Mayclin, 1978). The program planned to modify the survey approach, which was time-consuming and expensive, in other Region VII states by asking staff members of cooperating facilities to conduct the interviews.

Boland (1976) surveyed the continuing education needs of rehabilitation counselors. Responses to a mail questionnaire were obtained from 104 counselors and 19 supervisors in three Western states. Agreement between counselors and supervisors was found for areas of training need and included: psychological aspects of disability, test interpretation, and personality disorders. In addition, both groups named the workshop or seminar approach to training as their method of choice, with regular college/university courses as a second choice.

The Region IX RRCEP (Sullivan & McFarlane, undated) developed an eleven-page self-report instrument for surveying rehabilitation counselor training needs. The survey requested educational background, professional experience in rehabilitation, present caseload characteristics, previous training, general training needs, and immediate training needs. A study of Region IX state rehabilitation agency counselors revealed that 74.4 percent of the 330 respondents indicated that their last work experience was in noncounseling areas, while recent training was most frequently focused on administrative/agency structure and organization, and general treatment skills and knowledge (McFarlane & Sullivan, undated).

Each state rehabilitation agency is charged with the responsibility for identifying general and specific training needs of all agency personnel (Rehabilitation Services Administration, 1976). Various methods for implementing this responsibility are utilized by state agencies. Montana, for example, conducts employee evaluation and training need surveys. The performance evaluation report is a universal form which is completed after six months of employment and then every twelve months. This report includes ratings of work performance in general areas (e.g., job knowledge and quality of work) and supervisor comments. The training need survey consists of two parts. Part One lists knowledge areas which are rated by individual respondents in terms of importance, the need to increase professional effectiveness, and learning methods. Part Two asks respondents to identify areas of desired training, training methods, and training length.

The Utah rehabilitation agency conducts need assessment with a position-specific questionnnaire. It contains job tasks which the employee uses to make self-ratings of performance. Employees indicate the degree to which training for a number of topics is thought to be useful for increasing personal job effectiveness. Then the four leading topics in each of a number of categories are rank-ordered for supervisory review. The training needs and number of employees are then summarized by supervisors for review by an agency advisory committee. Employees also complete an Annual Development Plan which indicates personal development objectives and proposed learning methods.

Training Evaluation

Rehabilitation postemployment training evaluation is only beginning to develop. Most of the literature suggests that training evaluation is desirable, yet there appears to be resistance to conducting evaluation. Acree (1977) suggests that when agencies decide to become involved with evaluation, it is usually because it is required for funding or is viewed as helpful for management decisions.

The Eighth Institute on Rehabilitation Services (1970) lists a number of approaches for evaluating training: observation, personal interview, program administrative reviews, tests, reviews of case folders, and questionnaires. However, the greatest emphasis in the past has been on participant reaction to aspects of training (e.g., preparation of the instructor, relevance of the content, and the extent to which objectives were met).

Some participant reaction approaches are very good. The best participant reaction approach in rehabilitation training is the one developed by Browning and Foss (1977) called *Training Evaluation Kit (TEK).* *TEK* is a highly structured, systematic evaluation tool for determining participant reaction to training in terms of objectives, methods, and outcomes. Evaluation involves the learner and the trainer in listing objectives at the beginning of training and then rating the degree to which each was met on a scale of 1 to 4; rating training methods on a 1 to 4 scale in three areas—content, presentation, presentor; comparing the relevance of instructional units of the training session to each other; and indicating the degree of participant change in knowledge, behavior, attitudes, and motivation.

Some continuing education programs in rehabilitation (e.g., the rehabilitation administration programs at Seattle University and the University of San Francisco, and the RRCEP at the University of Northern Colorado) use an approach developed by the Education and Training Division of the Life Office Management Association (Fast, 1974). The technique involves identifying the instructor's objectives, and the participant's indication of those objectives which are important to him or her and their degree of importance (weights add to 100) before the training. Following the training, the participant indicates the degree of fulfillment for each objective identified as important on a scale of 0 to 10. The maximum score possible is 1,000 points. A positive feature of this approach is the possibility of adjusting the curriculum to learner-identified needs before and during training.

A national survey conducted by Browning and McGovern (1974) solicited opinions of rehabilitation training personnel relative to the technology of training. Evaluation was considered important but difficult. For the 86 respondents who were responsible for 575 short-term training programs serving approximately 12,000 trainees, direct observation and verbal reports were the methods most commonly used to evaluate training.

A follow-up study for short-term training (Perry, Browning & Rankin, 1975) indicates that participants think training influences them. Participants reported using resources identified during training, reading professional literature, and self-perceived changes in information, behavior, motivation, attitude, and interpersonal relationships.

Martin, Johns, and Bitter (1978) tried to put training evaluation in a larger perspective. For them, training evaluation involves both theoretical and practical considerations. The theoretical considerations involve determining the general training intent, specific needs for training, strategies for converting objectives into action, implementation, and outcomes. For each of these, there are practical considerations: *targets* (e.g., instructor(s), media resources, small group interactions, learner competencies, reports); *areas* (e.g., learner reaction to instruction, knowledge acquired, performance skills acquired, and results—the impact of learning on third-party beneficiaries); and *methods* (e.g., student feedback, independent observers, mechanical device recordings, and unobtrusive measures). Few, if any, rehabilitation training programs engage in such a comprehensive approach.

Browning (1970) edited a monograph containing six papers pertaining to theoretical positions, methodological approaches, and strategies applicable to the evaluation of rehabilitation short-term training. The paper in this monograph by Marvin C. Alkin suggests the need for training evaluation in five areas: systems assessment, program planning, program implementation, program improvement, and program certification. Jerome Moss, Jr., recommends that evaluation data include learner characteristics, program characteristics and costs, intervening variables, and outcomes. Leo O. Hammerlynck proposes that actual client behavior be used as a criterion for evaluating the effectiveness of short-term training.

Pre- and postmeasurement, though not a very strong research design, is becoming more frequently used to assess the impact of training on participants. Moriarty (1971) applied pre- and postattitude measures for short-term training of newly employed rehabilitation counselors. The training, which focused on attitudes toward people with disabilities, resulted in significantly improved attitudes of the counselors.

Similarly, Bitter (1978b) describes a two-week continuing education program for new rehabilitation counselors which applies pre- and postmeasures for content knowledge, job performance, and attitudes. Knowledge was measured with multiple-choice questions. Participants averaged 51 percent correct response on pretests and 79 percent on posttests. *Goal Attainment Scaling* (Goodyear & Bitter, 1974; Kiresuk, 1973) was used for assessing job performance of participants. Participants' supervisors rated them in four job areas: individualized written rehabilitation program development, client evaluation, counseling, and job placement. Five levels of job performance, using behavioral descriptions, were identified for each of the four job areas. The participant's supervisor rated the counselor while at the training session and again two months later. The ratings were converted to standard T scores, with a mean of 50 and a standard deviation of 10. Participants in the two-week training program were reported to have averaged 42 on performance preratings and 58 on postratings. Counselor attitudes were also measured using Form A of the *Attitude Toward Disabled Persons Inventory.* The participants' pretraining score average was at the 82nd percentile (when compared with norms for nondisabled males) and at the 87th percentile after training.

A pretest-posttest control group design was applied to a two-and-a-half-day orientation program for rehabilitation counselors at a state mental hospital (Tipton & Wenger, 1970). A semantic differential instrument was used. Results suggested that the training served best as a means for motivating counselors to work with psychiatric clients.

CURRENT ISSUES FOR REHABILITATION CONTINUING EDUCATION

At least four major issues currently face proponents of rehabilitation continuing education: certification and certification maintenance; approaches for assessing training needs; measuring training outcomes; and the need for long-range national and regional personnel planning.

Certification

Certification for rehabilitation counselors appears to have become a mainstay in the rehabilitation field. Counselors may, by taking a written examination, become certified. This means they have obtained a satisfactory score that, hopefully, reflects knowledge competence in the following areas:

- Rehabilitation philosophy, history, structure, and laws
- Medical aspects of disability
- Psychological aspects of the handicapping condition
- Occupational information in the world of work
- Counseling theory and techniques
- Community organization and resources
- Placement processes and job development
- Psychology of personal and vocational adjustment
- Evaluation and assessment
- Ability to utilize research findings and professional publications
- The delivery of rehabilitation services

It is likely, too, that rehabilitation legislation may require that rehabilitation counseling services be provided by persons who meet, or are under the supervision of persons who meet, nationally recognized professional standards (National Rehabilitation Counseling Association-American Rehabilitation Counseling Association, 1978).

The retention of professional certification by engaging in continuing education activities became a requirement on January 1, 1978. To maintain certification, professionals must either take 150 hours of approved continuing education during a five-year period or retake the examination. Though certification maintenance is desirable and necessary for promoting quality services, it is plagued with numerous process questions. Brockman (1978) raises some of them:

1. Limited continuing education resources in rehabilitation, particularly for rehabilitation facility staffs.
2. Insufficient alternatives for acquiring credits toward recertification, (i.e., either training or retest).
3. Cost for recertification processes.

Other concerns are: (1) a course approval process for recognizing the quality of learning for recertification; (2) the voluminous record keeping required for certification maintenance; and (3) the recertification of nonpracticing counselors (e.g., educators and administrators).

Assessing Training Needs

Though the assessment of training needs is generally recognized as important for identification of training topics and resources, there are differing viewpoints regarding whose responsibility it is and how it is conducted. Training needs assessment is most often conducted by the employer, but sometimes by training programs. It is this writer's opinion that the identification of needed training is a responsibility of employers based upon program and individual employee performance. Thus, determination of training needs requires program performance information and individual employee performance evaluation. Frequently, however, training needs are indicated by asking employees what they need or through surveys conducted by training programs; both methods result in a determination of interests. Training programs do have a role in training needs assessment. They can provide consultation to rehabilitation employers for establishing a systematic, objective process for identifying areas for improvement or development which can be helped by training and for establishing training priorities.

Measurement of Outcomes

As noted earlier in this chapter, rehabilitation continuing education evaluation is often of the participant reaction variety. It is, of course, the easiest to devise and conduct, and it generally satisfies constituencies.

However, it does little to provide information about the impact of training—on the learner, the agency, and the client. Bolton (1978) points out that there is a lack of knowledge for assessing counselor performance.

Kirkpatrick (1967) suggested four areas for evaluation—reaction, learning, behavior, and results—which offer some guidance for a changed and more meaningful emphasis. Experimental studies are, admittedly, difficult to achieve in training, and there is some resistance by public agencies and trainers to the investment of time which such evaluation takes. Yet, the application of research methodology is a worthy goal if we are to know the true value of continuing education efforts.

Training evaluation would be aided considerably if program objectives and training session objectives were expressed in outcome terms. Frequently, program objectives are stated as management, or enabling, objectives—for example, "to conduct six training sessions." Such statements say nothing about the impact of the training sessions (i.e., knowledge learned, job performance change, agency change, or client benefit). Everyone connected with rehabilitation continuing education —trainers, learners, employers, and funding agencies—deserves to know about the effectiveness of training.

National and Regional Planning

With an increased emphasis on postemployment continuing education for rehabilitation personnel, there is a need for increased attention to long-range national and regional planning for optimal utilization of training resources in the public rehabilitation program. Comprehensive regional training plans are suggested. Such planning begins with the identification of regional training goals which are related to national goals; more specific program objectives; and individual project goals, objectives, activities, and resources. Such planning, involving training programs and shared with them, can result in more effective and efficient use of limited resources.

SUMMARY

Rehabilitation continuing education, the postemployment development of rehabilitation personnel, has been receiving increasing emphasis since 1954. A number of federally supported programs now exist, including: state rehabilitation agency staff development programs, national and regional short-term training, Regional Rehabilitation Continuing Education Programs, Rehabilitation Research and Training Centers, and Rehabilitation Facility Administration training programs.

Continuing education can be for information, concept, skill, or attitude development. Many approaches are used. Though the one-time several-day approach to training is still very popular, more and more training activities are involving multiple sessions and multimethods, with particular attention to skill development and job application. Recent methodological examples for postemployment training include vertical training, community-oriented outreach training, internships, simulations, and telecommunications. Media instructional packages, directories of materials, and information centers are also increasing, thus making available additional resources to trainers.

Appropriate training is dependent upon adequate assessment for training needs. Though there are many approaches to assessing needs, there is still a great reliance on employee expression of training interest rather than program and employee evaluation. Similarly, training evaluation depends heavily on participant reaction rather than information gain, improved job performance, agency change, and client benefit. There is, however, a trend toward more rigorous evaluation of training effectiveness.

Current issues in rehabilitation continuing education include certification maintenance, approaches for assessing training needs and measuring training outcomes, and the increasing need for long-range national and regional personnel training planning.

Thus, continuing education has become recognized as increasingly important for the development of quality rehabilitation programing. In addition to the availability of more public funds for rehabilitation continuing education, many methodological advances are occurring. Hopefully, the ultimate beneficiaries are the recipients of more effectively and efficiently delivered rehabilitation services.

REFERENCES

Acree, D. Evaluation: Process or impact. In: Rehabilitation Aministration and Management Programs. *Staff Development Manual* (Second National Seminar on Rehabilitation Staff Development and Training, December 6–10, 1976). Norman, Okla.: University of Oklahoma, 1977.

Anthony, W. A., Dell Orto, A. E., Lasky, R. G., Power, P. W., Shrey, D. E., and Spaniol, L. J. The realities of competency-based rehabilitation counselor education: A response to Diamonti and Murphy. *Rehabilitation Counseling Bulletin,* 1977, *21*(1), 58–62.

Bitter, J. A. *Guide to Region VIII rehabilitation training needs assessment.* Greeley, Colo.: University of Northern Colorado Regional Rehabilitation Continuing Education Program, 1978a.

Bitter, J. A. Continuing education for new rehabilitation counselors. *Rehabilitation Counseling Bulletin,* 1978b, *22*(1), 74–77.

Blose, J. L., and Schill, S. J. Psychiatric internships for rehabilitation counselors. *Journal of Applied Rehabilitation Counseling,* 1977, *8*(3), 190–192.

Boland, J. M. *Comparison of rehabilitation counselor and supervisor perceptions of counselor needs and continuing education.* Ed.D. dissertation. Bozeman, Mont.: Montana State University, 1976.

Bolton, B. Methodological issues in the assessment of rehabilitation counselor performance. *Rehabilitation Counseling Bulletin,* 1978, *21*(3), 190–193.

Brammel, H. L. *Progress Report No. 13.* Denver: University of Colorado Rehabilitation Research and Training Center, 1978.

Brockman, R. L. Personal communication to Dr. Suzanne M. Bruyere, August 30, 1978.

Browning, P. L. (Ed.). *Evaluation of short-term training in rehabilitation.* Eugene, Ore.: University of Oregon Rehabilitation Research and Training Center, 1970.

Browning, P. L., & Foss, G. *Training Evaluation Kit.* Eugene, Ore.: University of Oregon Rehabilitation Research and Training Center, 1977.

Browning, P. L., & McGovern, K. B. Technology of rehabilitation short-term training. *Rehabilitation Counseling Bulletin,* 1974, *18*(2), 117–122.

Clark, B. S. Assessing needs: A competency-based model. *Awareness* (Region III Rehabilitation Continuing Education Program newsletter), 1977, *2*(2), 1, 6.

Cornell University (New York State School of Industrial and Labor Relations). A first: Work adjustment Region II. *Rehabilitation Management Training Newsletter from Cornell University,* 1977, 3(1).

Diamonti, M. C., & Murphy, S. T. Behavioral objectives and rehabilitation counselor education: A critique. *Rehabilitation Counseling Bulletin,* 1977, *21*(1), 51–57.

Dickerson, L. R., & Roberts, R. R. Inservice training of rehabilitation counselors in state agencies. *Rehabilitation Counseling Bulletin,* 1973, *17*(1), 22–28.

Eighth Institute on Rehabilitation Services. *Guidelines for staff development.* Washington, D.C.: Rehabilitation Services Administration, Department of Health, Education and Welfare, 1970.

Fargher, J. R. *Training needs assessment approaches for rehabilitation.* Greeley, Colo.: University of Northern Colorado Regional Rehabilitation Continuing Education Program, 1977.

Fast, D. A new approach to quantifying training program effectiveness. *Training and Development Journal,* 1974, *9*(28), 8–14.

Fourth Institute on Rehabilitation Services. *Training methods in vocational rehabilitation.* Washington, D.C.: Rehabilitation Services Administration, Department of Health, Education and Welfare, 1966.

Goodyear, D. L., & Bitter, J. A. Goal attainment scaling as a program evaluation measure in rehabilitation. *Journal of Applied Rehabilitation Counseling,* 1974, *5*(1), 19–26.

Kiresuk, T. J. Goal attainment scaling at a county mental health service. *Evaluation,* 1973, 1, 12–18.

Kirkpatrick, D. L. Evaluation of training. In: R. L. Craig & L. R. Bittel (Eds.), *Training and Development Handbook.* New York: McGraw-Hill Book Company, 1967.

Martin, W. E., Jr., Johns, A., & Bitter, J. A. Evaluation planning considerations for post-employment training of professionals in rehabilitation. *Rehabilitation Literature,* 1978, *39*(6–7), 180–185.

Mayclin, M. V. *Training needs assessment: Missouri rehabilitation facilities.* Columbia, MO: Region VII Rehabilitation Continuing Education Program, University of Missouri-Columbia, 1978.

McDonald, A. A., Sr., & Lorenz, J. R. Graduate curriculum and training delivery preferences of practicing rehabilitation facility administrators. *Journal of Rehabilitation Administration,* 1977, *1*(4), 12–22.

McFarlane, F. R., & Sullivan, M. B. *A study of educational and training needs of rehabilitation counselors.* San Diego: San Diego State University, Region Nine Rehabilitation Continuing Education Program, undated.

Miller, L. A., & Obermann, C. E. *Continuing education for rehabilitation counselors: A review and context for practice and research.* Iowa City: The University of Iowa, 1969.

Miller, L. A., & Roberts, R. R. *Understanding the work milieu and personnel in developing continuing education for rehabilitation counselors.* Iowa City: The University of Iowa, 1971(a).

Miller, L. A., & Roberts, R. R. *Rehabilitation counselor change associated with experimental continuing education programs.* Iowa City: The University of Iowa, 1971(b).

MITRE Corporation. *Telecommunications for vocational rehabilitation (Volume VI).* McLean, Va.: The MITRE Corporation, METREK Division, 1977.

Moriarty, J. B. Counselors (newly-employed): Effects of intensive short-term training on attitudes. *Research Directory of the Rehabilitation Research and Training Centers.* Washington, D.C.: Social and Rehabilitation Service, Department of Health, Education and Welfare, 1971.

National Rehabilitation Counseling Association-American Rehabilitation Counseling Association *The NRCA-ARCA News Report.* Washington, D.C.: National Rehabilitation Association, August 1978.

Pan, E., & Senkevitch, J. J. *Rehabilitation training materials study.* Washington, D.C.: The George Washington University, Rehabilitation Research and Training Center, 1975.

Pan, E., Senkevitch, J. J., & Fern, L. *A feasibility study for a National Rehabilitation Information Center.* Washington, D.C.: The George Washington University, Rehabilitation Research and Training Center, 1975.

Perry, S. A., Browning, P. L., & Rankin, R. J. *Rehabilitation short-term training: A follow-up study.* Working Paper No. 78. Eugene, Ore.: University of Oregon Rehabilitation Research and Training Center in Mental Retardation, 1975.

Rehabilitation Administration and Management Programs. *Staff development manual.* Norman, OK.: University of Oklahoma, 1977.

Rehabilitation Services Administration. *Audio-visual aids directory of the Rehabilitation Research and Training Centers.* Washington, D.C.: RSA, Department of Health, Education and Welfare, 1975.

Rehabilitation Services Administration. *Draft Rehabilitation Services Manual Chapter.* Washington, D.C.: RSA, Department of Health, Education and Welfare, 1976.

Rehabilitation Services Administration. *Evaluation of the Regional Rehabilitation Continuing Education Program.* Washington, D.C.: RSA, 1977.

RRCEP Directors. RRCEP directors discuss continuing education. *Journal of Rehabilitation,* 1975, *41*(6), 23–25, 30, 41, 47.

Sadlick, M., & Penta, F. Changing nurse attitudes toward quadriplegics through use of television. *Rehabilitation Literature,* 1975, *36*(9), 274–278.

Saxon, J. P. Intensive interpersonal communication training: An effective method for improving rehabilitation counselor functioning. *Rehabilitation Counseling Bulletin,* 1977, *21*(1), 47–50.

Steger, J. M. Rehabilitation counselor education and competency-based instruction. *Rehabilitation Counseling Bulletin,* 1977, *20*(4), 260–266.

Sullivan, M. B., & McFarlane, F. R. *Training needs identification and assessment of rehabilitation counselors.* San Diego: San Diego State University Region Nine Rehabilitation Continuing Education Program, undated.

Tipton, R. M., & Wenger, D. H. Evaluation of a short-term program for orientation of field counselors to psychiatric rehabilitation. *Journal of Applied Rehabilitation Counseling,* 1970, *1*(1), 10–15.

6

Impact of Psychosocial Research on Rehabilitation Services: A Selective Review*

JEROLD D. BOZARTH, PH.D.
JOHN R. BARRY, PH.D.

This chapter identifies the impact on rehabilitation services of some key psychosocial research themes in rehabilitation over the past few years. Areas covered include (1) theory and practice of rehabilitation counseling; (2) client attitudes toward themselves, their disability, and the rehabilitation process; (3) counselor attitudes; and (4) community attitudes toward the disabled. Utilization of psychosocial research is also discussed. The review was undertaken using the perspective of what the authors term a "Research Action Model" (RAM), which consists of three main steps: (1) development of research projects in a specific area designation; (2) translation of that research into pragmatic terms with dissemination to practitioners; and (3) efforts to promote utilization of these disseminated results by practitioners. Much of the psychosocial research reviewed here has indeed been utilized, particularly research conducted using the RAM approach and sponsored by the Rehabilitation Services Administration (RSA). There is, however, much complexity involved in the process of adoption/adaption and use. Federal legislation, federal funding, client advocacy demands, and current vogues are among the factors which have influenced the adoption of research findings.

Study of the psychosocial aspect of disability has long been an important part of the research tradition in rehabilitation. Research in this area has become more important with the 1978 congressional amendments in

*The authors appreciate the suggestions of Drs. Brian Bolton, Rick Roessler, and Thomas Backer in preparing this chapter.

rehabilitation services legislation. These amendments emphasize the goal of *independent living* for disabled individuals, thus making it much more important to increase our understanding of nonvocational areas. The aim of this chapter is to identify some of the principal psychosocial research themes in recent years and to discuss the practical impact of these investigations on rehabilitation services. Finally, barriers to more effective utilization of psychosocial research findings in rehabilitation will be examined.

DEFINITION OF THE TERM "PSYCHOSOCIAL"

The literature concerning psychosocial aspects of disability covers a wide range of topics (see, for example, Albrecht, 1976; Barker, Wright, Meyerson, and Glinick, 1953; Garrett and Levine, 1973; Malikin and Rusalem, 1969; McDaniel, 1976; Marinelli and Dell Orto, 1977; Neff, 1968, Safilios-Rothschild, 1970; Shontz, 1975; Stubbins, 1977; Sussman, 1965; and Wright, 1960). Type of disability, self-perceptions, societal attitudes, and a host of other variables are considered in this literature. With this diversity, just defining what we mean by *psychosocial* becomes a problem.

A major psychosocial research project now being conducted by the Arkansas Rehabilitation Research and Training Center (ARR&TC) utilizes a behavioral framework for examining psychosocial phenomena and intervention strategies for responding to psychosocial maladjustments. The ARR&TC definitions of the term *psychosocial* contain a common core component—*the disabled individual's ability to respond effectively to continually changing situational demands.* Several viewpoints in the literature which reflect this emphasis have been compiled by Roessler and Bolton (1978):

> Adjustment services are viewed as enabling the person to learn the behaviors and skills necessary to become a more fully functioning member of the community (Baker and Sawyer, 1973, p. V).
>
> The emphasis is on the development of effective means of coping with life problems as they unfold in the social context (Wahler, Delbridge, and Clubb, 1969, p. 124).
>
> The focus is on what people do in relation to the psychological conditions in which they do it (Mischel, 1973, p. 265).
>
> The desired outcome is that effective behaviors will lead to increases in positive reinforcement from the environment and the self without increases in rates of punishment (Adams, 1972, p. 18).

> A considerable amount of the rehabilitation process can be considered to be a learning situation. The disabled patient must learn new ways of behaving and new methods of responding that will take the place of behavior precluded by the disability (Trotter and Inman, 1968, p. 347).
>
> Learning the physical-medical aspects of life as a disabled person and learning new activities that are rewarding are the core of the rehabilitation process (Trieschmann, 1974, p. 556).

The definition of psychosocial research used in this chapter is consistent with these points of view. *Psychosocial functioning* is defined as "the degree to which a client demonstrates social and psychological adaptability which serves to enhance feelings of security, adequacy, functioning capability, emotional stability, and social interaction" (First Institute of Rehabilitation Issues, 1974, p. 6). The Sixth Institute of Rehabilitation Issues Prime Study Group on adjustment services was in the process of further examining psychosocial functioning at the time this chapter was written. The results of this institute are apt to include further refinement of the definition of psychosocial functioning (Rice, 1979).

The review in this chapter is intended to be *selective* rather than comprehensive in its presentation. Since any change in client behavior (e.g., work skills) also includes changes in psychosocial functioning, the term *psychosocial aspects of disability* could theoretically be expanded to cover almost any research on understanding of client change, how to promote it, and how to measure it. Consideration of psychosocial research could include cognitive processes, cognitive theories, learning, behavior, personality, motivation, and social psychological theory. It might include skills and motivations of people, or it might include consideration of the social environment. Indeed, the psychosocial aspects of any one disability could be a major thrust for organization of a comprehensive review. Research on language disorders, hemiplegia, blindness, deafness, cancer, or mental illness could each be examined within a psychosocial framework.

The expansiveness of the term *psychosocial aspects of disability* dictates selectivity and deliberate limitation. The much more restricted definition here will cover the following major areas: (1) theory and practice of rehabilitation counseling; (2) client attitudes toward themselves, their disability, and the rehabilitation process; (3) counselor attitudes; and (4) community attitudes toward the disabled. Utilization of psychosocial research will be the final subject of analysis.

It is also important to remember that a great deal of the research on counseling and psychosocial aspects occurs *outside* of the rehabilitation field. This poses difficulties in identification of that psychosocial research most pertinent to rehabilitation and adds to the problems of adaption of such research. This point will be discussed further in the last part of this chapter.

REHABILITATION SERVICE ADMINISTRATION (RSA) SPONSORSHIP OF PSYCHOSOCIAL RESEARCH

Rehabilitation research has been primarily sponsored by the federal government, mostly through the agency now called the Rehabilitation Services Administration (RSA). Federally sponsored psychosocial research over the last twenty years has been targeted at specific problem areas. These problem areas were determined, in part, by legislative mandate and, in part, by RSA policy makers, who received varying amounts of input from service delivery staff and administrators in the field. Recently consumers have begun to demand a voice in decisions about services and are now a force to consider (see the chapter on consumer advocacy). Each of these forces has helped to determine what research has been funded and how it has been applied to rehabilitation services.

Federal sponsorship of Research and Training Centers (RTC) has been one major instrument in facilitating rehabilitation research. One of these centers, the Arkansas Rehabilitation Research and Training Center (ARR&TC), has designated as a core area of research the psychosocial aspects of disability. Another center, the West Virginia Rehabilitation Research and Training Center (WVRR&TC), has hosted the Institute of Rehabilitation Issues Prime Study Group in adjustment services, which incorporates psychosocial functioning as part of its coverage.

The major focus of a five year RSA-funded project at the Human Resources Center, Programatic Research on Employment Preparation (PREP), is on the transition from school to work of severely disabled youth, studying four major areas: (1) independent living, (2) career education, (3) job placement, and (4) attitudes. There are three major work phases affiliated with each of these areas: applied research, pilot model development and evaluation, and research utilization. (Schroedel, 1978).

The RSA has sponsored a number of training programs for rehabilitation clients and counselors in the psychosocial area. Training strategies have been oriented toward particular problems of psychosocial adjustment. Roessler (1972) and Roessler and Bolton (1978, p. 53) list some of these problem areas and the training packages developed by several sources to aid psychosocial adjustment:

1. *Problem:* Inability to interact satisfactorily with others
   Training: "Interpersonal Skills"

2. *Problem:* Ineffective behaviors in important life situations
   Training: "Life Skills Modeling"

3. *Problem:* Low achievement need and drive
   Training: "Achievement Motivation Training"

4. *Problem:* Expectation of little control over one's fate
   Training: "Internal Control Training"

5. *Problem:* Minimal desire to establish personal goals and to devise ways to achieve those goals
   Training: "Capacity for Self-direction Training"

6. *Problem:* Poor physical fitness
   Training: "Physical Fitness Training"

The RSA has also sponsored at least eleven individual research and demonstration projects in this field between 1955 and 1973 (Crocker, Muthard, Reinhardt, and Wells, 1973). An additional eleven projects in the area of psychosocial disabilities were reported in professional rehabilitation journals between 1968 and 1973 (Muthard, 1974). Most of these efforts were directed toward the psychosocial aspects of a particular disability. In the past four years, at least six books dealing with "psychological aspects" have been written, edited, or updated (Albrecht, 1976; Malikin & Rusalem, 1969; Marinelli & Dell Orto, 1977; McDaniel, 1976; Shontz, 1975; Stubbins, 1977), most of them at least partly sponsored by the RSA.

Much of this review uses the perspective of an approach the RSA seems to have followed in its research and development grants program over the last several decades, which we will term the *Research Action Model (RAM).* This approach has three major phases: (1) the *development* of research projects in a specific area (e.g., psychosocial); (2) the *translation* of that research into pragmatic terms and principles, with targeted dissemination to practitioners; and (3) promotion of actual *utilization* of these principles by practitioners. In short, RAM is an applied research model.

The RSA's sponsorship of psychosocial research projects has led to application of many research findings in the psychosocial area, helping to close communication gaps between researchers and potential users.

Training packages or similar sets of systematic guidelines for practitioners are a common form for these transmissions. This appears true for many of the materials developed, for example, by ARR&TC. The utilization of research is often dependent upon the priority systems of practitioners and administrators, and upon the clarity of materials eminating from research endeavors. The RAM approach has increased the frequency of research materials which are viewed as understandable, relevant, and applicable. Thus, the RSA's efforts have served to influence those who receive research results as well as to increase production of usable findings and improve transmission media within certain subject areas.

COUNSELING

The profession of rehabilitation counseling has developed from the general counseling/psychotherapy field with its many diverse theoretical positions: psychoanalysis, client-centered, reality therapy, Adlerian, rational-emotive, and various behavioral orientations. The latter have been heavily based on learning theory. In this section, we will limit our discussion to the "self" theories and to behavioral approaches.

The "Self" Theories and Approaches

The work of Carl Rogers (1959) over the years is well known. Concepts such as client self-esteem, client responsibility, self-actualization, and nondirective interviewing were developed and popularized by Rogers and his colleagues. Most counselors, including rehabilitation counselors, demonstrate at least some awareness of these concepts in their methods of practice.

Rogers' (1957) postulates concerning the necessary and sufficient conditions of a therapeutic relationship were the basis for development of rating scales by Truax and Carkhuff (1967). These scales included definitions at each scale point for the interpersonal skill dimensions of accurate empathy, non-possessive warmth, and genuineness. Truax and Mitchell (1971) and Carkhuff (1969) have explored the effects of specific counselor interpersonal skills on many aspects of the counseling situation. Carkhuff (1972) proposed a human relations development model that goes considerably beyond the three interpersonal skill dimensions. Carkhuff (1969, 1972) and his colleagues have provided extensive research and training aids (books, manuals, films, and other audiovisual materials) to aid in the teaching of specific counselor behaviors within the Carkhuff model. Other individuals (Akridge, Means, Milligan, &

Farley, 1976; Gazda, Asbury, Balzer, Childers, Desselle, & Walters, 1973; Ivey, 1971; Snydor & Parkhill, 1973) have extended this model or developed alternatives.

These variations of the interpersonal skill dimensions training programs are widely used in rehabilitation counselor education programs. Specific packages for rehabilitation counselors include the treatment packages previously mentioned by Roessler and Bolton (1978) and the "Interpersonal Skills" training package (Akridge, Means, Milligan, & Farley, 1976).

The various levels of accurate empathy, nonpossessive warmth, and genuineness have related to the psychosocial adjustment of clients in psychotherapy (Truax & Mitchell, 1971), in many other counseling situations (Carkhuff, 1969), and in rehabilitation settings of all kinds (Anthony, Buell, Sharratt, & Althoff, 1972; Bozarth & Rubin, 1977). However, a recent review (Mitchell, Bozarth, and Krauft, 1977) of interpersonal skills research related to psychotherapy raises several concerns. Some of these are:

1. The hypothesis that high condition therapists' clients achieve more positive psychosocial adjustment has rarely been tested. High condition therapists used for research studies seldom score higher than minimal facilitative levels on the scales in question.
2. There is little direct evidence of the effectiveness of interpersonal skills training programs.
3. The results of research in the interpersonal skills area in psychotherapy is much more complex than originally thought.

Some have questioned the research evidence supporting the superiority of the human relations training approach (Lambert, DeJulio, & Stein, 1978). However, others (Anthony & Drasgow, 1978; Bozarth & Rubin, 1977) have demonstrated the effectiveness of higher condition counselors with varying populations, including rehabilitation clients. In general, while the efficacy of these concepts has not been strongly demonstrated according to some authors, the evidence is as great as that for any other approach (Smith & Glass, 1977).

Impact of "Self" Theories and Approaches

Application of concepts and training approaches in this area has been extensive. The majority of rehabilitation counselor education programs have implemented some variation of human relations training. Thus, most rehabilitation counselors have been exposed to at least one of the variations of this training. The training packages developed to increase "generic" counseling skills are available to rehabilitation counselor educators. As noted previously, one specific interpersonal skills package has been developed for rehabilitation counselors (Akridge, Means, Milligan, & Farley, 1976). The essence of the model has also been utilized in psychiatric rehabilitation (Anthony, Buell, Sharratt, & Althoff, 1972). One training package which incorporates an interpersonal skills dimension utilizing some of the principles postulated by Rogers, and incorporating specific materials related to rehabilitation counseling, has been developed and implemented (Rubin, Means, Rice, Bozarth, & Milligan, 1975). Research investigation concerning the use of this package by counselors suggests some effectiveness in improving service delivery (Farley, 1978).

Behavioral Approaches

Principles drawn from learning theory have long been advanced to explain personality and behavior change (Dollard & Miller, 1950; Rotter, 1954). More recently, a wide variety of behavioral methods was strongly embraced by clinical psychologists who were searching for alternatives to humanistic and psychoanalytical approaches. The learning theory rationale provided by Wolpe, Skinner, and their followers was simple to apply and had very concrete, limited goals which could be understood in motivational terms (Fordyce, 1974). Rather than seeking a massive character change, specific discrete behavior patterns were identified and techniques involving positive and negative reinforcement of responses were utilized to bring about particular behavior changes.

While these methods were initially used to deal with phobic reactions, they also lend themselves readily to many adjustment problems (for example, to induce a change in work habits, skill acquisition, and attitude change). For psychologists these methods have the virtue of being based on psychological learning theory and research, rather than on the philosophy of another discipline.

In rehabilitation, the promise of behavioral methods has been outlined by Meyerson, Michael, Mowrer, Osgood, and Staats (1960), Fordyce (1971, 1974), and Asken (1976). The simplicity of these approaches and their derivation from large bodies of psychological research on learning and motivation have resulted in their widespread adoption in rehabilitation. Their simple application and clear-cut, discrete (although small) units of accomplishments also are appealing to rehabilitation professionals. The service provider, as well as the client, can be repeatedly rewarded by the success of these methods in changing behavior (Lazarus, 1976).

Positive reinforcement, token economies, and several similar approaches have been used in the rehabilitation of clients with a variety of disabilities. For example, a successful program for complex skill training of public offenders on an individual basis is provided at Draper State Prison in Alabama. Research evaluation of this program suggests that the *combined* effects of an enriched rehabilitation effort and positive reinforcement techniques increase the rate of successful rehabilitation (Rehabilitation Research Foundation, 1968 and 1973).

Mischel (1973) suggests use of the behavioral method called *assertiveness training* for handicapped individuals, using role playing, self-reports and activity budget pretest and posttest measures. For handicapped and disadvantaged clients who have accepted society's evaluation of themselves as inferior, such training can be helpful in counteracting this negative self-image.

In a behavioral program described by Roessler and Bolton (1978), *coping* is stressed. Physical, intellectual, and emotional growth strategies are taught; very specific and detailed instructions are provided. These approaches have been tested in varied settings and have proven useful with clients having a wide variety of disabilities. For example, an evaluation of a personal adjustment training program conducted for rehabilitation clients at the Hot Springs Rehabilitation Center suggested that a program encompassing physical, intellectual, and emotional training produces improvement in specific physical, goal-setting, and interpersonal skills (Roessler, Bolton, Means, & Milligan, 1975). Utilization of a randomized experimental design in this study, with pretest and posttest measures, is reflective of the rigorous way this research is being conducted. In addition, the training packages developed by ARR&TC are predicated upon a behavioral approach, and the ARR&TC definition of psychosocial adjustment comes from a behavioral frame of reference.

The operant conditioning approach has been used to improve job placement procedures with psychiatric patients of the Hot Springs hospital (Azrin, Flores, & Kaplan, 1975; Jones & Azrin, 1973). In addition, Glaser and Backer (1974) report on a "blue ribbon project" of the Research Utilization Specialist in Virginia (one of nine funded on a demonstration basis by the RSA), who established a behavior modification training program for clients of the Woodrow Wilson Rehabilitation Center in his state.

Behavior modification programs have been used with nearly all psychosocial disability groups. Yates (1970) describes programs for disability classes as diverse as psychoses, alcoholism, drug addiction, and mental deficiencies.

Impact of Behavioral Methods

Application of behavioral methods has often been directly associated with rehabilitation facilities. A relatively "pure" form of behavioral application has occurred in facility settings, such as rehabilitation centers and psychiatric hospitals. However, the general behavioral approach to the diagnosis and treatment of behavioral problems permeates the entire rehabilitation process in both facilities and state Vocational Rehabilitation agencies.

Behavioral approaches have entered the rehabilitation counselor's domain in a somewhat piecemeal fashion. Contract negotiation with clients and the development of behavioral objectives are examples of applications in rehabilitation counseling; these are now extensive, but not as systematic as, for example, behavior therapy as a subfield of clinical psychology.

The impact of behavioral methods in rehabilitation counseling can be noted in many counselor reports delineating goals and often exists in the form of assessment procedures. The impact is also clear in the development of the behavioral training packages previously mentioned. This impact is difficult to assess precisely, however, because behavioral methods are often combined with other approaches and thus are not "pure" in form. The overall efficacy of these methods for changing complex behaviors also remains to be carefully evaluated (Belcastro, 1978). It seems likely that the behavioral approaches will join the large array of techniques from other schools of therapy and psychology (e.g., the psychoanalytic and the humanistic), which service providers utilize when the technique appears to fit the problem and when the service provider and the client agree that it may be helpful.

ATTITUDES

Defined as predispositions to respond, *attitudes* toward the self, toward significant others, and toward environmental factors are believed to guide and influence much of people's behavior. Many personality theorists feel that attitudes are a major component of personality and certainly influence the impression one makes on others (Wright, 1964). It is therefore not surprising that attitudes—of clients, counselor, and community—are believed to play an integral part in rehabilitation (Kutner, 1971).

Client Attitudes

At a global level, motivation has been considered a major factor in rehabilitation for many years (Lane & Barry, 1970). Clients are said to be motivated (or unmotivated) to realize their full potential in getting well and/or returning to work. The counselor may try to motivate the client, or may try to discover the client's existing motivations in order to energize the client toward self-help. The self-regard of the client is central to this entire procedure.

Client self-concept may be considered one of the many self-attitudes. Several research projects have examined the relation of a client's self-concept to rehabilitation objectives. Fitts (1972a, 1972b, pp. 32–33) has referred to the poor self-concept often characteristic of psychiatric clients. Fitts (1972b) speculates that self-concept differences within disability groups are likely to have the same significance as they do in any population. The evidence suggests that disabled clients report lower self-esteem than nondisabled persons, and that some disabling conditions have greater impact on self-concept than do others (Meighan, 1970; Safilios-Rothschild, 1970; Schurr, Joiner, & Towne, 1970; Shelsky, 1957; Smits, 1964; and Wright, 1960). Examination of data from a nationwide study of state agency rehabilitation counselors (Bolton, 1976; Bozarth & Rubin, 1977) identifies psychological adjustment (and the part that self-concept plays in such adjustment) as an important dimension for client improvement.

Another important attitude is the client's general feeling about work. There is widespread agreement that work is an important part of everyone's life (Neff, 1968). Holding a job provides the worker with a social and physical environment, with feelings of satisfaction and self-worth, and with financial support. Disabled clients' attitudes about self-sufficiency and their contributions to society are often noted in writings on rehabilitation but have not been systematically studied to date. Nevertheless, it seems self-evident that attitudes about self in relation to work have an impact on the rehabilitation process.

In general, attitudes toward self are a significant determinant of an individual's behavior. Through such behavior, self-attitudes are communicated to others, who may then tend to adopt similar attitudes about the individual. As with a self-fulfilling prophecy, a negative self-attitude is perceived by others with whom the client interacts. This perception then tends to result in negative evaluations of the client by others. The individual perceives this, and the negative self-attitude is thus reinforced. To effect change, it is necessary to break this circle of effects (Wright, 1960).

Counselor Attitudes

The relation of counselor attitudes to counseling effectiveness is another area which has had significant impact in rehabilitation counseling. In one study, Leviton (1973) contrasted the views of helpers and clients on different aspects of the helping relationship. On some issues they view things similarly (e.g., the professional control in rehabilitation). But in other ways, clients and their helpers are far apart in their viewpoints. Understanding these differences can help counselors to be more effective.

Work by McPhee (1967) and his colleagues also suggests the importance of the role of counselors' attitudes toward their clients' interpersonal skills. Studies of attitudes among mental health workers indicate that those

> . . . who are younger, the mainstream of American middle-class culture, more highly trained, and of greater social and professional status tend to be less socially restrictive and less authoritarian in their attitudes about mental illness and mental patients (Rabkin, 1977, p. 170).

Rabkin also reports therapists as being more receptive to mental patients who have certain characteristics:

> . . . patients who are young, physically attractive, well educated, members of the upper middle class, intelligent, verbal, willing to talk about and take responsibility for their problems, possessing considerable ego strength, and showing no signs of gross pathology are those who are welcomed as good therapeutic candidates (p. 173).

It is likely that similar counselor attitudes exist toward clients in rehabilitation. A finding which suggests that behavior which is socially visible and unpredictable is particularly objectionable to therapists (Rabkin, 1977, p. 174) is also applicable to rehabilitation counselors.

Thoreson and Kerr (1978) conclude, in an analysis of the healer-patient relationship, that the rehabilitation practitioner's attitude is often patronizing toward disabled individuals. These authors suggest that rehabilitation counseling, as a process of remediation, ignores the environment as a source of both difficulties and of improvement.

Community Attitudes

There has been much research on the subject of attitudes toward disability on the part of nondisabled community members. Roessler and Bolton (1978) have summarized the conclusions of such investigators as Barker, Wright, Meyerson, and Glinick (1953) and Siller, (1976):

1. Attitudes toward disabled persons, while highly varied, are frequently negative. Public, verbalized attitudes are on the average mildly favorable. However, indirect evidence suggests that deeper unverbalized attitudes are more frequently hostile.
2. Society's rejecting attitudes toward the disabled result in greatly restricted vocational and social opportunities.
3. The attitudes of disabled persons toward their own disabilities have been inadequately studied. Furthermore, the available evidence indicates that the subject is complex, e.g., Weinberg-Asher (1976) found that disabled persons perceived themselves in much the same way that able-bodied persons perceived themselves; but Schroedel and Schiff (1972) concluded that deaf persons manifest more negative attitudes toward deafness than do hearing persons.
4. Attitudes toward the disabled are multidimensional in structure, i.e., there are from 10 to 12 relatively independent attitudinal components that account for unfavorable reactions to disabled persons.
5. Attempts to modify negative attitudes toward the disabled have generally been unsuccessful.
6. The evidence is rather clear that the attitudes of parents toward their disabled children tend to be extreme more often than the attitudes of parents toward their normal children.

Yuker and his colleagues at Abilities, Inc. (Yuker, Block & Campbell, 1960; Yuker, Block, & Young, 1966) have developed a widely used global measure of attitude toward disability. This measure defines attitude as a single variable based on the notion that there is a measurable generality among the various attitudes toward different kinds of disabled persons. The scale has been used to study the generalized attitude toward disability by both disabled and nondisabled persons (Cordano & Shontz, 1969; Noonan, Barry, & Davis, 1970).

Others (e.g., Siller, Chipman, Ferguson, & Vann, 1976; Siller, Vann, Ferguson, & Holland, 1976) have examined attitudes toward specific groups of disabled people: the blind, deaf, obese, cosmetically impaired, and amputees. Visible impairments, particularly of the cosmetic kind, appear to stimulate "disgust at the thought of close physical contact" and "limited aversive feeling." Using factor analytic techniques, certain general variables appeared to underlie attitudes toward several, but not all, of the groups of disabled persons. Uneasiness and social embarrassment were evoked by all five groups. Differences in the structure of attitudes toward the disabled did not appear to be associated with age, sex, or education. These studies have helped to pinpoint differences in attitudes toward different kinds of disabilities, and to further define and delineate specific aspects of negative attitudes toward the disabled. As a result, those who work with the disabled can better understand their own feelings toward the disabled, as well as the feelings of the disabled toward themselves and attitudes of nondisabled people.

Goldberg (1977) believes that community attitudes perpetuate social stigma toward the physically disabled and may have more impact upon their social and psychological adjustment than does the severity of the disability. It is widely accepted that the disabled perceive the aversive feelings directed toward them by the general population. This perception is believed to reinforce a negative self-concept.

Research on community attitudes has often come from outside the rehabilitation field. Nevertheless, findings from these studies concerning community attitudes and attitudes of others toward the disabled can provide much information to the rehabilitation practitioner. Such research has provided a foundation for instruction in universities, as well as basic information to practitioners. In the area of counselor attitudes, research has pointed toward the interpersonal skills variables of accurate empathy, nonpossessive warmth, and genuineness.

Impact of Attitude Research

The application of research on attitudes is somewhat different than for research in other areas. Findings from studies in this area permeate many areas of the rehabilitation process; to date, no specific packages for counselors or clients have been produced. Thoreson and Kerr (1978) suggest some general strategies for changing attitudes toward disabled people:

1. Redefinition of acceptance of disability to mean tolerance of disability;
2. Redefinition of role relationships in such a way as to treat a disabled person because he is human, not because he is "sick";
3. Redefinition of "handicap" in terms of the environment; and
4. Redefinition of problems of disabled individuals as problems not unlike those which all people face (p. 21).

Thoreson and Kerr also suggest some ways to implement these strategies, including: "consciousness-raising," "the training of rehabilitation counselors in the arts of environmental design and consultation," and "determining of means of breaking down employment barriers to the severely disabled" (p. 25). Specific training materials for these purposes have yet to be developed, however.

Speculation that the healer-patient relationship is laden with patronizing attitudes toward disabled individuals suggests a need for research on psychosocial variables. The postulate of Thoreson and Kerr (1978) that the acceptance of disability is intrinsically derogating is also a prime research topic.

In general, the impact of research findings about attitudes may be less tangible than in other areas of study. The extent to which practitioners and administrators have utilized much of the knowledge about attitudes toward the disabled is not widely reported. The strategies noted by Thoreson and Kerr (1978) may provide an initial base for more systematic and applied research in the future. It may be that more recent focus on the *severely* disabled and consideration of rehabilitation beyond the vocational area will enhance the impact of such research in the future.

KNOWLEDGE UTILIZATION STRATEGIES

The RSA at the federal level, supplemented by activities in certain states, has long made vigorous efforts to support the field application of rehabilitation research. All of these efforts, and others funded by the RSA, have provided the support for the dissemination and utilization of psychosocial research. These efforts include:

1. A Visiting Consultant Program to provide technical assistance to rehabilitation agencies (Butler, 1975).
2. Project RULE (Research Utilization Through Learning Experiences), which has funded site visits by rehabilitation professionals to innovative programs in other settings (Kunce & Hartley, 1975).
3. Four Research Utilization Laboratories (RULS) in Chicago, New York, Virginia, and Texas (the work of the Chicago Laboratory is reported in Soloff, Goldstein, Pollack, & White, 1975).
4. The National Research Utilization Specialist (RUS) Demonstration Program in nine state VR agencies (Hamilton & Muthard, 1975).

5. The National Rehabilitation Information Center at Catholic University in Washington, D.C.
6. The longstanding project of the Oklahoma Clearing House Information Exchange to disseminate current information on rehabilitation, often before its formal publication in established journals.

Regardless of which utilization mechanism we are discussing, however, there are certain unique aspects of the psychosocial area that require attention where utilization efforts are concerned. First, much psychosocial research is completed *outside* the rehabilitation area and may not easily be transferred to rehabilitation problems. Second, this outside research is usually not completed using the RAM approach and may often be more basic than applied in nature. Findings thus may be irrelevant for any immediate application, or at least require much translation and repackaging. Third, such research often does not involve a "hard product" and may produce more questions than answers; this is perhaps more true in the psychosocial area than in many others.

Research in the psychosocial domain especially is affected by other research findings from multiple fields. Knowledge utilization strategies for such findings must always be open to continuous change in responding to these realities, with flexible rather than rigid application.

The following two examples are offered to provide a further idea of how knowledge utilization strategies can be applied in the psychosocial area:

Application Example 1—Personal Adjustment Skills

Several aspects of psychosocial difficulties of clients appear to involve socialization and motivation skills. The lack of personal adjustment and problem-solving skills are noted as integral psychosocial limitations for many rehabilitation clients (Bolton, 1976; Roessler, 1972). The availability of other systematic packages—e.g., for group training (Lasky, Dell Orto, & Marinelli, 1977; Means & Roessler, 1976) and for interpersonal skills training (Carkhuff, 1969)—provide initial intervention strategies for such psychosocial difficulties. The Personal Achievement Skills (PAS) package was developed as a systematic approach to group counseling to provide "treatment through training" procedures for social and motivational skill building. This program is described in more detail by Roessler and Bolton (1978, pp. 93–110).

PAS is a systematic training package which uses a group counseling format. The basic concepts are taught didactically, and then clients practice the seven major life skills within a group setting. PAS generally requires forty hours to complete; there is both a leader's manual and a workbook for participants.

Steps taken to develop, disseminate, and promote utilization of PAS were the following:

1. Relevant research findings and details about systematic training packages were identified.
2. The PAS training package was developed.
3. The package was evaluated in several trial settings.
4. The package was introduced to the field and demonstrated by trained leaders.
5. Continued evaluation of the effectiveness of the package was built into most of the training sessions.
6. Managers and trainers in the field settings began to utilize the package when it appeared to be effective and appropriate to their clients' needs.

Research on the PAS package suggests that it is effective in improving self-perceptions and life skills of rehabilitation clients (Roessler & Bolton, 1978). Evaluative studies have included: (1) a compilation of assessments of PAS by rehabilitation counselors (Roessler & Green, 1974); (2) appraisals by teacher and aide observations of high school students (Roessler & DeWeese, 1975); (3) evaluations of PAS by rehabilitation clients in the rehabilitation center work-adjustment program (Roessler, Cook, & Lillard, 1976, 1977); and (4) assessment of PAS blind rehabilitation clients in a personal adjustment program (Roessler, 1978).

Clients' self-report data and evaluation by experimental studies thus indicate the utility of PAS in work-adjustment settings. Roessler and Bolton (1978) summarize the main findings about PAS in work-adjustment programs at a rehabilitation center.

1. More PAS participants than controlled subjects reported improvement in life perspective.
2. PAS participants reported significantly greater gain "pre" to "post" on vocational maturity, vocational functioning, and interpersonal maturity.
3. Self-reported evidence of goal attainment occurred predominantly with the PAS group.
4. Data suggested the PAS group developed a more realistic perception of the benefits of work.
5. The PAS program was rated as useful, stimulating, and well organized by program participants.

6. No differences were found between PAS participants and controlled subjects on counselor-leader ratings of period adjustment or improvements in adjustment (pp. 106–107).

The PAS package has now been utilized by agencies and rehabilitation facilities in most Southeastern and Southwestern states with uniformly positive feedback.

Application Example 2—Facilitative Case Management Module

Another training package developed to improve effectiveness for dealing with psychosocial factors is the Facilitative Case Management Module. This package consists of a leader's workbook, a participant's workbook, a typescript of a client tape, and the audiotape of the counselor-client session (Rubin, Means, Rice, Bozarth, & Milligan, 1975). This training package was developed to aid counselors to improve their rehabilitation counseling skills. The sequence of the development of this package was as follows:

1. Theoretical and research reports were reviewed, and a basic approach was developed in a way which was applicable to improving rehabilitation counselor performance (Bozarth & Rubin, 1972).
2. Counselor-client audiotapes of sessions were collected from a national sample of rehabilitation agency counselors (Bozarth & Rubin, 1977).
3. Transcripts of demonstration segments were developed from the counselor-client audiotapes (Bozarth & Rubin, 1972).
4. These segments were presented as examples, with comments about the application of the model (Bozarth & Rubin, 1972).
5. The model was further refined during presentations to rehabilitation counselors in over twenty states.
6. The systematic package was developed for application in the field (Rubin, Means, Rice, Bozarth, & Milligan, 1975).
7. This package was presented to agency counselors throughout the country by training personnel of ARR&TC.
8. Counselors and/or supervisors who were trained with the package then offered the same training program to counselors in their respective states.

9. Systematic evaluations of participants' reactions to the program were gathered.

Training in this package has been completed by participants in over twenty-one state rehabilitation agencies and university rehabilitation counselor education training programs. Systematic feedback from participants of these programs reflects general satisfaction with the relevancy and value of the program (Farley, 1976a). Rubin (1979) also reports consistent positive evaluation of the program by participants who have gone to continuing education programs coordinated by the University of Tennessee.

In addition, Farley (1978) reports results which indicate that the training module has positive effects on "rehabilitation counselor cognitive development, affectiveness reaction, and on-the-job performance" (p. 100). An earlier study by Farley (1976b) reveals that counselor trainees rated the program highly in terms of its appropriateness and relevancy for rehabilitation counselors.

CONCLUSIONS

This chapter has reviewed several areas of psychosocial research application and impact: (1) theory and practice of rehabilitation counseling; (2) client attitudes toward themselves, their disability, and the rehabilitation process; (3) counselor attitudes; and (4) community attitudes. The role of research utilization activities was also discussed. The review was undertaken from the perspective of what the authors have called a Research Action Model (RAM), which consists of conducting research in a specific area, translating that research into pragmatic terms with dissemination to practitioners, and promoting utilization of these principles by practitioners.

Psychosocial research has had a major impact on the theory and practice of rehabilitation counseling. In particular, research related to self theories, the human development model, and behavioral methods has had considerable practical application. Research on self theories has extensively influenced rehabilitation counseling practice and served as a foundation for conceptualizing human development models. These models have resulted in training packages, which include systematic training procedures to be utilized by rehabilitation counselors and counselor educators. Research in the behavioral realm has been directly applied in rehabilitation facilities and in the field. Behavioral techniques have permeated many rehabilitation counselors' functions in both state rehabilitation agencies and private settings (e.g., goal setting and client-counselor contract negotiation).

Extensive research has taken place in the areas of counselor attitudes, client attitudes, and community attitudes toward rehabilitation and the disabled. While these research findings permeate many areas of rehabilitation functioning, specific training packages have not been developed from them. The research findings in this area offer more of a foundation for the development of strategies which may lead to more systematic and applied research in the future. Research in this area has not often followed the RAM approach. This is usually due to the more basic nature of such research.

Knowledge utilization efforts for psychosocial research face several unique problems: (1) the complexity of much psychosocial research does not always lend itself to rapid transmission in knowledge utilization paradigms; (2) many factors which induce change have nothing to do with research findings; and (3) research may be utilized only after a problem becomes familiar to the public. For example, one obvious influence on rehabilitation services has been that of federal legislation. Furthermore, such legislation is seldom predicated upon research findings.

Creating legislation entails input from many sources. Special interest group pressures and administrative considerations are influences which often—in fact, mostly—have a greater impact on legislation and policy than does research. Another factor which influences change, but has little to do with research, is client advocacy groups. These groups may demand specific services which may result in the adoption of new techniques in response to their demands.

The *familiarity* of a problem to the public is sometimes a prerequisite to making changes in practice already suggested by research. For example, the Vietnam War was accompanied by an increase in the number of spinal cord injured and drug abusers. Research findings already available on how to provide effective rehabilitation services for these groups were suddenly put into action because there was a demand from these clients and from the public for increased services.

From this review, it appears that there has been a considerable amount of psychosocial research that has led or is leading to measurable impact on rehabilitation service delivery. Despite the barriers to research application we have just noted, and indeed limits in the current state of our knowledge regarding psychosocial aspects of disability, we agree with Margaret Mead that

> Knowledge joined to action . . . knowledge about what man has been and is . . . can protect the future. There is hope, I believe, in seeing human adventure (the search for man) as a whole and in the shared trust that knowledge about mankind, sought in reverence for life, can bring life (Mead, 1972, p. 296).

The rapid transmission of research findings on psychosocial aspects of disability and adjustment to it can, it is hoped, increase our knowledge and be joined to action in order to bring about a better life for the handicapped.

REFERENCES

Adams, H. *Psychology of Adjustment.* New York: Ronald Press, 1972.

Akridge, R. L., Means, R., Milligan, T., & Farley, R. C. *Interpersonal skills training basic helping skills for rehabilitation workers.* Fayetteville, Arkansas: University of Arkansas, 1976.

Albrecht, G. (Ed.). *The sociology of physical disability and rehabilitation.* Pittsburgh: University of Pittsburgh Press, 1976.

Anthony, W. A., Buell, G., Sharratt, S., & Althoff, N. E. The efficacy of psychiatric rehabilitation. *Psychological Bulletin,* 1972, *78,* 447–456.

Anthony, W. A., & Drasgow, J. A human technology for human resource development. *The Counseling Psychologist,* 1978, *7*(3), 58–65.

Asken, M. J. Behavioral techniques and orthopedic disability: A review. *Rehabilitation Psychology,* 1976, *23,* 41–64.

Azrin, N., Flores, T., & Kaplan, S. Job-finding club: A group assisted program for obtaining employment. *Behavioral Research Therapy,* 1975, *13,* 17–27.

Baker, N. J., & Sawyer, H. *Adjustment services in rehabilitation: Emphasis on human change.* Auburn: Auburn University, Rehabilitation Services Education and Department of Vocational and Adult Education, 1973.

Barker, R. G., Wright, B. A., Meyerson, L., & Glinick, N. R. *Adjustment to physical handicap and illness:: A survey of the social psychology and physique and disability* (Rev. ed.). New York: Social Science Research Council, 1953.

Belcastro, F. P. Use of behavior modification with visually handicapped subjects: A review of research. *Education of the Visually Handicapped,* 1978, *9,* 114–118.

Bolton, B. Case performance characteristics associated with three counseling styles. *Rehabilitation Counseling Bulletin,* 1976, *19*(3), 464–468.

Bozarth, J., & Rubin, S. E. *Facilitative management in rehabilitation counseling: A case book.* Champaign, Ill.: Stipes, 1972.

Bozarth, J., & Rubin, S. E. Empirical observations of rehabilitation counselor performance and outcome: Some implications. *Rehabilitation Counseling Bulletin,* 1977, *19*(1), 294–298.

Butler, A. J. Visiting consultant program for research utilization. *Rehabilitation Counseling Bulletin,* 1975, *19,* 405–415.

Carkhuff, R. R. *Helping and human relations: A primer for lay and professional helpers* (Vols. 1 and 2). New York: Holt, Rinehart & Winston, 1969.

Carkhuff, R. R. New directions in training for the helping professions: Toward a technology for human and community resource development. *The Counseling Psychologist,* 1972, *3,* 12–30.

Cordano, L. L., & Shontz, R. E. Psychological determinants of self-evaluations. *Journal of Counseling Psychology,* 1969, *16,* 575–578.

Crocker, L. M., Muthard, J. E., Reinhardt, E. W., & Wells, S. A. *An index to rehabilitation and social service projects* (Vol. II). Gainesville, Fla.: University of Florida, 1973.

Dollard, J., & Miller, N. E. *Personality and psychotherapy: An analysis in terms of learning, thinking, and culture.* New York: McGraw-Hill, 1950.

Farley, R. *An attitudinal evaluation of the facilitative case management program* (Research Report). Fayetteville, Ark.: University of Arkansas, Arkansas Rehabilitation Research and Training Center, 1976a.

Farley, R. *The evaluation of training.* Unpublished manuscript, University of Arkansas, 1976b.

Farley, R. *Facilitative case management: An evaluation of a short-term in-service training program for vocational rehabilitation counselors.* Unpublished doctoral dissertation. University of Arkansas, 1978.

First Institute of Rehabilitation Issues, *Measurement of outcomes* (Share). Paul T. Bassett, Morgantown, W. Va.: West Virginia Research and Training Center, 1974.

Fitts, W. H. *The self concept and psychopathology.* Monograph No. 4. Counselor Recordings and Tests, Nashville, Tenn., 1972a.

Fitts, W. H. *The self concept and behavior: Overview and supplement.* Monograph No. 7. Counselor Recordings and Tests, Nashville, Tenn., 1972b.

Fordyce, W. E. Behavioral methods in rehabilitation. In W. S. Neff (Ed.), *Rehabilitation psychology.* Washington, D.C.: American Psychological Association, 1971.

Fordyce, W. E. Behavioral science and rehabilitation. *Rehabilitation Psychology,* 1974, *21,* 82–85.

Garrett, J. R., & Levine, E. S. *Rehabilitation practices with the physically disabled.* New York: Columbia University Press, 1973.

Gazda, G. M., Asbury, F. R., Balzer, F. J., Childers, W. C., Desselle, R. E., & Walters, R. P. *Human relations development: A manual for educators.* Boston: Allyn & Bacon, 1973.

Glaser, E. M., & Backer, T. E. *Evaluation of the National Research Utilization Specialist Demonstration Program, 1969–1974.* Los Angeles: Edward Glaser & Associates, 1974.

Goldberg, R. T. Rehabilitation research on disability. *Journal of Rehabilitation,* 1977, *42,* 14–18.

Hamilton, L. S., & Muthard, J. E. Research Utilization Specialists in vocational rehabilitation: Five years of experience. *Rehabilitation Counseling Bulletin,* 1975, *19,* 377–386.

Ivey, A. *Micro-counseling: Innovations in interviewing training.* Springfield, Ill.: Charles C. Thomas, 1971.

Jones, R. J., & Azrin, N. H. An experimental application of a social reinforcement approach to the problem of job finding. *Journal of Applied Behavioral Analysis,* 1973, *6,* 345–353.

Kunce, J. T., & Hartley, L. B. Planned interpersonal informational exchanges: The RULE project. *Rehabilitation Counseling Bulletin,* 1975, *19,* 443–446.

Kutner, B. The social psychology of disability. In W. S. Neff (Ed.), *Rehabilitation Psychology.* Washington, D.C.: American Psychological Association, 1971.

Lambert, M. J., DeJulio, S. S., & Stein, D. M. Therapist interpersonal skills: Process, outcome, methodological considerations, and recommendations for future research. *Psychological Bulletin,* 1978, *85,* 467–489.

Lane, J. M., & Barry, J. R. Recent research on client motivation. *Rehabilitation Research and Practice Review,* 1970, *1,* 5–26.

Lasky, R., Dell Orto, A., & Marinelli, R. *Structural experiental therapy applied to rehabilitation* (SET-R). Paper presented at the annual meeting of the American Personnel and Guidance Association, Dallas, 1977.

Lazarus, R. S. *Patterns of adjustment.* New York: McGraw-Hill, 1976.

Leviton, G. Professional and client views on rehabilitation issues. *Rehabilitation Psychology,* 1973, *20,* 1–80.

Malikin, D., & Rusalem, H. (Eds.). *Vocational rehabilitation of the disabled: An overview.* New York: New York University Press, 1969.

Marinelli, R., & Dell Orto, A. (Eds.). *Psychological and social impact of physical disability.* New York: Springer, 1977.

McDaniel, J. *Physical disability and human behavior* (2nd ed.). New York: Pergamon Press, 1976.

McPhee, W. M. *Interpersonal relationships in rehabilitation counseling: A literature review.* Salt Lake City: University of Utah Regional Rehabilitation Research Institute, 1967.

Mead, M. *Blackberry winter, my earlier years.* New York: Simon & Schuster, 1972.

Means, B., & Roessler, R. *Personal achievement skills leader's manual and participant's workbook.* Fayetteville, Ark.: Arkansas Rehabilitation Research and Training Center, 1976.

Meighan, T. *An investigation of the self concept of blind and partially seeing adolescents and of the relation of their self concepts to academic achievement in language and paragraph reading.* Unpublished doctoral dissertation, Catholic University, Washington, D.C., 1970.

Meyerson, L., Michael, J., Mowrer, O., Osgood, C., & Staats, A. Learning, behavior, and rehabilitation. In L. Lofquist (Ed.), *Psychological research and rehabilitation.* Washington, D.C.: American Psychological Association, 1960.

Mischel, B. Toward a cognitive social learning reconceptualization of personality. *Psychological Review,* 1973, *80*(4), 252–283.

Mischel, M. H. Assertion training with handicapped persons. *Journal of Counseling Psychology,* 1973, *25,* 238–241.

Mitchell, K. M., Bozarth, J. D., & Krauft, C. C. A reappraisal of the therapeutic effectiveness of accurate empathy, non-possessive warmth, and genuineness. In A. S. Gurman & A. M. Razin (Eds.), *Effective psychotherapy: A handbook of research.* New York: Pergamon Press, 1977.

Muthard, J. E. *Vocational rehabilitation index: 1974.* Gainesville: University of Florida Rehabilitation Research Institute, 1974.

Muthard, J. E. Personal communication, January 8, 1979.

Neff, W. S. *Work and human behavior.* New York: Atherton, 1968.

Noonan, J. R., Barry, J. R., & Davis, H. C. Personality determinants in attitudes toward visible disability. *Journal of Personality,* 1970, *38,* 1–15.

Rabkin, J. C. Therapists' attitudes toward mental illness and help. In A. S. Gurman & A. M. Razin (Eds.), *Effective psychotherapy: A handbook of research.* New York: Pergamon Press, 1977.

Rehabilitation Research Foundation. *The Draper E & D Project: An experimental manpower project for training and placement of youthful inmates.* Final Report to U.S. Department of Labor Manpower Administration, Washington, D.C.: Government Printing Office, 1968.

Rehabilitation Research Foundation. Phase III Final Report, *Experimental manpower laboratory for corrections.* Washington, D.C.: U.S. Department of Labor Manpower Administration, 1973.

Rice, D. Personal communication, January 3, 1979.

Roessler, R. Human dignity: An attainable goal. *Rehabilitation Research and Practice Review,* 1972, *4*(3), 1–10.

Roessler, R. Personal achievement skills training with the visually handicapped. *Rehabilitation Counseling Bulletin,* 1978, *21,* 106–112.

Roessler, R., & Bolton, B. *Psychosocial adjustment to disability.* Baltimore: University Park Press, 1978.

Roessler, R., Bolton, B., Means, B., & Milligan, P. The facts of physical, intellectual, and emotional training on rehabilitation clients. *Journal of Applied Rehabilitation Counseling,* 1975, *6*(2), 106–112.

Roessler, R., Cook, D., & Lillard, D. *Effects of systematic group counseling in work adjustment training period research report.* Fayetteville, Ark.: Arkansas Rehabilitation Research and Training Center, 1976.

Roessler, R., Cook, D., & Lillard, D. Effects of systematic group counseling in work adjustment clients. *Journal of Counseling Psychology,* 1977, *24*(4), 313–317.

Roessler, R., & DeWeese, M. *Personal achievement skills training in a classroom setting.* Unpublished paper, Fayetteville, Ark., 1975.

Roessler, R., & Green, P. *An evaluation of personal achievement skills by rehabilitation personnel* (Research Report). Fayetteville, Ark.: Arkansas Rehabilitation Research and Training Center, 1974.

Rogers, C. R. The necessary and sufficient conditions of therapeutic personality change. *Journal of Consulting Psychology,* 1957, *21,* 95–103.

Rogers, C. R. A theory of therapy, personality, and interpersonal relationships, as developed in the client-centered framework. In S. Koch (Ed.), *Psychology: A study of science* (Vol. 3). New York: McGraw-Hill, 1959.

Rotter, J. B. *Social learning and clinical psychology.* New York: Prentice-Hall, 1954.

Rubin, S. E. Personal communication. January 8, 1979.

Rubin, S. E., Means, B. L., Rice, B. D., Bozarth, J. D., & Milligan, G. T. *Facilitative case management: Instructors manual.* Fayetteville, Ark.: University of Arkansas, Arkansas Rehabilitation Research and Training Center, 1975.

Safilios-Rothschild, C. *The sociology and social psychology of disability and rehabilitation.* New York: Random House, 1970.

Schroedel, J. G. *Attitudes towards persons with disabilities: A compendium of related literature* (Human Resources Center Project PREP). Long Island, N.Y.: Human Resources Center, 1978.

Schroedel, J. G., & Schiff, W. Attitudes towards deafness among several deaf and hearing populations. *Rehabilitation Psychology,* 1972, *19,* 59–70.

Schurr, K., Joiner, L., & Towne, R. Self-concept research on the mentally retarded: A review of empirical studies. *Mental Retardation,* 1970, *8,* 39–43.

Shelsky, I. *The effect of disability on self-concept.* Unpublished doctoral dissertation, Columbia University, New York, 1957.

Shontz, F. *The psychological aspects of physical illness and disability.* New York: Macmillan, 1975.

Siller, J. Attitudes toward disability. In H. Rusalem & D. Malikin (Eds.), *Contemporary vocational rehabilitation.* New York: New York University Press, 1976.

Siller, J., Chipman, A., Ferguson, L. T., & Vann, D. H. Attitudes of the nondisabled toward the physically disabled. In *Studies in reactions to disability* (Vol. XI). New York: School of Education, New York University, 1976.

Siller, J., Vann, D. H., Ferguson, L. T., & Holland, B. Structure of attitudes toward the physically disabled. In *Studies in reactions to disability* (Vol. XII). New York: School of Education, New York University, 1976.

Smith, M. L., & Glass, G. V. Meta-analysis of psychotherapy outcome studies. *American Psychologist,* 1977, *33,* 752–760.

Smits, S. *Reactions of self and others to the obviousness and severity of physical disability.* Unpublished doctoral dissertation, University of Missouri, 1964.

Snydor, G. L., & Parkhill, N. L. *The analysis of human behavior: A program manual.* Mindon, La.: Human Resources Development Training Institute, 1973.

Soloff, A., Goldstein, L., Pollack, R., & White, B. Research utilization laboratory. *Rehabilitation Counseling Bulletin,* 1975, *19,* 416–424.

Stubbins, J. (Ed.). *Social and psychological aspects of disability.* Baltimore: University Park Press, 1977.

Sussman, M. (Ed.). *Sociology and rehabilitation.* Washington, D.C.: American Sociological Association, 1965.

Thoreson, R. W., & Kerr, B. A. The stigmatizing aspects of severe disability: Strategies for change. *Journal of Applied Rehabilitation Counseling,* 1978, *9*(2), 21–26.

Trieschmann, R. Coping with the disability: A sliding scale of goals. *Archives of Physical Medicine and Rehabilitation,* 1974, *55,* 556–560.

Trotter, A., & Inman, D. The use of positive reinforcement. *Physical Therapy,* 1968, *48*(4), 347–352.

Truax, C. B., & Carkhuff, R. R. *Toward effective counseling and psychotherapy: Training and practice.* Chicago: Aldine, 1967.

Truax, C. B., & Mitchell, K. M. Research on certain therapists' interpersonal skills in relation to process and outcome. In A. E. Bergin & S. L. Garfield (Eds.), *Handbook of psychotherapy and behavior change: An empirical analysis.* New York: Wiley, 1971.

Wahler, H., Delbridge, C., & Clubb, C. *Needed: Competence rehabilitation.* Proceedings of the ninth annual research meeting of the Department of Institutions, State of Washington and the University of Washington, Research report, *2*(2), April 1969.

Weinberg-Asher, N. The effect of physical disability on self-perception. *Rehabilitation Counseling Bulletin,* 1976, *20,* 15–20.

Wright, B. A. *Physical disability: A psychological approach.* New York: Harper & Row, 1960.

Wright, B. A. Spread in adjustment to disability. *Bulletin of the Menninger Clinic,* 1964, *28,* 198–208.

Yates, A. J. *Behavior therapy.* New York: Wiley, 1970.

Yuker, H. E., Block, J. R., & Campbell, W. J. *A scale to measure attitudes toward disabled.* Albertson, N. Y.: Human Resources Foundation, Abilities, 1960.

Yuker, H. E., Block, J. R. & Young, J. H. *The measurement of attitudes toward disabled persons.* Albertson, N. Y.: Human Resources Foundation, Abilities, 1966.

7

Developing Evaluation Standards for Vocational Rehabilitation*

LINDA BARRETT, M.H.A.
SUSAN SHEA, M.C.P.

The 1973 Rehabilitation Act contains, among its many other provisions, a requirement that evaluation standards be devised and implemented to measure the performance of the Vocational Rehabilitation (VR) program in achieving its mandate.

In this chapter, the authors report on the development of two types of performance measures of importance in vocational rehabilitation: standards for evaluation of federal/state VR programs and standards for measuring the effectiveness of individual projects funded by the Rehabilitation Services Administration. The rationale for development of standards and their use are also discussed.

These performance measures have important implications for state rehabilitation agency administrators, service deliverers, and project staff. The proposed program *evaluation standards would institute a revised reporting system throughout the state agencies and the federal administration. This, in turn, would generate information allowing for measuring the achievement of overall program goals and for explaining the factors contributing to their achievement. Such feedback would be expected to result in program modifications to enhance future performance. The proposed* project *standards, on the other hand, would require a new reporting system designed to uniformly collect comparable information on the diverse training, service, and research projects supported through the discretionary fund programs funded by the Rehabilitation Services Administration. In addition to facilitating project management, this data base would provide impact assessment information for improving the functioning of the program authorities and ultimately the basic VR program.*

*Based on a study conducted by Berkeley Planning Associates under contract # HEW 105–76–4116 with the Rehabilitation Services Administration.

THE ROLE OF STANDARDS

This chapter discusses the development of two types of standards of importance to vocational rehabilitation: standards for evaluating the state VR programs and those for evaluating projects funded by the Rehabilitation Services Administration. Included in the ensuing discussion is the role standards play in program evaluation, the proposed system of standards for the VR basic programs, and the measures recommended in assessing their accomplishment. The actual data sources for these measures are omitted here for brevity (Berkeley Planning Associates (BPA), November 1978). However, the approach to analyzing the program standards is discussed in terms of both state performance and the system of supportive evaluation used to explain differences in performance. The next topic is the approach to developing standards for the projects supported by RSA discretionary funds. This section discusses the design issues considered, the standards system proposed, and the implications for use by the projects and their program authorities in the RSA.

Although developed for difrerent purposes, the two sets of standards are similar in that they both express and allow for achieve minimal costs. If no standards emphasize outcome, the program may permit concern for client outcome to become subsidiary to cost concerns. If outcome standards do not establish quality criteria, volume of clients processed may supersede quality of service and outcome.

Given the role of standards as behavioral incentives, there are other concerns. If there are too many standards, covering too many elements of a program, there will be no clarity for program direction, and attention may become too diffused. Administrators will be required to try to meet norms for elements which may be less critical than others, and which, in fact, may not make a positive contribution to the ultimate goal of the process (i.e., gainful employment of clients).

While it is clear, from the discussion of the role of standards, that comprehensiveness is critical for a useful evaluation system, it is also apparent that this cannot be achieved through a proliferation of the number of standards which measure overall program goals. In essence, a *standard* is an acknowledged program objective—a criterion or norm against which performance is assessed. It expresses an expected level of performance whose achievement is "desired," "good," or "appropriate."

It may be argued that standards themselves should meet certain criteria if they are to be effective. Standards used in program evaluation should focus not only on the impact, or degree of effectiveness of the program for individuals, but also on coverage, or the number of clients served. A system of evaluation standards for program performance thus should address effectiveness and efficiency and relate to coverage and impact issues.

In addition to their function in an evaluation system, standards have another dimension—that of representing the goals of a program, the direction in which it desires to move, and the conditions which indicate success for the program. Supplementing the more objective goals traditionally viewed as VR program goals (e.g., competitive employment, increased economic independence, retention of benefits), Backer (1977) suggests a variety of additional outcome measures to be considered in evaluating program success. These range from client assessment of satisfaction with the services, their utility, and their outcome to employer satisfaction and case review of counselor performance.

It can be seen how standards, incorporated with an implicit or explicit reward or sanction system, may become behavioral incentives; program administrators, presented with a set of standards against which performance will be measured, may begin to move programs in the direction implied by the set. For instance, if standards emphasize the costs of providing services, administrators may be expected to aim for achieving minimal costs. If no standards emphasize outcome, the program may permit concern for client outcome to become subsidiary to cost concerns. If outcome standards do not establish quality criteria, volume of clients processed may supersede quality of service and outcome.

Given the role of standards as behavioral incentives, there are other concerns. If there are too many standards covering too many elements of a program, there will be no clarity for program direction, and attention may become too diffused. Administrators will be required to try to meet norms for elements which may be less critical than others, and which, in fact, may not make a positive contribution to the ultimate goal of the process, i.e., gainful employment of clients.

While it is clear from the discussion of the role of standards that comprehensiveness is critical for a useful evaluation system, it is also apparent that this cannot be achieved through a proliferation of the numbers of standards which the program must address. Rather, the select number of standards, established because they represent the appropriate focus for program evaluation, and because they form a cohesive base for program direction, must be incorporated into a comprehensive planning and evaluation framework. This is the only way to combine the need for appropriate program direction with a sufficiently thorough evaluation framework in order to identify the "why" of a standard's achievement or failure (i.e., the cause-effect relationships among elements of the program contributing to performance on the standards).

The context of standards includes not only the client service part of the system but also the organizational and administrative structure in which it is housed; the planning and financial, research and evaluation program development functions which support it; and the factors which impinge on the system from outside. The supportive evaluation structure into which the standards are set permits each of these elements to be considered in relation to the established standards. Differences in performance on the standards can be analyzed in terms of differences in administrative structure, in fiscal and cost variables, and in elements of the process (service mix, caseload management) to determine the factors responsible for poor, adequate, or good performance. It is this structure that places the standards in a context which makes them more than a measurement technique, and makes them a basis for program improvement. Performance on the standards is assessed, relationships between this performance and program inputs and processes (and outside factors) are explored, and program improvements can be made.

STANDARDS FOR EVALUATING VR PROGRAMS

The Rehabilitation Act of 1973 (Public Law 93–112) called for the development of program evaluation standards for the VR program. Their development has been a continually evolving process since the mandate of the act and the subsequent publication of standards in the *Federal Register* in December 1975. Reactions to the standards initially promulgated (JWK International, 1975; Rubin, 1975; The Urban Institute, 1976; Walker and Associates, 1976) centered on several issues:

- Did the standards cover the right elements of the program?
- Were some important aspects of the VR service delivery process omitted? Alternatively, were some of the elements included not sufficiently important for the establishment of a standard? Were the measures and data elements associated with the standards accurate and valid reflections of accomplishment of the intent of the standards?
- Did the performance levels establish appropriate expectations for state VR agencies?
- Who should be responsible for implementation of the standards in terms of data collection and reporting? What was to be done with

the data reported? What types of feedback should states receive on their performance?

- What actions would be taken to improve performance?

The system of standards proposed for the basic VR program contains three elements: performance standards, procedural standards, and elements of supportive evaluation. The specific standards proposed for each are presented in Table 1.

PERFORMANCE STANDARDS

Performance standards measure the achievement of a desired outcome or mission of VR (e.g., competitive employment closures). Explicit performance level expectations are set, with adjustments for client difficulty. Data elements on these standards (the actual information submitted) are reported annually for each state, mainly by RSA through routine data systems. The exception in the reporting responsibility takes the form of state-administered uniform closure and follow-up surveys of clients, designed to capture many of the concerns expressed in earlier reviews of outcome measures (Backer, 1977; Rubin, 1975). These surveys measure client satisfaction with various aspects of the VR program and their personal outcome, the utility of VR services, and the degree to which VR should be credited with responsibility for gainful activity, as well as the retention of benefits, both functional and economic.

Table 2 presents the data elements for each of the eight performance standards.

Procedural Standards

Procedural standards address the protection of client interests by ensuring that certain key processes are adhered to and monitored. No standardized performance level is set, however, due to legitimate individual differences among clients. Thus, data elements consist of stipulated procedures for state agencies to execute on some regular basis (e.g., annual reviews of a sample of cases to assess whether timely movement through VR has occurred). These procedures will form the basis for agency decisions to make appropriate changes in practices, where current processes are not in keeping with client interests and positive program performance.

TABLE 1
The Program Standards

Performance Standards

1. VR shall serve the maximum proportion of the potentially eligible target population, subject to the level of federal program funding and priorities among clients.
2. The VR program shall use resources in a cost-effective manner and show a positive return to society of investment in vocational rehabilitation of disabled clients.
3. VR shall maximize the number and proportion of clients accepted for services who are successfully rehabilitated, subject to the meeting of other standards.
4. Rehabilitated clients shall evidence increased economic independence.
5. There shall be maximum placement of rehabilitated clients into competitive employment. Noncompetitive closures shall represent an improvement in gainful activity for the client.
6. Vocational gains shall be attributable to VR services.
7. Rehabilitated clients shall retain the benefits of VR services.
8. Clients shall be satisfied with the VR program, and rehabilitated clients shall appraise VR services as useful in achieving and maintaining their vocational objectives.

Procedural Standards

9. Information collected on clients by the R-300 and all data reporting systems used by RSA shall be valid, reliable, accurate, and complete.
10. Eligibility decisions shall be based on accurate and sufficient diagnostic information, and VR shall continually review and evaluate eligibility decisions to ensure that decisions are made in accordance with laws and regulations.
11. VR shall ensure that eligibility decisions and client movement through the VR process occur in a timely manner appropriate to the needs and capabilities of the clients.
12. VR shall provide an Individualized Written Rehabilitation Program for each applicable client, and VR and the client shall be accountable to each other for complying with this agreement.

Supportive Evaluation Elements

1. Outreach and referral practices
2. Staff mix
3. Staff training
4. Administrative and organizational structure
5. Administrative costs, fiscal, and budget elements
6. Caseload size
7. Caseload balance
8. Caseload management: continuity, frequency of contact, supervision, monitoring service delivery
9. Job placement activity
10. Service mix, including postemployment services
11. Reliability of service delivery
12. Service costs
13. Use of similar benefits
14. Closure appropriateness

TABLE 2
Summary Table of Data Elements Recommended as Measures of the Eight Performance Standards

Standard	*Data Elements*
#1 Coverage	(i) Comparison of caseload served to expenditures (ii) Clients served per 100,000 population
#2 Benefit-cost and cost effectiveness	(i) Expenditure per competitively employed closure (ii) Expenditure per 26 closure (iii) Benefit-cost ratio (iv) Discounted net present value
#3 Rehabilitation rate	(i) Percent 26 closures
#4 Increased economic independence	(i) Percent 26 closures with weekly earnings at/above federal minimum wage (ii) Comparison of earnings of competitively employed 26 closures to earnings of employees in state (iii) Comparison of earnings before and after VR services (iv) Comparison of 26 closures with public assistance as primary source of support before and after VR services
#5 Competitive employment	(i) Percent 26 closures competitively employed (ii) Percent 26 closures with hourly earnings at/above federal minimum wage (iii) Percent 26 closures with competitive outcome or with noncompetitive outcome and noncompetitive goal (iv) Percent noncompetitively employed 26 closures showing improvement in gainful activity
#6 Causality	(i) Comparison of earnings change from referral to closure of 26 closures to earnings change of a control group
#7 Retention of benefits	(i) Percent 26 closures retaining earnings at follow-up (ii) Comparison of 26 closures with public assistance as primary source of support at closure and at follow-up (iii) Percent noncompetitively employed 26 closures retaining closure skills at follow-up
#8 Client satisfaction and utility appraisal	(i) Percent closed clients satisfied with overall VR experience (ii) Percent closed clients satisfied with specific aspects of VR (iii) Percent 26 closures judging services received to have been useful in obtaining their job/homemaker situation (iv) Percent 26 closures judging services received to be useful in current performance on the job/homemaker situation

Although an instrument is available (McFarlane, 1978; BPA, July 1978) and recommended for state use, the adoption of the standardized case review instrument will be voluntary, and states will be allowed to develop their own instrumentation as long as the needed items are included.

Supportive Evaluation Elements

Supportive evaluation elements are aspects of the VR process for which data are collected and analyzed, not necessarily on a routine basis, to help explain differences in performance on the standards and to help identify what improvements should be made to enhance performance on standards. This would include cost data, organizational and management data, and other items. Collection of these data might take a number of forms: Program Administrative Reviews, special audits, RSA data-reporting systems, case reviews, and others. Supportive evaluation will be addressed in greater detail in the section on analysis.

APPROACH TO ANALYSIS

The heart of the standards system will be the *analysis phase.* One of the most serious failings with the current standards, particularly as perceived by state agency personnel, has been the lack of use of and impact from the data reported by the states on their performance on the standards (Rubin, 1975). The lack of an analysis plan, the incapacity to carry out analysis, and the lack of vital feedback to the states from analyses of their performance have rendered the current standards a rather vacuous reporting exercise. Here we briefly outline the basic structure of the analysis, which will be an essential component of the standards system. The analysis of state agency performance on the standards will take place at two levels: basic assessment of agency performance and supportive evaluation of differences in agency performance.

The basic assessment of agency performance requires both a basis for the assessment—i.e., the establishment of performance level expectations—and consideration of the need for adjustments to state performance data to compensate for important differences in agency contexts, thus making performance data comparable across states. Following our recommended approaches to comparability adjustments and the establishment of performance levels are presentations of our approaches to the basic assessment of agency performance and to supportive evaluation for the standards.

Recommendation for Comparability Adjustments

The need for comparability adjustments that will account for basic differences in state performance on the standards and make valid comparisons among them has been supported by the research of many program analysts (Armstrong, 1973; Backer, 1977; Bellante, 1973; Conley, 1973; Noble, 1974; Scheinkman, 1975; Sermon, 1972; Serot, 1972; Westerheide, 1974; Worrall, 1975, 1978; Wright, 1972). In our review of these efforts, we examined the possible sources of need for adjustments (e.g., the environment, the disabled population, agency funding, and the number and difficulty of clients resulting from client selection), as well as the types of comparability adjustments available (e.g., disaggregated performance standards, self-adjusting performance standards, single index adjustments, and composite index adjustments) and those actually in use by various agencies (BPA, July 1978).

Our analysis has identified only one type of adjustment as potentially appropriate; thus, a client difficulty index, patterned after Sermon (1972), has been proposed to take into account differences across states in the type of clients served. The index identifies important client characteristics and, based on their relative difficulty in terms of achieving successful outcomes, adjusts state performance measures accordingly.

Use of this index will be tested during the demonstration period and a final decision made on its usefulness for understanding state performance.

Recommendation on the Approach to Performance Levels

Once a state's performance on a given standard is known, a method is needed to determine whether it meets, exceeds, or falls below some accepted level of performance. In general terms, the method recommended is based on a "progress norm" approach, which sets an expectation not for an arbitrary static level of performance but, rather, for an expected level of progress from year to year. Expected performance for the coming year is based on states' relative and historical performance. The recommended approach also provides that each state play a role in defining "reasonable expectations" with regard to expected performance. In other words, once RSA establishes its level of expected performance for individual states, states are given the option to respond to these achievement expectations and to present evidence supporting a case for modification where warranted. It is *not* the recommendation that RSA implement a performance expectation methodology simply to have states ultimately set their own goals. It is important that each state agency realize that RSA has an information system that provides RSA with baseline information on historical and relative performance, from which judgments concerning future achievement and agency expectations can be made. It is equally important, however, that states have the opportunity to inform RSA of unusual situations or of previously unaccounted for obstacles to achievement. This particular approach was selected because it minimizes many of the pitfalls inherent in static reporting systems (BPA, June and July 1978). It also sets a definite direction that states are to respond to and work toward, rather than simply "grading" states' performance after the fact.

The actual method for setting expectations for the coming year's performance is as follows:

- Using the mean of national performance on any given data element as the norm for establishing categories of performance, the states will be classified as having high, medium, or low performance. States scoring above the mean of a given data element will be classified as high performers; states scoring in the range between the mean and one standard deviation below the mean will be classified as medium performers; and states scoring below one standard deviation below the mean will be classified as low performers.
- The rate of improvement nationally will be calculated for the data element over the previous year.
- States classified in the high-performance category will be expected to increase 75 percent of the national rate of performance change on any data element.
- States falling in the medium-performance category will be expected to improve 125 percent of the national rate of performance change on any data element.
- States classified in the low-performance category will be expected to improve 150 percent of the national rate of performance change. (It should be pointed out that "150 percent of the national rate of performance change" sounds larger than it actually is. For example, for Standard #1, Data Element (ii), 150 percent of the national rate of performance change equals an increase of 35 clients per 100,000 population.)

What is the overall outcome and purpose of this performance level approach? As stated earlier, having information on individual agency and national performance levels will establish a sound baseline estimate of what can be expected. The negotiation process between RSA and individual states will further adjust this figure to what we have called reasonable expectations of performance. At that point, states will have a clear statement of what is expected of them with regard to all performance standards and, more specifically, the data elements upon which the standards are built.

Finally, such a system will provide a warning or flagging mechanism, specifying those areas of agency performance that fail to meet negotiated expectation levels. As a result of this system, further evaluation, such as supportive evaluation, can take place with a keener focus and direction. Actually, this performance system provides not only information on historical and relative performance but also the first steps in an analysis dealing more directly with specific agency shortcomings and the degree to which these shortcomings are problematic.

Basic Assessment of Agency Performance

Tables 3 through 5 provide the information needed by RSA and state agency management staff to obtain an overview of agency performance in comparison with other states, in comparison with previous periods, and in terms of established performance level expectations, respectively. The appropriate tabular presentations are illustrated with these dummy tables. Table 3 illustrates how agency data on a given data element can be presented to show unadjusted data, adjusted data, and ranking of each agency on both unadjusted and adjusted figures. Table 4 compares the performance of each state to previous periods as a preliminary to presentation of data on state performance compared to established performance level requirements. Table 5 compares each

TABLE 3
Dummy Table of State Agency Performance and Rank: Adjusted and Unadjusted, 1978

Standard #3, Data Element (i): $\frac{\text{\# 26 closures}}{\text{\# of 26 + 28 + 30 closures}}$

Agency	*Unadjusted Performance*	*Rank*	*Adjusted Performance*[a]	*Rank*
State A	41%	21	56%	24
State B	59%	14	79%	12
State C	82%	9	72%	15

[a] Adjustment here is purely hypothetical, exemplifying whatever adjustment formula is ultimately developed.

TABLE 4
Dummy Table of Change in State Agency Performance:
Fiscal Year 1977–78

Standard #2, Data Element (ii): Total Agency Expenditure per Rehabilitation

Agency	*Adjusted Performance 1977*	*Adjusted Performance 1978*	*Percent Change 1977–78*[a]	*Average Percent Change 1972–77*[a]
State A	$3,722	$3,657	+2	+8
State B	$2,802	$2,676	+5	–5
State C	$6,782	$10,136	–33	+15

[a]Positive (+) indicates *decreased* costs.

state agency's performance to performance levels set for the standards. This set of tables would be presented for each data element of each standard; where separate performance levels are set for severe and nonsevere client populations, a separate set of tables would be presented for these two subpopulations in each state agency.

Supportive Evaluation

The supportive evaluation framework should ensure that standards have a positive impact on program performance by providing an ability to pinpoint causes for problems in performance, identify factors leading to enhanced performance, and thus isolate appropriate policy recommendations and program actions that can be taken by state agencies, RSA, or Congress.

The steps involved in this type of program evaluation research are very familiar to the experienced analyst but perhaps not so to the

TABLE 5
Dummy Table of Expected Versus Actual Performance, 1978

Standard #4, Data Element (i): Percent 26 Closures with Wage at/above State Minimum Wage

	1977 Performance		*1978 Performance*		
Agency	*Actual*	*Classification*	*Expected*	*Actual*	*Ratio of Actual to Expected Performance*
State A	58.3%	medium	67.1%	68.3%	1.02
State B	79.1%	high	86.2%	84.0%	.97
State C	41.9%	low	46.9%	47.0%	1.00

program manager or policy maker. Although the steps in analysis can be outlined, the substance of the required analyses cannot be firmly laid out in advance, nor can the extensiveness of the activity of any given step be predetermined. These will depend on the particular issues raised by the nature of the standards' data each year. For example, if in a given year all states meet the performance expectations for competitive employment closures, and all states achieve performance in a very narrow range, then evaluation of state differences, the causes of the differences, and the ways to improve performance will be inappropriate. Thus, although it is tempting to wish to provide a "recipe" for the total supportive evaluation analysis, this cannot be done. The main ingredient will be the analysts themselves, who must be soundly grounded in both analytic techniques and program issues to be able to detail each year's analytic plan. Whereas, then, we cannot prescribe the analyses to be performed, we can present a picture of the basic steps in analysis.

Simple table analyses form the first step in identifying patterns that explain differences in agency performance on the standards. These analyses serve to initially test hypotheses of what might account for the differences between "successful" and "unsuccessful" agencies and thus what might improve the performance of the program. For example, if we wish to understand differences in agency costs per successful rehabilitant, or in costs per competitive employment closure, we might test, via supportive evaluation, whether different organizational structures would explain different costs—perhaps umbrella agencies have higher overall costs, or cannot meet performance level expectations on the standards, and thus should be discouraged through policy statements. A simple table of the following kind could form a preliminary test of this hypothesis:

	Umbrella Agencies	*Independent Agencies*
Agencies meeting standard	10%	76%
Agencies not meeting standard	90%	24%

In this example, an apparent relationship exists between structure and success in regard to the standard in question, indicating the desirability of further exploration using more sophisticated analysis. The bivariate analysis stage would consist of a series of such tables for each data element. The results of these preliminary analyses would be used to determine what factors receive further consideration for potential program changes or policy actions.

Although bivariate analyses are extremely instructive and are more readily understandable to many program managers than other, more sophisticated forms of analysis, they are incomplete if relied upon solely. There may well be two or more factors acting in concert to explain differences in agency performance, and the interactions among factors will be hidden unless multivariate forms of analysis are used. Thus, in our example of cost per competitive employment closure, it is very likely that not only administrative structure but also service mix, use of similar benefits, and several other factors play roles. Multivariate regression analysis is recommended as the appropriate technique for supportive evaluation on the standards. Such analyses will often be quite technical, but because they are in depth and account for the broadest possible range of factors that might be affecting performance on the standards, they can serve to sort out which elements of the VR service process (inputs, processes, outcomes) are related to high program performance and where interventions will be fruitful.

EVALUATION STANDARDS FOR DISCRETIONARY PROJECTS

Since the enactment of Public Law 93-112, most of the focus in the development of standards for VR has been on standards for the basic program of the federal/state system (BPA, January 1977). Some preliminary work on the development of project standards was done by The Urban Institute (1976), expanding on research in related areas (Glaser and Taylor, 1973). During BPA's contract to revise and refine the VR program evaluation standards, parallel efforts were undertaken to develop standards for projects in the discretionary programs funded under the Rehabilitation Act of 1973 as amended (*Federal Register,* 1975).

These programs represent a wide range of activity in training, service, research, and innovation and expansion, as indicated by the list of programs, including their authorizing legislation and regulation sections, shown in Table 6.

The problem of developing a standards system that serves such a varied collection of projects is challenging—one that requires a flexible approach and thoughtful application of the standards during implementation. Thus, BPA has recommended a generic approach to standards for the evaluation of these programs and projects, a system that

TABLE 6
Discretionary VR Projects

Activity	*Act*	*Regulations*
Program and project evaluation	Sec. 401	§1362.90
Rehabilitation research and demonstration	Sec. 202	§1362.60, 1362.61
Rehabilitation research and training centers	Sec. 202(b)(1)	§1362.62
Rehabilitation engineering centers	Sec. 202(b)(2)	§1362.63
End-stage renal disease	Sec. 202(b)(2)	§1362.65
International program for research demonstration, and training	Sec. 202(b)(5)	§1362.66
Rehabilitation training	Sec. 203(a) Sec. 400(a)(2)	§1362.70–1362.76
Helen Keller National Center for Deaf-Blind Youth and Adults	Sec. 305	§1362.80
Special projects and demonstrations: Improved services to the severely handicapped	Sec. 304(b)(1)	§1362.40
Special projects and demonstrations: Spinal cord injury	Sec. 202(b)(3) Sec. 304(b)(2)	§1362.64 §1362.40
Special projects and demonstrations: New approaches to service delivery; making recreational activities accessible to the handicapped	Sec. 304(b)(2)	§1362.41
Special projects and demonstrations: Grants for services for handicapped migratory agricultural workers or seasonal farmworkers	Sec. 304(c)	§1362.42
Projects with industry	Sec. 304(d)	§1362.43
Client assistance projects	Sec. 112	§1362.45
Rehabilitation facility assistance grants	Sec. 301(d) Sec. 301(b) Sec. 301(c) Sec. 302(c) Sec. 302(b) Sec. 304(e)	§1362.50 §1362.51 §1362.52 §1362.53 §1362.44 §1362.102
Innovation and expansion	Sec. 120, 121	§1361.15

is based on the fundamental principles of program evaluation. This system is based on the importance of goal setting and the measurement of the achievement of proposed project objectives. We emphasize that the determination of the appropriateness of objectives and measures should be made by RSA and the relevant project authorities. However, the overall evaluation framework, grounded in project participation and self-evaluation, should apply to all discretionary programs.

Issues in the Development of Project Standards

In considering the development of standards for the discretionary programs of RSA and their individual projects, a number of design issues must be taken into account.

Standardization of Projects

Do standards imply standardization of projects? These projects and programs of projects are areas where innovation and experimentation, outside the traditional VR delivery system, are encouraged. If the effect of standards is to standardize projects, then much of the anticipated value of such projects may be lost.

Risk

Many projects, particularly research projects, involve risk. Projects are undertaken to learn or to develop something, and sometimes the projects "fail," by criteria that favor the clear-cut, the concrete, the doable, or the usable. Research that succeeds only in generating previously unasked questions, or in increasing the investigator's own store of experience, may well be as important in the long run as that which produces a product. If standards are to stress achievement of objectives, there is concern that there would be a disincentive to fund "risky" projects. For research projects, where there is much to be learned even if final results are not as hypothesized, there is concern that the standards allow for risk and that they not concentrate on comparison of outcomes across dissimilar projects.

Suppression of Fringe Research

If one accepts Kuhn's distinction between "normal" and "revolutionary" research and his concept of paradigm overthrow (Kuhn, 1970), it probably follows that a more systematic and rigid method of assessing research would discriminate against unusual, untried, system-shaking research—even though this, in the end, is the vehicle by which science succeeds in solving puzzles to normal science and in explaining more of the world. Research-funding agencies are usually more concerned with cumulative, shared, demonstrable knowledge and refinement of existing techniques than with research into basic theory.

Loss of the Happy Accident

Fleming was not out to invent penicillin and Priestley was not looking for oxygen when those famous experiments were under way. Discoveries may not lie in the realm of intentions. For research to be "successful," the ability to reassess directions in midstream and the freedom to pursue hunches may be as important as the ability to follow through with a technically competent research design. A standardized research assessment instrument may discriminate in favor of the latter.

Who Should Do the Evaluation?

The Urban Institute (1976) strongly recommended that individuals outside the projects do the evaluation. RSA Regulations for Program and Project Evaluation state that "contracts for the study of program activities conducted under the Act may only be awarded to agencies or organizations which are not immediately involved in the administration of the program or project to be evaluated" (§1362.90). Outside evaluation affords objectivity and can complement evaluation done by the project itself. Yet, for more than 2,000 projects, some with very low funding levels, a complete outside evaluation, to be done every year, is probably not feasible. The standards should enable project evaluation —inside or outside—by providing evaluation information.

General Standards versus Project-Specific Standards

The final, obvious dilemma in project standards design is that of generic versus project-specific standards. To generate specific standards for the more than 2,000 current and ever-changing individual projects is to tailor standards for more than 2,000 evaluations, a vast and infeasible endeavor. On the other hand, to design one set of performance standards for all 17 or so program areas, with their many diverse projects, seems problematic. Any manager could easily explain nonperformance, since general standards would inevitably fail to take into account some unique but important design elements or special conditions. The design of project standards is thus a difficult task, a design problem very unlike the development of performance standards for the basic VR program.

A Three-Phase Project Standards System

The approach to project evaluation and project standards reflects evaluation concerns over time: at the beginning of a project, during implementation, and at project completion or application for refunding.

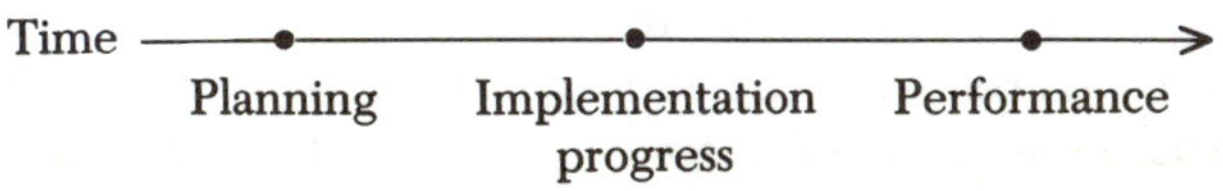

Table 7 presents the 20 proposed project standards as they correspond to these phases. These standards are all essential to carrying out evaluation studies. In his seminal program evaluation text, Suchman (1967) has described the evaluation process and illustrated it as follows:

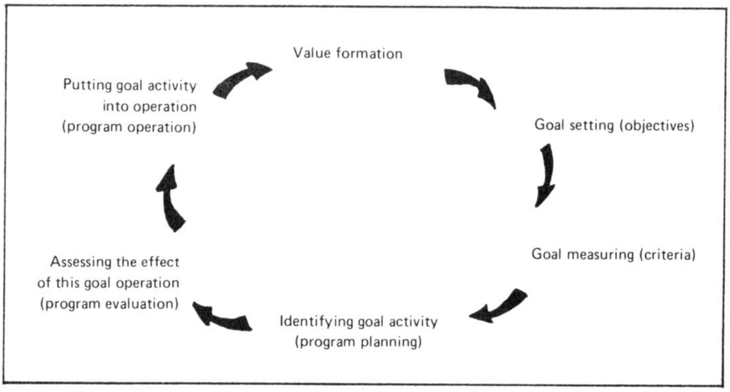

The stages of this process correspond to our three phases as follows: *project planning standards* require value formation (problem identification), goal setting (objectives), goal measuring (criteria), and identifying goal activity (description of the model and program planning); *project progress standards* reflect changes and impacts while putting goal activity into operation; and *outcome evaluation standards* allow for the assessment of the effect of the goal operation. Our standards system thus corresponds to the chronological and logical model illustrated by Suchman.

Standards for Project Planning

Standards for project planning (Standards 1 through 9) convey what a proposed project intends to accomplish, how it intends to do so, and for whom project benefits are intended. These standards are not concerned with setting priorities among proposed projects. Although standards for project design can aid RSA in choosing among projects, they do not supplant the need for RSA's judgment in choosing among project designs. These standards also do not intend that certain developmental steps be taken to force procedural homogeneity on projects or to specify the quality and level of desirable outcomes. Most projects are experimental and intentionally innovative in the methods and techniques used to attain goals. However, the project plan should ensure that certain conditions or standards are met.

The standards require projects to describe their designs and to suggest outcome measures of their success in attaining objectives that contribute to the attainment of overall legislative objectives and VR

TABLE 7
Proposed Project Standards

Standards for Project Planning

1. Projects should clearly state the rehabilitation problems and target groups that their objectives will address.
2. Projects should state their relevance to authorizing legislation and to VR program goals and policies.
3. Projects should state their goals and indicate the measurable objectives they propose to attain.
4. Projects should describe the limitations to the achievement of objectives and indicate how they might be overcome.
5. Projects should indicate their organizational plan.
6. Projects should describe the proposed training approach or service delivery system or research design; this should include the data collection or record-keeping plan, types and sources of data and records, and a plan for periodic evaluation.
7. Projects should present a detailed work plan to achieve project objectives.
8. Projects should present their budgets and indicate estimated costs for the achievement of objectives in the work plan.
9. Projects should present a plan for the utilization and dissemination of findings.

Standards for Project Progress Reporting

10. Projects should note changes in definition of objectives, in project design and organization, or in schedules for objective achievement.
11. Progress reports should show the project's progress with respect to significant milestones identified in the planning stage.
12. Projects should describe steps in data collection or record keeping for training activities and service delivery systems as well as the research methodologies in research projects; any changes in these or in the design should be documented.
13. Projects should conduct internal evaluations upon completion of major operational phases.

Standards for Outcome Evaluation

14. Projects should demonstrate whether and how the innovative and/or experimental methods and techniques underlying their design represent a potential improvement in the VR system.
15. Projects should describe their impacts on legislative objectives and VR program objectives and policies.
16. Projects should describe the attainment of internal project goals and objectives.
17. The evaluation should include a description of constraints on the achievement of objectives and the difficulties of implementation.
18. Projects should describe the final project design or model, including the project's final organization plan, in such detail that it can be replicated.
19. Projects should submit a statement of project costs.
20. Evaluations should include a report on the utilization and dissemination of findings.

program goals. Thus, standards for project planning will facilitate both self-evaluation and outside project evaluation, since both progress and performance may then be assessed in light of objectives defined in planning the project. As such, project planning standards serve the purpose of guiding project staff in designing projects to attain well-defined goals and objectives.

Standards for Project Progress Reporting

Formative evaluation of project progress in meeting interim goals is important for management and evaluation. Many projects will change in design somewhat as they are implemented. Innovative projects may develop new goals or change delivery models. Progress reporting (Standards 10 through 13) has two major functions in this scheme: to monitor achievement of the plan and to record changes and adjustments so that an accurate and realistic project assessment is possible later.

Standards for Outcome Evaluation

Evaluation standards (Standards 14 through 20) are measures of achievement gauged by some optimal level and quality of outcomes. This set of generic standards will focus on the qualitative and quantitative dimensions of outcomes, as identified by the projects themselves. The intent is to concentrate on the impact or results of a project rather than exclusively on processes or inputs. The performance standards suggested here center on the following: To what extent have projects attained their objectives? How appropriate were their methods and procedures? What relevance do project accomplishments have to VR program goals and the legislative objectives? What impacts on the VR system have resulted or are expected to result as a consequence of project activities?

Table 8 illustrates the relationship of the standards throughout the life of a project. Reading across the table allows comparison of related standards in the three phases of reporting.

Implementing the Project Standards System in RSA

The preceding section described the overall information requirements for projects that constitute the standards reporting system and provide the basis for systematic RSA evaluation of projects. However, information alone will not constitute an evaluation system. Corresponding to the project information, there should be a system of evaluation, in place in RSA, to review and evaluate the information collected and to carry out both project and program evaluations based on the standards.

TABLE 8
Relationships Within the Project Evaluation System

Standards for Project Planning	*Standards for Project Progress Reporting*	*Standards for Outcome Evaluation*
Establish these conditions during planning . . .	. . .in order to assess progress and . . .	. . .in order to evaluate results.
1. Rehabilitation problems and target groups addressed		14. Potential improvement in the VR system
2. Relevance to authorizing legislation and to VR goals and policies		15. Impact on legislative objectives and VR goals and policies
3. Goals and measurable objectives	10. Note changes in definition of objectives 11. Progress reports should indicate achievement of objectives	16. Show achievement of internal project goals and objectives
4. Limitations to achievement of goals		17. Description of constraints and difficulties of implementation
5. Organizational plan	10. Note changes in organization, in project design, in the model itself	18. Describe final project model
6. Project set-up and/or research design and data collection plan, including plan for periodic evaluation (of project progress)	12. Describe data collection, record keeping, and research methodology, documenting any design changes 13. Conduct internal evaluations upon completion of major phases	(data for evaluation)
7. Detailed work plan	10. Note changes in schedule for objective achievement	
8. Budget, estimated costs		19. Submit a statement of project costs
9. Plan for utilization and dissemination of findings		20. Report on utilization and dissemination of findings

Project Officers' Use of the Standards

The *project officer* is the individual RSA officer in charge of monitoring a particular effort. This officer will receive the evaluation information prepared by the projects. The project officer will evaluate the material by use of a checklist for assessing the degree to which projects have fulfilled the standards. The checklist will have a section for comments, allowing project officers to record extra information and to note changes in the project over time. This checklist will serve the dual functions of (1) providing RSA with a review process that ensures attention to all aspects of the projects' standards reports and (2) providing standardized, quantifiable information, which, when aggregated, can provide evaluation results within and across project areas.

RSA's and Program Authorities' Use of Project Standards

This section addresses the issues of evaluating the programs of projects and how the standards provide information for program authorities' use. There are four major ways in which the standards information may be useful for RSA and RSA's program authorities:

1. The standards themselves provide descriptive information that may be aggregated to show policy-relevant program information, such as the extent to which different client groups are emphasized in the grant programs.
2. The RSA project officer's review of the standards, recorded on the proposed scales, would provide an indication of the adequacy of project plans and of progress within and among project programs.
3. Comparison with planned and actual achievement, to be done by project officer review, would provide RSA with the impact assessment information desirable for planning and evaluation purposes and for reporting to Congress and to DHEW.
4. The standards would provide an essential data base for periodic evaluation of the success of projects and program authorities in achieving their overall missions in rehabilitation.

The first possible use of the standards would be to provide standardized descriptive information across the entire program. There are many data requests in the project standards that refer to policy issues and questions that currently are answered in part, but in an unsystematic way, by other related RSA reporting procedures. By calling for standardized information on a broad range of descriptive topics, the project standards would enable RSA to report more comprehensively on a number of different items for which information is regularly requested (RSA, 1976). As has been previously pointed out, most of the project standards are directly related to information needed for planning and evaluation and, therefore, will not burden projects with additional information requirements, except for the requirement to prepare the information on the standardized form.

The second use of the standards would be as indicators for use in monitoring projects' and programs' performance in implementing their plans and in meeting the needs for evaluation information. The scales used in the project officer checklist are in a form that can be directly keypunched; computer analysis of project and program performance on the standards can then be easily carried out. For instance, the following aggregate measures of program performance might be developed:

- For project planning—percent of projects in the program with measurable objectives or percent of projects in the program with top-rated approach
- For project progress—percent of projects on schedule, percent of projects within budget, or percent of projects with new goals

These are only suggestions of the types of aggregate indicators that RSA might choose to examine when analyzing the project standards checklist information.

The third way in which the standards information might be used by RSA and the program authorities is in assessing achievement, through the use of the information collected on the objectives achievement and cost data forms. As discussed before, the final step in completion of this form occurs at the end of the grant period, and information for all phases is retained on one form, for comparison purposes. Four major data items that might be useful in assessing project outcomes for each program are as follows:

- Percent of projects in program meeting their goals
- Degree of goal attainment for the projects, for programs of projects, and overall across grants
- Percent of projects judged to have fully justified costs
- Percent of projects judged to have made a reasonable contribution to goals of program

Interim project and cross-project reports on achievement could assist in deciding whether to continue, contract, or expand the funding of particular projects and programs.

The fourth way in which the standards would be useful is by providing necessary data for evaluating the overall project authority and program funding the various projects, as required by Congress and as needed for good management of the overall rehabilitation mission of RSA. Currently, such evaluations are usually done through one-time evaluation contracts with outside research organizations. The principal purpose of such program evaluations should be to determine whether the overall achievement of the program—as represented by the aggregate achievement of the individual system—justifies program costs and achieves the legislative and strategic mandate for the program. This issue is quite distinct from, though partially dependent upon, whether individual projects are achieving their goals. Questions must be raised about whether the right kind of goals are being articulated for potential grant applicants, whether the best projects for meeting the program's goals are being funded, whether projects once funded are receiving the necessary federal support to maximize effectiveness, and whether the achievements of the projects are being disseminated or utilized by the rest of the rehabilitation system. Frequently, so much energy must be invested in simply determining whether the projects funded met their individual goals that there is little opportunity for asking these broader questions about the overall program and project authority. The proposed standards provide the critical data base about projects for such program evaluation, so that the evaluation can go on to try to answer the broader questions about the overall worth of the program efforts.

Because the concept of project standards is such a new one within RSA, and because implementation of the standards in the various project areas will require review, within each program area, of the applicability and special measures needed, the aggregate measures proposed here are only illustrative. More definite aggregate measures should be defined as the program areas themselves begin to adapt the standards to their own program information and evaluation requirements. The implementation of the project standards and an evaluation system based on these standards will be a developmental process; application to an individual RSA program, or across programs, will require tailoring the standards requirements to the individual needs of programs. Although the standards information may vary considerably across programs, the overall framework and standardized review process for RSA will ensure both the installation of a program evaluation process in the projects and the gathering of information for comparing programs' progress and contribution to the achievement of the objectives that they have specified in reference to RSA's legislative mandate.

As indicated by the preceding discussion, the approach to developing standards for the state agencies' basic rehabilitation programs differs considerably from the approach to standards for RSA's discretionary projects. The former presents program evaluators with the ability to measure each state's performance against the philosophical goals held in common through legislative direction; the latter enables projects to self-assess their goal achievement and subsequently to permit project authorities to assess the project's contribution to furthering the goals of the program. Together, the program standards and project standards provide interested parties—state and federal administrators, program analysts, legislators, and consumers—with information central to present accountability and future improvement of the program.

REFERENCES

Armstrong, Philip A. *Weighted Case Closure Systems: An Analysis of Sermon's Method Applied to Counselor Activities.* Washington, D.C.: The Urban Institute, 1973.

Backer, Thomas E. "New Directions in Rehabilitation Outcome Measurement." In Pan, Elizabeth, ed. *Emerging Issues in Rehabilitation.* Washington, D.C.: Institute for Research Utilization, December 1977.

Bellante, Donald M. "A Multivariate Analysis of a Vocational Rehabilitation Program." *The Journal of Human Resources* VII (2):19, 1973.

Berkeley Planning Associates. *Critique of the Current Standards.* Report to U.S. Department of Health, Education and Welfare/Rehabilitation Services Administration (U.S. HEW/RSA), January 1977.

Berkeley Planning Associates. *Criteria for Standards Development.* Working Paper 1 to U.S. HEW/RSA, February 1977.

Berkeley Planning Associates. *Alternative Conceptual Approaches to Standards.* Working Paper 2 to U.S. HEW/RSA, March 1977.

Berkeley Planning Associates. *Specification of Candidate Areas for Standards, and the Conceptual Approach Underlying the Standards System.* Revised Working Paper 3 to U.S. HEW/RSA, August 1977.

Berkeley Planning Associates. *Recommendations for VR Program Evaluation Standards.* Report to U.S. HEW/RSA, September 1977.

Berkeley Planning Associates. *Data Items Associated with Standards: Availability of Data, Validity of Data, Pretest Results, and Study of Composite Measure.* Working Paper 4 to U.S. HEW/RSA, March 1978.

Berkeley Planning Associates. *Project Standards for Vocational Rehabilitation: A Generic Approach.* Report to U.S. HEW/RSA, March 1978.

Berkeley Planning Associates. *The VR Evaluation Standards: A System for Data Collection, Validation, Processing and Analysis.* Revised Working Paper 5 to U.S. HEW/-RSA, June 1978.

Berkeley Planning Associates. *The VR Evaluation Standards: A Guide for Implementation.* Working Paper 6 to U.S. HEW/RSA, July 1978.

Berkeley Planning Associates. *Proposed Demonstration Projects to Assist in Further Development of the VR Evaluation Standards.* Working Paper 7 to U.S. HEW/RSA, September 1978.

Berkeley Planning Associates. *The VR Evaluation Standards: Final Report.* Report to U.S. HEW/RSA, November 1978.

Berkeley Planning Associates. *Project Standards for RSA Discretionary Programs: Final Report.* Report to U.S. HEW/RSA, December 1978.

Conley, Ronald. "Weighted Case Closures." *Rehabilitation Record,* Washington, D.C., 1973.

Federal Register. "Implementation Provisions, Vocational Rehabilitation Programs." DHEW, OHD and SRS, Washington, D.C., November 1975.

Glaser, Edward M., and Taylor, Samuel H. "Factors Influencing the Success of Applied Research." *American Psychologist,* 28(2):140–146, 1973.

JWK International Corporation. *Vocational Rehabilitation Performance Standards Study (Part I: Analysis Details).* August 1975.

Kuhn, Thomas S. *The Structure of Scientific Revolution.* (2nd ed.). University of Chicago Press, Chicago, 1970.

McFarlane, Fred R., and Brenes, Lana C. *Case Review Schedule,* RCEP IX Rehabilitation Counselor Program, San Diego State University, September 1978.

Noble, John H., Jr. *Incentive Matching: An Option for Improving State Rehabilitation Performance.* Paper prepared for Workshop on Rehabilitation Program Evaluation and Outcome Assessment, Tufts University, Washington, D.C., 1974.

Rehabilitation Services Administration. *Forward Plan and FY 1978 Budget Request.* Memo to Assistant Secretary for Human Development from Commissioner of Rehabilitation Services, U.S. HEW/OHD/RSA, May 28, 1976.

Rubin, Sanford E. (ed.). *Studies in the Evaluation of the State Vocational Rehabilitation Agency Programs (The New Orleans Report).* University of Arkansas, Arkansas Rehabilitation Research and Training Center, Arkansas Rehabilitation Services, November 1975.

Scheinkman, Norman, et al. *The Unsuccessful State Vocational Rehabilitation Client: An Analysis.* Menomonie, Wis.: Research and Training Center, University of Wisconsin, 1975.

Sermon, Duane T. *The Difficulty Index—An Expanded Measure of Counselor Performance.* Research Monograph No. 1. St. Paul, Minn.: Division of Vocational Rehabilitation, State of Minnesota, March 1972.

Serot, David E. *Indices of Cost, Output, and Productivity for Use in Evaluating Rehabilitation Service Programs.* Berkeley, Calif.: Institute of Urban and Regional Development, 1972.

Suchman, Edward A. *Evaluative Research: Principles and Practice in Public Service and Social Action Programs.* New York: Russell Sage Foundation, 1967.

Urban Institute, The. *Final Report on Refinement and Expansion of the General Standards for the Evaluation of the Performance of the Vocational Rehabilitation Program.* Washington, D.C., November 1976.

Urban Institute, The. *Final Report on Standards for Vocational Rehabilitation Projects.* Washington, D.C., November 1976.

Walker and Associates, Inc. *Review of Current General Standards.* Minneapolis, Minn., September 1976.

Westerheide, William J., Lenhart, Lowell, and Miller, M. Clinton III. *Field Test of a Services Outcome Measurement Form: Case Difficulty.* Monograph No. 2. Oklahoma City, Okla.: Department of Institutions, Social and Rehabilitation Services, State of Oklahoma, 1974.

Worrall, John D. "Correlates of Success and Prediction of Outcomes." In Berkowitz, Monroe et al., eds. *An Evaluation of Policy Related Rehabilitation Research.* New York: Praeger, 1975.

Worrall, John D. "Weighted Case Closure and Counselor Performance." *Rehabilitation Counseling Bulletin,* 21:324–325, June 1978.

Wright, George N., Reagles, Kenneth W., and Thomas, Kenneth R. "Who Are the Tough Rehabilitation Cases?" *American Archives of Rehabilitation Therapy,* 21:2–5, March 1972.

8
New Directions in Rehabilitation Outcome Measurement*

THOMAS E. BACKER, PH.D.

This chapter is about measuring what happens to an individual who receives vocational rehabilitation services. It describes the main outcome measurement systems now used in the state–federal rehabilitation system and in private facilities; research and development regarding improved methods of outcome measurement; the problems associated with getting these new methods installed in rehabilitation service delivery organizations; and ways to overcome some of these difficulties.

The chapter is aimed at rehabilitation counselors, administrators in vocational rehabilitation agencies and decision makers in policy organizations. The impact that outcome measurement approaches have on counselors' *daily working lives and job satisfaction, as well as recommendations about what individual counselors can do* themselves *to promote improvement in the existing outcome measurement system, are covered.*

The treatment of underlying problems and resistance to change in outcome measurement would be of interest to decision makers *in policy organizations. The section dealing with current research and knowledge gaps should be useful in setting priorities for future research, as should the recommendations made regarding national-level efforts in outcome measurement.*

Rehabilitation is not a light switch, either "on" or "off." Anyone who has worked in the field knows this, yet that's exactly how rehabilitations have been recorded since the 1920s. In state vocational rehabilitation

*This chapter is based on a monograph of the same title that appeared as one of a series called "Emerging Issues in Rehabilitation," published by the Institute for Research Utilization (Washington, D.C., 1977) with funding support by the Rehabilitation Services Administration. The author wishes to thank the following individuals who contributed to the preparation of the earlier monograph: Dr. John Barry, Mr. Paul Bassett, Dr. Brian Bolton, Ms. Margaret Brown, Dr. Herbert Dorken, Dr. Dennis Dunn, Mr. Bertrum Griffis, Mr. Eric Lucero, Dr. John Muthard, Dr. Elizabeth Pan, Ms. Susan Stoddard, Dr. Fredric Schlamp, Dr. Carolyn Vash, Mr. Robert Walker, and Mr. Marvin Weisinger.

(VR) agencies and most private facilities, the criterion of individual client, counselor, and program success has been the famous—or infamous—Status 26 "closed-rehabilitated," which simply means that at the end of the rehabilitation process the client was gainfully employed. How much effort it took to make the placement and how successful the rehabilitation—kind of job obtained, how long it will last, client's degree of satisfaction with the job and with the rest of his or her life, etc.—are simply not reflected in this system of measurement. In this chapter, recent developments in outcome measurement approaches will be reviewed, and these methods will be appraised in the context of the impact outcome measures have in rehabilitation practice. Finally, some resources and guidelines for action in improving outcome measurement technology will be given.

There have, of course, been advantages to using the Status 26 criterion of rehabilitation success. This criterion places the focus on vocational goals, and until recently getting the handicapped back into gainful employment was considered the main, often the only, goal of all rehabilitation facilities.

The status of "closed-rehabilitated" is conceptually simple and can be measured concretely. For this reason, it has been possible to document the number of rehabilitations achieved by the state-federal VR system, and this has been a key political strength in obtaining federal funding. Congresspersons and taxpayers alike are impressed with "the numbers"—clear indications that large numbers of handicapped people have been returned to gainful employment and are contributing to the economy—a consequence of rehabilitation services they received at the taxpayers' expense. The concept of "quantity" of people who get a job is easy for political decision makers to grasp: "quality" moves into a domain that is harder to explain.

Finally, in comparison with other service delivery programs, a key strength of the rehabilitation outcome measurement approach is that a concrete criterion has in fact existed. In many other areas of the human services, it has not been possible to criticize specific outcome criteria because none existed, only vague statements of "goals." Even today, as other service delivery systems are beginning to come to grips with accountability issues, rehabilitations's outcome measurement system is arguably the best.

Times have changed since the 1920s. The way we now think about rehabilitation and its goals, as perceived by rehabilitation professionals, agency decision makers, legislators, and even the general public, is very different. The system for delivering rehabilitation services is itself quite different. Modern technology has overtaken rehabilitation just as it has every other human service delivery field, and the rising clamor for services, plus the mandate of rehabilitation to get into areas of service delivery it hasn't had to cover before, has greatly increased the scope and complexity of the system. Rehabilitation personnel are better trained and more able to cope with the delivery of a broad range of services to handicapped individuals. As a result, there has been a snowballing of problems in the traditional outcome measurement system, such as the following:[1]

- A tendency to emphasize numbers, not quality of rehabilitation. Under such conditions, the criterion can become an end in itself.
- A tendency to handle simple rehabilitation cases requiring little of the counselor's time in order to increase number of cases closed ("creaming").
- A tendency to place clients before they are ready to enter the job market, in order to achieve another Status 26 closure.
- In other situations, a tendency to keep clients in the rehabilitation process, delaying closure in order to meet next year's quota.
- Difficulty in providing an even flow of work in a local rehabilitation agency, because Status 26 record keeping is so imprecise.
- Difficulty for specialized counselors who handle more complex client problems than does the average counselor, and difficulty for generalists, especially in rural settings, who handle everyone.
- An inability to give credit to counselors for work on cases closed, not rehabilitated, but where there has been meaningful improvement in the client's life or future potential for vocational adjustment.
- A tendency, therefore, for counselors to be less motivated to go after challenging cases or ones where it is understood from the start that complete rehabilitation cannot occur.
- Inhibition of feedback to counselors, since the main record system is not oriented toward estimation of the quality of either services or outcomes.
- De-emphasis on nonemployment-related factors, such as activities of daily living, although these variables are known to be important to ultimate vocational rehabilitation.
- A tendency for counselors to guard information about job openings, since a colleague may make closures that a "helpful friend" might otherwise have made.

- Under pressure for numbers, counselors may suggest inappropriate jobs for clients.
- Impedance of program evaluation efforts or other means of stimulating program improvement, since it is not possible to get accurate data about current levels of performance.

The litany of problems is familiar and requires no further discussion. What this recitation really suggests is that the system of outcome measurement currently employed in American rehabilitation service delivery settings is being used for purposes for which it was never intended, and therefore it is not working well. Who could expect it to? The service delivery system, and the people within it, both clients and counselors, have changed, but the outcome measurement technology has not. Case difficulty and service quality constitute categories of fugitive data in rehabilitation, but it is not fair to criticize the system for this shortcoming: It was never designed to provide that kind of information.

Many of these same difficulties apply not just to individual counselors but to rehabilitation facilities which provide services to state VR agencies.

A more responsive system for outcome measurement must take account of a number of conditions prevailing in vocational rehabilitation at the present time:

- A focus on services to the severely disabled, as mandated by the Rehabilitation Act of 1973.
- A heavy emphasis on accountability—evaluation of services was also mandated by the 1973 Rehabilitation Act—with the resultant need for routine gathering of relevant infomation about the nature and quality of services provided.
- An increasing emphasis on the psychosocial aspects of rehabilitation and an intensified awareness of the importance to all individuals of the quality of working life and life satisfaction in general.
- Rising expectations for services, in conjunction with a proliferation of services available.
- Better-trained, more skill-diversified rehabilitation personnel.
- The problem of disincentives—factors which discourage disabled persons from participating in vocational rehabilitation—especially in states where it is more attractive financially for a disabled person to stay on state disability.

For the past few years, a good deal of research and local experimentation has aimed at improving the antiquated outcome measurement system we now have. Many books and articles have appeared on this subject, particularly in conjunction with the increasing emphasis on program evaluation. In consequence, there is by now considerable new knowledge available about how to improve outcome measurements in rehabilitation. In this chapter, some of the most important components of that body of knowledge will be presented.

DEFINING THE TERRITORY

The major objectives of this chapter are:

- To understand the barriers and resistances to change in vocational rehabilitation outcome measurement systems.
- To present and describe alternatives for improvement in this system, including available technology for increasing the quality of outcome measurement, and including research now underway to provide better alternatives in the future.
- To present resources for obtaining further information about this potentially usable technology.
- To present both policy and grass roots level recommendations about how to initiate change in outcome measurement at different levels in rehabilitation organizations.

Therefore, this chapter can be seen both as a review of the current state of the art and as an effort to promote knowledge utilization in the outcome measurement field.

Audiences

The three main target audiences for this discussion are vocational rehabilitation counselors, administrators in local and state rehabilitation agencies and private facilities, and decision makers in policy bodies such as the Rehabilitation Services Administration (RSA), Council of State Administrators of Vocational Rehabilitation (CSAVR), Council on Accreditation of Rehabilitation Facilities (CARF), National Accreditation Council (NAC) for the blind, and national rehabilitation and professional associations, such as the American Rehabilitation Association (ARA) and the National Rehabilitation Association (NRA).

We will not emphasize the information needs and policy options of consumers of improved services—disabled people themselves—or researchers, whose principal aim is to generate new knowledge. These two audiences are surely important, and researchers may find parts of this volume of considerable help in their own work, but we have chosen to concentrate on developing materials useful to the first three groups mentioned.

Focus of the Chapter

We will focus on outcome measurement at the individual level. That is, we will look only at those measurement techniques suitable for determining what happens to one individual in his or her movement through the rehabilitation system. Measures of groups and program effectiveness will be left to discussions in the field of program evaluation.

Overview of the Chapter

The next two sections discuss how outcome measurement is conceptualized and used by each of the three main audiences mentioned. The following section describes current parameters of outcome measurement in rehabilitation, including relevant federal standards. It also analyzes some of the reasons why changing the rehabilitation outcome measurement system has been so difficult.

Following this is a "catalog" of recently developed measures of rehabilitation outcomes that may have potential for improving the overall systems. The focus is on systems for weighted closure.

Next are discussed research studies now underway to improve outcome measurement systems, gaps in the body of knowledge that still need to be closed, and the impact of outcome measurement on counselors, administrators, and policy makers.

The next section presents information resources for getting up-to-date knowledge on new and improved methods of outcome measurement plus prescriptive guidelines for what counselors, administrators, and policy makers can do, in their own bailiwicks, to promote change.

The final section makes a few predictions about what the future may bring, including how changes in outcome measurement may fit into other developing trends in rehabilitation.

OUTCOME MEASUREMENT: AN OVERVIEW

Outcome measurement has to do with systematic means for discovering how disabled clients change as the result of their participation in vocational rehabilitation. While the traditional parameter of change is whether or not the client gets a job, there is general agreement today among practitioners, as substantiated in the literature, that outcome measurement has to do more generally with measuring changes in clients' economic, physical, and psychosocial functioning, as well as in their vocational functioning and potential.

The First Institute on Rehabilitation Issues (Bassett, 1974, pp. 5–6) established definitions for four main areas of client change:

- *Vocational Functioning and Potential*—The degree to which a client demonstrates capacity to appraise realistically his/her own vocational potential and to exhibit the physical and emotional endurance necessary to achieve vocational objectives.
- *Economic Independence*—The degree to which the client can function independently in society without reliance on public support for income and social services.
- *Physical Functioning*—The degree to which a client demonstrates the capacity for reduction of symptoms, improved physical tolerance, development of practical compensatory mechanism, and increased endurance.
- *Psychosocial Functioning*—The degree to which a client demonstrates social and psychological adaptability which serve to enhance feelings of security, adequacy, functioning capability, emotional stability, and social interaction.

There is now increasing interest in the study of multiple outcomes, covering some or all of the above areas of client change. This reflects a fundamental alteration in the philosophy. The change of legal mandate for rehabilitation services is an important determiner of the kinds of rehabilitation outcome measurement devices that are of interest. Clearly, if all four areas of change defined above are regarded as relevant to appraising rehabilitation services, traditional Status 26 outcome measurement is no longer effective—for it covers only one aspect of the total field.

Another dawning realization, although not one discussed much in the literature up to this point, is that outcome measurement systems serve different purposes for different individuals or groups within the rehabilitation service cycle. These differences necessitate either a flexible system which can encompass the needs of all those who must use the information or else parallel or tandem systems that separately produce the data needed for decision making and action.

For counselors, the main uses of outcome measurement data are to give information for direct use with given clients (e.g., corrective feedback to modify a treatment plan in midcourse); for improvement of services rendered to clients similar to the individual on whom feedback was provided; for general professional development for performance appraisal, either by oneself as an independent professional or by one's immediate supervisor.

Administrators and policy makers, on the other hand, are more likely to be concerned with setting policy in regard to how outcomes are to be measured rather than with using individual case outcome data themselves. They will be interested in outcome measurement strategies, as applied in the aggregate, for use in program evaluation. Rehabilitation supervisors would be most likely to use individual case data in training and performance evaluation.

The current outcome measurement system began with a program reporting need. State VR agencies were required to indicate how federal funds were spent to rehabilitate clients. In the days when a more limited range of vocational rehabilitation services was provided, and where only a limited range of clients was served (i.e., those with some clearly specified physical handicaps, but also with clear potential for getting a job if provided with appropriate training or assistive devices), the Status 26-style outcome measurement system may have been reasonably appropriate. In today's rehabilitation system, it obviously is not.

For administrators and policy makers, a system which focuses only on employment status at the end of the rehabilitation process provides performance data too crude for use in making program improvements or for justifying funding or continuation of a particular service delivery effort. The information is equally limited for dealing with the needs of individual counselors, who may not be able to benefit from performance feedback if all they know is whether a client has held down any job for a given period of time.

Sadly, though, this is the system that basically still exists in state vocational rehabilitation agencies and in most private facilities. Despite all the research and innovative practice undertaken in recent years, and an advancing state of knowledge about outcome measurement systems, what is known is much greater than what has been applied. There are new programs in some states (e.g., California, Florida, Oklahoma) in which revised outcome measurement systems have been experimented with, but even in these cases there is still a basic need to comply with the demands of the federal-state reporting system. This is most unfortunate, for the means by which outcome measures are taken have a great deal of impact on counselor, client, and the entire rehabilitation system *because they help to define the reality of rehabilitation services.* Some specific types of impact are as follows:

- Outcome of service is a fundamental part of any management information system; thus, the means used to gather such data have an impact on the entire VR organization.
- There is an impact on clients psychologically and behaviorally.
- Whatever outcome measures are taken will be used in performance review of employees, leading to consequences in terms of career advancement, motivation, and other factors.
- With the increasing pressure for program evaluation and accountability, more rehabilitation agencies are installing formal program evaluation systems, which will be significantly affected by whatever outcome measurement methods are used.
- There is an impact on the training of new counselors, since some of the philosophy and practice of outcome measurement will filter down to university training programs.

The Institute on Rehabilitation Issues (Bassett, 1974) expands on this list of basic impacts in a compilation of "reasons for outcome measurement." A list of these reasons is as follows:

- Assess counselor performance
- Improve caseload management
- Program development to a special target group
- Evaluate substate service performance in areas
- Provide budget justification
- Reduce dissatisfaction
- Minimize conflict in client assessment of services
- Collect data showing state agency performance
- Make aggregate profiles of special target groups
- Show utility of demonstration projects, pilot projects, and research utilization
- Measure performance over time/trend series
- Measure impact of alternative case service delivery and administrative approaches
- Measure recovery or reduction of cost of social security and trust funds and SSI programs

- Respond to rehabilitation constituency
- Provide basis for audit and program administration reviews used in evaluating legislative proposals and amendments
- Make cross-program and cross-agency projections and comparisons
- Devise long-range projections of economic and social indicators
- Devise cost-benefit ratios used in lobbying efforts at all levels, used in specific client appeals on service outcome

It is in this context of very broad potential impact throughout a VR organization that the alternative systems for outcome measurement presented in this review must be evaluated.

CURRENT PRACTICE

The Status 26 closure as a basic measure of vocational rehabilitation outcome is a well-entrenched part of the VR establishment. It exists within a welter of reporting requirements that include other statuses as well for coding purposes: carrying clients through the rehabilitation process, into referral to another agency, to closed-not-rehabilitated, and so on.

Considering the number of years this system has been in operation, it has generated remarkably few political and funding difficulties. As remarked in Bassett (1974, p. 1), "Many vocational rehabilitation agencies have never been challenged in legislative or budget processes to elaborate upon the 26 closure." The present system is one legislators are used to. Case closures can be easily translated into dollar values. More abstract measures of "quality of life" cannot, at least at the present time.

In the present system, individual counselors keep records of their clients' progress through the rehabilitation process. This information is aggregated in the form of caseload reports; unit reports, prepared by a local rehabilitation agency office, for example; district office reports; and ultimately state agency reports. States then interact with RSA regional and federal offices in order to provide required information about case outcomes.

RSA has issued federal standards in the form of a June 1971 *Vocational Rehabilitation Manual,* which dictates procedures by which case statuses are generated. Form RSA-300 accumulates basic information about each case closure and is used in measuring the effectiveness of the rehabilitation program as a whole and by target group populations; in describing client characteristics and program-related experiences to Congress, state legislatures, and various public and private agencies and organizations interested in the vocational rehabilitation of the handicapped; and in providing specific answers to questions frequently raised for budgetary, legislative, administrative, and informational purposes. The form provides a way to record what happens to each client from first contact to final closure. The R-300 form is thus a basic component of the overall VR management information system, which guides funding and other types of interaction between the RSA and the state VR agencies.

At present, the 26 closure encompasses the following: closed in competitive employment, full time, economically independent; closed in competitive employment, less than full time, sheltered employment; homebound employment; unpaid family worker; and homemaker. This range of subclasses within Status 26 creates some problems, since there is a substantial difference between full-time and part-time work, worker and homemaker, and so on.

Reporting requirements have changed somewhat since passage of the 1973 Rehabilitation Act. Evaluation of the effectiveness of services is now mandated. Needs of the severely handicapped are emphasized, and measurement systems are called for that will be sensitive to outcomes in these cases. Individualized rehabilitation plans must be written for each client to specify goals and how these will be achieved. Also, the VR agency's role in providing services to individuals dependent on public support was continued, and is to be evaluated in terms of reduction of dependency.

To further detail what VR agencies are now required to do in the way of program evaluation, Congress directed the Secretary of HEW to publish a set of standards providing for a multicriteria approach to evaluating VR services. These nine standards, which have been frequently revised since their initial issuance by RSA are:

1. To insure that the rehabilitation program is serving the eligible disabled population and to insure that these services are provided in an equitable manner;

2. To insure that rehabilitated clients are placed in gainful employment suitable to their capabilities;

3. To insure that undue delays are avoided in providing clients with VR services;

4. To insure that available resources are utilized to achieve maximum operational efficiency;

5. To insure that manageable-sized caseloads are maintained;
6. To insure that clients closed-rehabilitated retain the benefits obtained from the rehabilitation process;
7. To insure that the need for post-employment services is satisfied;
8. To insure that agencies consistently identify reasons why clients are not successfully rehabilitated;
9. To insure that the client is satisfied with the vocational rehabilitation services as developed with the counselor.

Federal reporting is supposed to be done in the context of these standards, although there have been difficulties because the standards have changed so frequently. There is some evidence that states continue to report in the old R-300 terms rather than converting to the new system. State VR agencies are also required to submit a report, the "A-1 report," each year detailing their future plans for service delivery to various types of clients. This reporting requirement still needs to be coordinated with the nine standards.

Making such broad-gauged standards workable is no easy job. In addition to its own efforts and CSAVR's, the RSA has also awarded contracts—first to the Urban Institute and now to Berkeley Planning Associates (Berkeley, California)—to undertake further refinements in the standards. Berkeley Planning Associates issued a working paper (1977) which reviews literature relevant to the nine standards and gives some idea of future directions in their evolution.

For private facilities, a similar set of evaluation standards has been devised by the Commission on Accreditation of Rehabilitation Facilities (CARF), as presented in their *Standards Manual for Rehabilitation Facilities.*[2] The principal components of these standards are as follows:

1. The evaluation system shall provide for a statement of purposes, program goals and objectives.
2. There shall be a relationship between the statement of purposes, program goals and objectives, who is served, and services provided.
3. Statements of goals and objectives must be achievable, measurable, and the attainment of all objectives should enable the program goals to be achieved.
4. The facility's evaluation system shall provide for measures of effectiveness.

5. The facility's evaluation system shall provide for measure of efficiency.
6. There shall be a system to describe and monitor who is being served by the facility.
7. The evaluation system result shall be communicated to appropriate parties to be utilized in facility decisionmaking.
8. Appropriate information on results shall be made available in an understandable fashion to the governing body and staff of the facility and to the public, including purchasers, contributors, and consumers.
9. The facility shall have a mechanism to provide for continuous review of the adequacy of its evaluation system.

The common threads in these two sets of standards are their advocacy of developing *means for specifying criteria* and *means for gaining knowledge through the evaluation process that can be used not only in judging program worth but also in making program improvements.*

One need look no further than these two sets of standards for program evaluation in rehabilitation organizations to understand that current case closure methods are wholly inadequate for meeting informational needs. This realization helped spur the formation of groups such as the First Institute on Rehabilitation Issues, which focused on measurement of outcomes, and the funding of research projects designed to facilitate the development of better outcome measurement systems. The latter will be described below. Sadly, there have been few fundamental improvements as yet.

Why is there such resistance to change? The motivation for rehabilitation agencies—and, indeed, for RSA at the federal level—to maintain the status quo is particularly powerful because of the extraordinary political success that has been enjoyed by rehabilitation over the years. As Moriarty (1977) observes, rehabilitation services have been supported broadly across the spectrum of political ideology from ultraliberal to arch-conservative. Richard Nixon, the first president ever to veto VR legislation, was careful to point out that he did so over technical matters, not substantive ones. When Congress overrode the veto, it did so by one of the largest majorities in its history. With this kind of track record, based in part on the easy measurability of the Status 26 case closure, small wonder that there is a vested interest in protecting the current system.

However, relative advantage alone is not the sole motivation. It is becoming increasingly evident that whatever the positive payoffs from this system, there are also a number of significant negatives. Therefore, we must seek additional mechanisms of explanation for the current state of affairs in outcome measurement.

One obvious factor is *habit.* In the literature on organizational change, it is noted that people have natural resistance to changes in accustomed methods of operation. This reflects more than just the desire to keep on doing something that has been reasonably successful, but also a human need to gain security and predictability in everyday affairs and to avoid the stress that inevitably comes with change.

The habit vectors would be particularly strong, since there have been so many other changes in the system recently. Rehabilitation services at the federal level have been organized, reorganized, and then reorganized again. State VR agencies have been compelled to undertake new activities—with the inevitable unsettling effects on staff at all levels. An increasing amount of time is taken up with routine record keeping and evaluative data gathering, and this in itself induces resistance to new outcome measurement systems which might further burden staff already overworked with paperwork.

This effect has been noted in the literature on program evaluation as well. People tend to be wary of evaluation systems partly because they fear that their installation will result in an increase in workload without any measurable advantage accruing to individual staff. This fear has a basis in reality. Outcome measurement or evaluation systems are often designed without proper concern for those who will be directly affected by their implementation.

Moreover, when it was noted that the outcome measurement system in VR is the most fully developed in all the social services, another source of resistance to change was identified. The more entrenched a system is, the more difficult it is to change.

There is also a certain amount of *suspiciousness* about new techniques, particularly those based on research. The gap between researchers and practitioners in the human services is well known and has often been documented in the rehabilitation field. Anything that grows out of a research study is viewed with some tentativeness as far as its potential applicability in the real world is concerned. Again, such reservations are often justified. A system which may work well in a controlled research study may be impractical or even counterproductive to use out on the firing line of service delivery agencies.

A final and very important aspect of resistance to change in the outcome measurement system is a *fear* of accountability. One of the psychological advantages of Status 26 is that it permits a lot of deliberate ambiguity. There are aspects of the performance of counselors, groups of counselors, programs, and entire state agencies which can never be tracked down precisely because they are obscured in the way outcomes are measured.

If a precise system of outcome measurement is introduced, the result would be a clear pinpointing of who is serving what kinds of clients, at what cost, and with what ultimate outcomes in terms of rehabilitation, not only to gainful employment but also to jobs with career potential, good salaries, and related impacts on physical and psychosocial functioning.

The sheer cost of making a nationwide change in the system for reporting outcomes of rehabilitation should not be disregarded. Even minor alterations can be expensive. The kind of overall revision contemplated in this review would entail expenditures of millions of dollars at the federal, state, and local levels. In an era when fewer dollars are available for human services, this can hardly be an appealing prospect —particularly if it occurs in the context of suspicion about whether or not the results will be worth it.

Human service professionals tend to have a strong internal conviction that the services they are providing are worthwhile, because they are dedicated to helping people and are professionally trained to do that job. The realization that all systems and the individuals within them can be improved, which is so fundamental to program evaluation, is not easily assimilated into this belief system. The result is that many professionals resist evaluation or outcome measurement because they think it is unnecessary. They know they are doing a good job and don't need a "fancy system of numbers and data forms" to prove it.

NEW OUTCOME MEASURES: A CATALOG

There have been many attempts to develop new outcome measures for rehabilitation services over the past few years. This chapter will not attempt a comprehensive review of them. For that purpose, the reader is referred to Chapter 4 of Bennett and Weisinger's *Program Evaluation: A Resource Handbook for Vocational Rehabilitation* (1974). In this volume, the authors culled 146 outcome measures from some 75 studies in the VR field. However, many of these measures are relevant only to programs, not to individual clients, and will not be discussed here. Much of the discussion that follows (including many of the evaluative comments) has been taken from Bennett and Weisinger's compendium, supplemented by other sources (including another review by Weisinger [1975]). The reader should note that there are a number of studies in progress, some of which may be published after the time of this writing. Literature reviews are always out of date by the time they are published, so the listing that follows should be thought of primarily as a mechanism of access, not an exhaustive compendium.

To set the stage for this discussion, following is a list of client variables typically assessed through outcome measures administered during or following rehabilitation services:

- Client's income (annual, monthly, or by household)
- Hours worked per week
- Job retention
- Job benefits
- Advancement potential of job
- Type of job (in relation to the client's training, past experience, and aspirations)
- Client's welfare status
- Amount of average welfare grant
- Change in client's skills as the result of rehabilitation
- Employer satisfaction with the client's work performance
- Employee satisfaction with job received
- Client's satisfaction with the rehabilitation process
- Psychological characteristics related to successful vocational and life adjustment
- Improvement in physical functioning
- Improvement in psychosocial functioning in relation to self, family and community
- Ability to maintain self independently
- Ability to perform the activities of daily living
- Upward mobility rating
- Attendance and punctuality at work
- Work quality

Most of the measures that follow are concerned with changes in these variables. The operational word is *change;* rehabilitation benefits have to do with changes in clients' lives as a result of the VR process.

It should be noted that these indicators vary widely in the degree of subjective measurement they require (e.g., from amount of income earned—highly objective—to employer's satisfaction with client work performance—highly subjective). In the literature on how people change as a result of psychotherapy, it has been found that subjective measures do *not* relate highly to more objective behavioral measures of outcome. What clients or counselors/therapists *say* and how clients *behave* may not be as highly related as common sense might suggest. This finding should be taken into account when appraising the potential of any given rehabilitation outcome measure. One obvious solution to this problem is *mutiple measurement*—reliance on not one but a number of variables for assessing client change. Among the recently developed outcome measures are the following:

- *Job Satisfaction and Family Functioning*—Not widely used in rehabilitation, this measure has been misused in evaluating program effectiveness. Lack of job satisfaction can lead to job termination but may or may not be related to the quality of VR services provided. The family function variable on this test is difficult to measure. (Schneiderman, 1972)
- *Rehabilitation Service Satisfaction Questionnaire*—A device for assessing clients' views of service effectiveness, which was still in the experimental stages in 1973. (Muthard and Miller, 1968; Rubin, 1973)
- *Scale of Rehabilitation Gain*—This scale attempts to assess effectiveness of VR services by assimilating diverse factors of physical and emotional health, work adjustment, and life activities. (Reagles, Wright, and Butler, 1970)
- *Rehabilitation Services Satisfaction Survey*—This scale measures the client's opinion of how good the VR program was. The results tend to measure how well the client liked the counselor. (Tenth Institute on Rehabilitation Services, 1972)
- *Measure of Employment Satisfaction*—An accepted, established scale measuring client satisfaction with employment. (Weiss, 1967)
- *Measure of Employment Satisfactoriness*—An accepted, established scale measuring the employer's satisfaction with the client. (Gibson et al., 1970)
- *Job-Relatedness to Vocational Training*—A scale measuring relevancy of training to employment. (Wheeler, 1971)
- *Structured Case Review*—This measure establishes standards for good counselor performance and then permits examination of a counselor's or program's case records to determine how well the standards have been met. (Muthard and Miller, 1966)

• *Pre- and Post-Treatment Structured Interview*—The value of this experimental approach to measuring VR outcomes is entirely dependent on how well the interview is planned and conducted. (Rubin, 1973)

• *Oklahoma RRRI Consumer Measurement Scale*—This scale attempts to measure client satisfaction on nine dimensions: speed of service, medical services, training services, employment satisfaction, participation and planning, counselor effort in placement, agency policies, physical facilities, and personal treatment. It does not provide for premeasuring to allow evaluation of client change. Most items are highly subjective. (Cited in Bassett, 1974)

• *West Virginia Follow-up Kit*—This how-to-do-it kit contains instructions for sampling, data collection, table construction, data analysis, and reporting on rehabilitation variables. A questionnaire for use with employers is included. It provides information regarding status of the client after closure on employment status, satisfaction with VR services and job, interpersonal relations on the job, personal work characteristics, characteristics of family, and contribution made by the VR agency to present vocational status. (Cited in Bassett, 1974)

• *Rhode Island Attitude Survey*—This instrument assesses client attitude change from initial interview to closure. A total of 96 subjective items reflect client attitudes toward disability and rehabilitation services. (Cited in Bassett, 1974)

• *New Jersey Client Satisfaction Scale*—This questionnaire is composed of thirteen items to measure client satisfaction with vocational rehabilitation, public assistance status, job history, and present occupational status. There is no premeasure to allow for assessment of client change. (Cited in Bassett, 1974)

• *Counselor Productivity Index*—The work of Serot (1972) to develop a counselor benefit index and a counselor cost index can be adapted to produce an index of overall counselor productivity. Rubin and Reagles (1976) suggest that such a device may be useful for counselor performance appraisal.

Weighted Closure Approaches

The most promising area for exploration in new methods of outcome measurement is that of the *weighted closure.*[3] This approach is designed to reflect the reality that some clients are harder to assess, harder to train, and harder to place than others. Many of these measures also acknowledge that rehabilitation gain may be made on more than the dimension of placement; thus, points can be awarded for gains the client may make in psychosocial functioning and other areas.

The weighted closure approach to outcome measurement has advantages for both counselors and program administrators. One key merit for agency decision makers is that the method permits some influence over counselor motivation to serve certain kinds of clients, simply by varying the weighting factors. As the IRI study group (Bassett, 1974) concludes: "The weighted closure approach is considered by many to be the best available answer to the problem of service criteria, adequacy of counselor performance and of cost-benefit analysis" (p. 32).

However, a number of important caveats are also offered in the Bassett report. First, there have been numerous difficulties in experimental applications of weighted closure systems thus far. Many have fallen short of the desired improvements in outcome measurement predicted by their inventors, often resulting in findings no more precise or helpful than what was available previously through use of the old-fashioned Status 26 system. Second, most of the systems are quite complex to use and do not meet the criteria of efficiency and minimum disturbance of the service delivery system.

There are several fundamental concepts inherent in most of the weighted closure systems to be described below:

- The idea of *rehabilitation gain*—that success is not a dichotomous variable (e.g., placed on a job versus not placed) but a continuous variable along which client improvement falls depending on the *degree* of success.

- The notion that improvement takes place not only in vocational terms but also in terms of economic independence, physical functioning, and psychosocial functioning.

- The notion that fair and effective measurement of outcome requires *weighting* the difficulty of cases against some norm so that counselors are not penalized for taking the time required to deal with the most difficult-to-rehabilitate clients.

Following are some weighted closure systems now being developed or in experimental use.

• *Rehabilitation Difficulty Score*—This screening device singles out difficult cases and uses available data related to outcome with disadvantaged clients. Its utility as a closure device has yet to be demonstrated. Kunce and Miller (1972) completed a study with a simplified version using R-300 data which had a common sense relationship to employment. (Kunce et al., 1969)

• *Weighted Closures*—The purpose of this approach is to develop relative weights for significant client variables. Validity and reliability are not well established because data from clients' records have often been missing for the cases processed. (Berkowitz, 1972)

• *Florida Difficulty Index*—This index has four basic elements: amount of time client was in rehabilitation process (Statuses 10–26); average case service cost; average number of case services provided; and Sermon's Composite Case Difficulty Index is compared against annual averages and composite difficulty score computed. This scale has been found to agree closely with counselor estimates of case difficulty. (Florida Division of Vocational Rehabilitation, 1973)

• *Oklahoma System Service Outcome Measurement Form*—In a three-year study designed to measure case difficulty in client change, five areas of client functioning are being considered: physical, educational, economic, vocational, and psychosocial. Case difficulty is computed by relating eight demographic variables to successful closure. (Cited in Bassett, 1974)

• *Human Service Systems Scale*—Developed in Wisconsin, this device attempts to measure the degree of change experienced by clients served through various human service agencies in five areas described by Maslow in his hierarchy of needs: physiological, safety and security, love and belongingness, self-esteem, and self-actualization. The instrument is machine scorable. (Reagles and Butler, 1976)

• *Virginia Rehabilitation Gain Schedule*—This instrument purports to measure work status, economic dependency, and psychological well-being with eighteen objective, multiple-choice questions. Orientation is to the disadvantaged/disabled client, and the scale may have limited application to the severely disabled and/or middle-class client. (Cited in Bassett, 1974)

• *Goal Attainment Scaling*—Developed by the Program Evaluation Resource Center in Minneapolis, this technique is applicable to a wide variety of human service activities. It identifies behaviorally defined goals and outcomes for clients on a simple scale ranging from most unfavorable outcome to best-anticipated outcome. Each area is identified by the counselor, often with input from the client, and weighted as to importance. Simple mathematical procedures are provided for weighting and for computing total outcome score.

Goodyear and Bitter (1974) report a study of the use of GAS at a rehabilitation hospital in Colorado. They concluded that GAS was a useful technique for measuring client change as a result of rehabilitation counseling services conducted in a rehabilitation setting. The Research Utilization Laboratory at the Jewish Vocational Service in

Chicago has produced a manual (1976) for applying GAS in rehabilitation settings. It includes step-by-step training in how GAS works and concrete examples of how the approach can be applied with VR clients. Further information on GAS in VR settings (e.g., how it relates to the CARF standards) is given in the January 1977 issue of RUL's Lab Notes.

The RUL manual includes the rationale used to select GAS as the preferred approach for responding to certain outcome measurement problems:

1. It can be used to measure a client's progress, a counselor's skill development, an agency's efficiency, or any number of things.
2. Scales are completely individualized, to reflect *realistic* possibilities for each client or operation one wants to measure rather than predetermined requirements.
3. GAS does not determine the methodology used to reach the goals that are chosen.
4. GAS can generate numerical scores if desired, but it can also be used more informally.
5. GAS can be used as a communication tool with clients, between agencies, with clients' families, or within an agency.
6. GAS does not have to be used with every client. It can be used with a random sample, with clients selected because they might benefit from its structure, with clients referred from a particular source, or with those chosen by some other criteria.
7. GAS has been thoroughly tested in the mental health field, and there have been extensive studies made of it by its originators.
8. GAS is compatible with management by objectives, can be computerized if desirable, and fits into other systems easily.

• Miller and Barillas' Weighting System—This approach weights closure on the basis of success ratios established for age, education, disability class, and type of previous service, based on the assumption that clients vary in their problem complexity. (Miller and Barillas, 1967)

• Wallis and Bozarth (1971) determined that this weighting system offered no better assessment than the present closure goal, allowing one credit for each 26 Closure.

• *Case Difficulty Index*—This approach is based on data about what percentage of cases in different disability classifications do not get rehabilitated, statistically converted into a difficulty factor for each individual case closure. It is currently in use in New Jersey, Florida, and Minnesota. (Sermon, 1972)

• *Service Outcome Measurement Form*—This is a sixteen-scale *device* for computing rehabilitation outcome in social, physical, emotional, and vocational terms and determine the relative difficulty of various cases. (Westerheide, Lenhart, and Miller, 1975)

• *Actuarial System for Weighting Case Closures*—Noble's approach uses the federal minimum wage as the standard against which to judge achievements by the state-federal program. A case is rated positively to the extent that it achieves or exceeds the standard and, conversely, receives negative weight to the degree that it fails to achieve the standard. The national experience with the VR program in facilitating employment for disabled clients is the actuarial basis for estimating the probabilities of success and failure. (Noble, 1973)

• *Difficulty Index*—This device relies on the counselor's estimated difficulty of rehabilitating persons with various disabilities in terms of time and effort. Paired comparison and semantic differential techniques are used, but all judgments are made in reference to standard closure critieria. (Silver, 1969)

• *Vocational Adequacy at Closure Measure*—This measure involves differential weights for work status at closure; DOT job code at closure; weekly earnings at closure; and closure code. A related scale, Vocational Adequacy at Follow-Up, involves employment at follow-up; work status improvement from closure; job satisfaction; and counselor estimate of success. (Eber, 1966)

• *Pattern-Probability Approach*—This approach involves computing a probability index of expected case difficulty based on biographical variables. The index can be used to weight case closure. (Bonge, 1975)

There are many interesting differences among these weighted case closure indexes. For example, some are based on traditional concepts of vocational outcome in rehabilitation, while others encompass nonvocational goals. Some are atheoretical, while one, the Human Service Scale, does have an underlying theoretical rationale.

Westerheide, Lenhart, and Miller (1975, p. 60) have developed a useful set of criteria which a measure of case difficulty and client change should meet:

1. Change should be measured for all clients regardless of closure status;
2. The measure should require no changes in the service delivery system;

3. The measure should not require sophisticated electronic data processing equipment;
4. The measure should be easily interpreted;
5. The measure should not require extensive in-service training;
6. The measure should not require more than ten minutes of the counselor's time per case;
7. The measure should yield reliable information when used across agencies, programs, and counselors; and
8. The content of the measure should reflect the real world concerns and goals of vocational rehabilitation.

These criteria can be used in evaluating any of the preceding outcome measures.

Westerheide and Lenhart (1972) have also defined questions that should be asked in a comprehensive, employability-based outcome measurement system. They suggest that an outcome measurement device administered to clients at the beginning of the rehabilitation process, again at the end, and later for follow-up, would be very useful.

In 1974, the Institute on Rehabilitation Issues Study Group on Outcome Measures decided that the then-available systems could not be endorsed as replacements for the standard Status 26 system. This situation probably still holds true today, for none of these systems has yet been subjected to a widespread national test of validity, reliability, and cost-effectiveness. However, there are a number of promising methodologies described above which could be tested and developed through further work and applied as a means of improving the present outcome measurement system.

RESEARCH AND RESEARCH GAPS

A number of research and demonstration projects now underway are designed to grapple with the problems of vocational rehabilitation outcome measurement. Following the discussion of potential new directions here, we will identify a number of gaps in the body of research knowledge to which studies and future investigations will need to be addressed.

One of the most comprehensive efforts to develop criteria for measuring outcomes is the Rehabilitation Indicators Project, located at the New York University Medical Center, Institute of Rehabilitation Medicine. The project is directed by Drs. Leonard Diller, Wilbert Fordyce, and Durand Jacobs, and is coordinated by Margaret Brown.

The purpose of the project, which was first funded in October 1974, is to develop a generic language—called Rehabilitation Indicators or RI's—that can be used to describe a rehabilitation client's capacities, behaviors, and relevant social or physical environment. These indicators can be used to describe as broad or narrow a range of goals and subgoals as are needed by varying clients at different kinds of rehabilitation centers.

The investigators assert that their RI's, when fully developed, will be useful not only in VR organizations but also in related service delivery environments, such as developmental disabilities and mental health. Through comparison of descriptions of actual behavior and goals, marked on the same indicator, the outcomes of rehabilitation can be described. Four types of rehabilitation indicators have been developed by the investigators:

- *Status* RI's describe conditions such as "living arrangement" and "employment status."
- *Activity pattern* RI's describe recreational, self-care, educational, and other activities selected by the client in day-to-day living.
- *Skill* RI's describe behavioral tools that constitute client strengths and problems (e.g., "walking up/down stairs," "reading the newspaper").
- *Environmental* RI's describe aspects of the physical, social, and personal environment that act as barriers or supports to clients in reaching their individual goals.

The investigators have conducted a number of meetings involving more than seventy-five rehabilitation professionals and consumers from across the United States in gaining input to develop these Rehabilitation Indicators. Current project activities are focusing on field testing of the RI's, which will be studied in cross-sectional and longitudinal analyses in many types of rehabilitation agencies and facilities.

There are several unusual features of the RI's which mark this long-term research effort as potentially quite relevant to outcome measurement. One is that the descriptors are relatively value free. They describe behavior and environmental conditions, leaving judgments to those who use the RI's. Second, this large-scale field research is likely to produce results more strongly and broadly validated than is typical. Third, RI's are being developed in nonvocational areas such as social and independent living skills.

At the West Virginia R&T Center, Dr. Joseph Moriarty and his colleagues have been aiding RSA in refocusing on measures of outcome in the use of RSA standards. The R&T Center has published a number of documents related to program evaluation, including reports interpreting the nine federal evaluation standards for professionals in rehabilitation settings.

At the Arkansas R&T Center, Dr. Stanford Rubin received an RSA grant in 1974 to coordinate a program of activities for program evaluation under the Rehabilitation Act of 1973. Two national training conferences in program evaluation were held in 1974 and 1975, and ten regional program evaluation field studies were conducted. The field studies, which were carried out in each HEW region, covered such areas as client follow-up and client satisfaction with the written rehabilitation plan and other agency services. For example, Region V was responsible for a study of the durability of results from rehabilitation services—whether rehabilitated clients hold on to their jobs over time, make satisfactory upward career progress, and so on. A report on the project is available from the Clearinghouse of Rehabilitation Material at Oklahoma State University.

In Minneapolis, Robert Walker of Evaluation Systems has developed a training package for rehabilitation facilities to help meet the CARF Section Nine Program Evaluation Standards. Facility staff, once put through this program, can have significantly increased capacity to carry out evaluation activities. Defining mission, goals, objectives, and specific evaluation measures, and then placing these into a context of practically feasible assessment, are involved in this procedure. Although not formal research in the traditional sense, Walker's work represents an excellent practical application of knowledge about evaluation and outcome measurement. The process used, a "package" of staff training activities, could be adapted for implementing any outcome measurement system.

Dr. Frederick Collignon and his colleagues at Berkeley Planning Associates have researched outcome measurement—related to employment, homemaking, and nonemployment impacts—from an economic perspective through grants from RSA since 1971. Their work has produced a number of planning and evaluation tools, principally for use in programs rather than individual facilities.

Research activities also are being conducted at the R&T Center at the University of Wisconsin-Stout, and efforts related to outcome measurement are planned at the newly established RRRI at the University of Michigan, which has a primary responsibility in the program evaluation area.

Weighted closure methods have been talked about for a long time. One of the earlier cogent discussions is by Muthard (1965). Miller and Barillas (1967) were perhaps the first to develop and report a method for estimating case difficulty. Since then, investigators such as those whose work is reviewed here have continued efforts in this area. The approaches have ranged from simple case difficulty weighting to complex actuarial and probability theory applications. Currently field testing of some of these methods is going on, but no one has yet emerged with a clear enough record of validity and utility to permit its outright recommendation as a replacement for the current technology. Reviews of weighted closure methods, in addition to the one provided in the preceding chapter, have been given in Bassett (1974), Walls and Tseng (1976), and Bennett and Weisinger (1974).

Despite all of these research activities, a number of problems and gaps in research knowledge remain:

- Most developers of alternative systems of outcome measurement have made the basic assumption that *one* measurement system should be devised and made flexible enough to accommodate the information needs of all. This assumption is a testable hypothesis. The needs of today's complex rehabilitation service delivery service *might* be much better met if a *series* of parallel or tandem outcome measurement technologies were developed. It may be more efficient for counselors to have one kind of outcome data fed back to them, while program decision makers get another.
- Bolton (1974) has questioned whether it is appropriate to aggregate outcome measures of vocational and nonvocational rehabilitation goals. It may be that a multidimensional model is appropriate and that there is some degree of independence between the variables that contribute to success in getting a job and the variables that contribute to improved psychosocial or physical functioning. This again constitutes a testable hypothesis, but one with important implications for outcome measurement models developed in the future.
- Regardless of what kind of system is developed, when one moves beyond the simple matter of whether a client is employed thirty days after rehabilitation closure, one must consider *how* to get ratings of client success. Some objective data are available (e.g., earnings, number of hours worked per week, and so forth). However, estimates of psychosocial or physical functioning almost always require an outsider's judgment—counselor, employer, family member—or the client's self-observation. Then the question of *rater bias* becomes highly relevant.

• There is a need to relate outcome measurement systems to the methods used to assess counselor performance. Too often, the latter are stated in vague, general terms or are related too much to administrative procedure and too little to the realities of serving clients.

• The influences of both the rehabilitation system and the community environment in which it exists need to be considered in relation to outcome measurement data. "Community" includes both the work organization in which a person is placed and the community at large, including the client's place of residence.

• A particularly troublesome problem is that of criteria: what *is* a rehabilitation success? Where psychosocial factors are concerned, how should we think of the measures we take—in psychodynamic terms or in concepts more applicable to the situation of work?

• There is a need to devise ways of bringing *client input* into the process, such as can be done with Goal Attainment Scaling. Such an approach requires research investigation in order to learn the best way for clients to have input that will not disrupt the operation of the system and to understand how making this input can lead to clients' taking increased responsibility for their own goals.

• Investigation is needed into how evaluation systems can be *speeded up* to provide quick feedback to those who need outcome information.

• Cost-benefits of outcome measurement systems need to be investigated carefully to learn which alternatives are most *economical* in different types of settings. This has to do with characteristics of the *agency* as much as the outcome measurement method.

• Efficient methods for *collecting follow-up data* need to be developed. To date, follow-up research has concentrated on telephone surveys, mail surveys, and personal interviews. Each method has advantages and disadvantages, and research is needed on how to increase the quality of follow-up data gathered by any approach and how to decide which method is most cost-effective for a given situation.[4]

• Knowledge of what client characteristics bear on outcome needs to be integrated into the procedures used to gather outcome data and the assumptions underlying them.

• What Joseph Kunce has called "statistical overkill" may lead to significant results using high-powered technical methods but little generalizability to everyday practice. Therefore, researchers must think of measures which are practical and whether the inclusion of certain secondary factors substantially improves the validity of conclusions drawn about outcomes.

- Most weighted closure systems have used the traditional criterion of employment to validate the new procedure. Some investigators (e.g., Miller and Barillas, 1976; Sermon, 1972; Wallis and Bozarth, 1971) have attempted to operationalize case difficulty in terms of the probability of achieving a Status 26 closure with a given client. Weighted closure systems based on this concept are suspect, for they are utilizing a shaky criterion to begin with.
- Few studies have been conducted to develop measures of near-term outcomes, that is, client changes *during* the rehabilitation process.
- Outcome measures need to be couched in terms of what clients can do and how clients and counselors can work together to produce these proficiencies, not in medical or psychiatric terms.
- There is always a question as to whether the outcomes measured are indeed the result of rehabilitation services. Spontaneous changes do occur in clients' lives, and they may interface with service resources. At the same time, there are ethical prohibitions to the use of control groups in true experiments that might otherwise be used to deal with this problem.

IMPACT OF OUTCOME MEASUREMENT: COUNSELORS

Any outcome measurement system has an impact on the work lives of counselors in a rehabilitation agency—a fact frequently ignored in the design and implementation of such systems. Yet the long-term prospects for success depend on whether a method is perceived to have more positive than negative effects on counselors. Development of a system that is responsive to counselor needs and expectations can proceed only through good understanding of how outcome measurement interfaces with the individual counselor.

Although counselors, like other professionals in the human services, may be threatened to some extent by outcome measurement, most can also perceive advantages to having a system for providing good outcome data. On the one hand, counselors may be afraid to have their failures displayed to their colleagues and supervisors, fearing punitive consequences if their "numbers" don't come up to par. Moreover, most service delivery professionals follow to some extent the medical model, in which there is an implicit assumption that dedicated professionals will and do provide helpful services and that, therefore, evaluation of outcome is a waste of time. On the other hand, if outcome measurement provides more information than just whether the client got a job, a counselor may find the system useful for working with clients and for understanding what impact his or her efforts have on a client's progress.

Vash (1978) notes that, as with most professional job roles, rehabilitation counselors can learn as much from their errors as from their successes. The more specific the feedback, the more learning can take place, and an outcome measurement system which is truly sensitive to this need is likely to be met with more acceptance.

Outcome measurement procedures have fairly predictable psychological consequences for the counselors living under them. A good system can provide counselors with motivation to work harder and benefit from feedback in terms of learning new skills and improving the ones they already have. A bad system can generate fear, particularly with respect to performance appraisal by superiors, or salary and promotional purposes. Any outcome measurement system also has a physical impact on counselors—the time and paperwork involved in keeping records used to compile outcome measurement data.

Finally, outcome measurement systems inevitably have an impact on clients as well. The counseling relationship can be a very nourishing one for many clients, and foreseeing the end of it as a by-product of measurement and feedback can be quite threatening. However, building in the concept of movement into full independence from the counselor at the start of the service process, and including it in the individualized treatment plan, can help to defuse some of this client anxiety.

IMPACT OF OUTCOME MEASUREMENT: ADMINISTRATORS AND POLICY MAKERS

Any outcome measurement system has predictable consequences on VR agency administrators and policy makers in RSA and other federal bodies. For administrators, one of the chief impacts concerns regular reports, which must be made for funding and program review purposes. The nature of the outcome measurement system in use can have an important impact on what political advantage a state VR agency or private facility may enjoy with its funding sources, as well as providing information usable for improving the system and its efficiency of operation. Outcome measurement also has a distinct impact on the program evaluation system of an agency and its management information system, if there is one.

At the policy level, outcome measurement data often can be used to make decisions about new programs, modifications or terminations of old ones, and about priorities for service delivery. Knowing what happens to people who go through a rehabilitation system can be illuminating in deciding how that system ought to be run in the future. Therefore, policy decisions may be greatly influenced by the kind of outcome data that are available.

TAKING ACTION

Information Resources

For those who wish to know more about outcome measurement systems in vocational rehabilitation in the United States, there are a number of resources that may be tapped. One of the most important is the Research Utilization Laboratory (RUL) at the ICD Rehabilitation and Research Center in New York City, an RSA-funded information retrieval and dissemination service in the program evaluation field. The RUL will answer information requests based on staff knowledge and on a considerable library of materials in the field, many of which are relevant to outcome measurement.

The RUL serves in this capacity in conjunction with several other RSA-funded efforts concerned with program evaluation. The Arkansas R&T Center has taken charge of evaluation in state agencies and has as a specialty area outcome measures. The West Virginia R&T Center is principally concerned with self-evaluation tools for use in rehabilitation settings. The Regional Rehabilitation Research Institute at the University of Northern Colorado has done research regarding program objectives, outreach, service delivery components of vocational outcomes, and other areas that would be relevant to outcome measurement. Finally, the University of Michigan RRRI will be concerned with program evaluation models and will have responsibility for information dissemination. Contact can be made with any of these organizations for retrieving desired information related to outcome measurement.

Secondary resources are the indexes to RSA-sponsored research and demonstration which provide basic citation data and brief abstracts for hundreds of research and demonstration projects completed under RSA funding over the past several years. Copies of these indexes are available in large university libraries and may also be obtained by request to RSA.

More general resources in the program evaluation field include the Evaluation Research Society and the Evaluation Network, two recently founded national professional organizations devoted to the subject of program evaluation in organizational settings. Although the primary focus of these two organizations is not on outcome measurement in rehabilitation, this subject is of interest to a certain segment of the membership, and much of the materials and information these organizations may be contributing would be relevant. The same may be true for the Center for the Study of Evaluation in the School of Education, UCLA, or the Center for Social Policy Evaluation at the Graduate School of Education, Harvard University. Those specifically interested in Goal Attainment Scaling as an outcome measurement technique can contact the Program Evaluation Resource Center in Minneapolis, an organization founded by Dr. Thomas Kiresuk, GAS's co-inventor.

A great variety of books, monographs, and journal articles related to outcome measurement have already been mentioned in this. Some key references which provide a general review of the outcome measurement field include: Chapter 4 in Bennett and Weisinger (1974), which is the most comprehensive compendium of program evaluation outcome measurement-related measures in existence; Bassett (1974), which is possibly the most up-to-date policy statement about outcome measurement in rehabilitation; *Recommended Standards for Closure of Cases* (Seventh Institute on Rehabilitation Services, 1969), a report from a study group on uniformity of standards in the determination of services to clients; Westerheide and Lenhart (1972); and Walls and Tseng (1976). The Westerheide and Lenhart review includes a particularly good synopsis of research on how client characteristics bear on outcomes.

Reviews in the related area of placement include Dunn et al. (1974) and Zadny and James (1976). The West Virginia R&T Center publishes a newsletter, *Rehabilitation Tomorrow,* which often contains material related to evaluation. Of even more significance is the *PA/VR Newsletter,* published by the ICD Research Utilization Laboratory. Each issue of this newsletter may contain helpful materials for those interested in either evaluation or outcome measurement.

Knowledge Utilization/ Organizational Change Resources

For those policy makers and administrators ready to consider developing and installing a new outcome measurement system, there are resources available which deal with the application of new knowledge and with making successful organizational changes. The most comprehensive reference work now in existence on knowledge utilization is *Putting Knowledge to Use: A Distillation of the Literature Regarding Knowledge Transfer and Change,* published by the Human Interaction Research Institute (1976). A key reference on the utilization of evaluation findings is Davis and Salasin (1975), and an excellent synopsis of important principles of knowledge transfer is Glaser (1973).

What the Counselor Can Do

Innovative outcome measurement systems can be used by individual counselors even if not installed formally in the organization in which they work, as a means of increasing self-appraisal and spurring their own growth as professionals. Simple forms can be devised and used as record-keeping systems for each counselor's work. Eventually the successful use of such systems on an individual level can lead to increased interest regarding their use in an agency.

Counselors can also take responsibility for stimulating a flow of information and active consideration of new systems for outcome measurement. If there are deficiencies in the present system, study them and gather evidence about the impact they are having on rehabilitation services. Then these findings can be presented in staff meetings or professional association meetings as a way of stimulating change. The amount an individual counselor can do to promote system change may be small, but opportunities do sometimes arise.

What Administrators Can Do

Administrators in state VR agencies and private settings can do much to implement improved systems of outcome measurement without waiting for changes in the national reporting system. These new systems can serve well for counselor self-improvement and performance appraisal and can provide useful information for program improvement.

Field trial and limited experimentation are necessary before full implementation. Administrators should remind themselves not to leap into use of a new system just because it is trendy. Also, outcome measurement systems will be more effective and more efficiently used if there are corresponding changes in the reward system for counselors as the result of changes in the way success in rehabilitation is appraised.

What Policy Makers Can Do

At the national level, there are a number of actions that could help to spur development of new and improved outcome measurement systems:

- Sponsor sessions and development of materials on outcome measurement, perhaps using as one model Robert Walker's material on program evaluation for rehabilitation facilities.
- Sponsor publications and newsletters in the outcome measurement field.

- Hold a national conference to clarify standards for measuring outcomes in rehabilitation, including policy makers, researchers, administrators, counselors, and disabled persons.
- Encourage examination and possible adaptation at the national level local or statewide tested systems which seem to have worked.
- Sponsor a national commission or task force to determine what improvements ought to be made in outcome measurement systems at all levels, and then develop a plan to implement them.
- Develop and implement a system of outcome measurement as a pilot project in collaboration with selected graduate students and faculty in a rehabilitation counselor training program, to assist in assessing the value of the system before expansion on a regional or nationwide basis.
- Facilitate cross-talk with other human service agencies in regard to outcome measurement issues. For example, Goal Attainment Scaling, one of the most promising innovations in outcome measurement discussed in this chapter, was originally developed under funding support from the National Institute of Mental Health. Instrumentation developed for use in personnel service programs with disadvantaged clients by the Employment and Training Administration, U.S. Department of Labor, would be another particularly likely source (see Backer, 1979, for a recent review).

Although it is beyond the scope of this chapter to analyze in any detail what research should be done and in what sequence, it does seem appropriate to remind the reader that proposed new research must be *coordinated* with past and ongoing efforts and must be adequately funded. Projects such as the New York University effort to develop Rehabilitation Indicators—a multiphase, national-scope undertaking—are probably what is most needed at this point in time. Developing new standards and techniques regarding outcome measurement which can be applied at the national level simply can't be done on a shoestring; the complexities are too great. It takes projects which have the necessary luxuries of large staffs, ample startup time for conceptualization, and resources for wide consumer involvement and field testing to create new methods that are credible and will, in fact, have good potential for use.

RSA at the federal level needs to serve in an overall coordinating role to minimize overlap and duplication if several such efforts were funded. The national commission on outcome measurement suggested above might be employed as a policy guidance body to advise RSA on such matters.

Finally, policy makers need to attend to changes in the VR legislation necessary for accommodating methods of outcome measurement. The present law seems to reinforce the traditional concepts (e.g., Status 26) rather strongly, and unless modifications in the law are made, it is unlikely that any new system will have a substantial impact. State VR agencies and private facilities will continue—in order to have funds with which to serve their clients—to follow the guidelines of record keeping and reporting suggested in legislation and administrative regulations surrounding it. When changes in the "rules of the game" are made, changes in agency and facility behavior can more reasonably be expected to occur.

THE FUTURE

The consensus of opinion seems to be that modifications in rehabilitation outcome measurement systems will eventually be made, but they will be small at first, and made slowly. An important attitude change that may help to increase the impact of future work in this area is for counselors, administrators, policy makers—and researchers—to start regarding the improvement of outcome measurement technology as everybody's business.

One way to solidify such an attitude change, and to provide a mechanism for carrying out suggestions made in the preceding chapter, would be for RSA to sponsor the creation of an independent Center on Rehabilitation Outcome Measurement. This center could develop, either using in-house staff or outside subcontractors, outcome measurement materials, publications, and newsletters. It could sponsor a national conference on outcome measurement and set up pilot projects for testing innovative approaches. Its advisory body could be the previously suggested National Commission on Outcome Measurement, which might include rehabilitation administrators, from both state VR agencies and private facilities, RSA representatives, VR counselors, and disabled consumers of VR services. Representation could also be provided from groups such as CSAVR, NRA, ARA, NRCA, and consumer advocacy organizations. Such a center could well provide the coordinated national effort which now seems so much needed to bring to a "critical mass" progress which is being made in the outcome measurement field.

Perhaps of critical importance is the fact that such a center would provide a focus for many diverse efforts and create a sense of visibility and purpose that would in itself increase the motivation for change. The well-entrenched outcome measurement system may not readily change under an impetus of any lesser intensity.

Pressures for evaluation and accountability, and for increasing services to the severely disabled, are likely to increase from the federal level. These pressures will serve as motivators for promoting faster changes in outcome measurement over the next few years. As new systems and resources develop, further changes will be easier to make. Ultimately, as Brian Bolton has pointed out, outcome measurement needs to be excellent because *prediction* of what will happen to a given client is at the heart of the rehabilitation process. Only by gathering good information about how clients have fared in the past can we build a knowledge base for the future.

NOTES

[1]See Vialle (1968) for a fuller discussion of some of these factors.

[2]CARF has just published a new manual, *Program Evaluation in Vocational Rehabilitation Facilities,* which supersedes the publication described here. Unfortunately, the new manual was not available for review when this chapter was prepared.

[3]Case difficulty indexes will be considered here as a special case of weighted closure.

[4]A manual on follow-up procedures is currently being prepared by ICD/RUL.

REFERENCES

Backer, T. E. *Client Assessment: A Manual for Employment and Training Agencies.* Washington, D.C.: Employment and Training Administration, U.S. Department of Labor, 1979.

Bassett, Paul T. *Measurement of Outcomes: A Report from the Study Group on Measurement of Outcomes.* First Institute on Rehabilitation Issues; Denver, Colo.; April 15–17, 1974. Institute, West Virginia: Research and Training Center, 1974.

Bennett, Eleanor C., and Weisinger, Marvin. *Program Evaluation: A Resource Handbook for Vocational Rehabilitation.* New York: ICD Rehabilitation and Research Center, 1974.

Berkeley Planning Associates. *VR Program Evaluation Standards: A Critique of the State of the Art.* Berkeley, Calif.: 1977.

Berkowitz, M. *Weighted Closures.* New Brunswick, N. J.: Bureau of Economic Research, Rutgers University, 1972.

Bolton, Brian. *Introduction to Rehabilitation Research.* Research Report ARRTC No. 798. Fayetteville, Ark.: Arkansas Rehabilitation Research and Training Center, University of Arkansas/Arkansas Rehabilitation Services, February 1974.

Bolton, Brian (ed.). *Handbook of Measurement and Evaluation in Rehabilitation.* Baltimore, Md.: University Park Press, 1976.

Bonge, D. *Placement: A Practical Measure for Comparing the Effectiveness of Rehabilitation Service Units.* Research Report ARRTC No. 293. Fayetteville, Ark.: Arkansas

Rehabilitation Research and Training Center, University of Arkansas/Arkansas Rehabilitation Services, November 1975.

———. *A Pattern-Probability Approach to Predicting Client Outcome.* Research Report ARRTC No. 923. Fayetteville, Ark.: Arkansas Rehabilitation Research and Training Center, University of Arkansas/Arkansas Rehabilitation Services, December 1975.

Commission on Accreditation of Rehabilitation Facilities. *Program Evaluation in Vocational Rehabilitation Facilities.* Tucson, Arizona: Author, 1974.

Davis, H. R., and Salasin, S. E. "The Utilization of Evaluation." In: Elmer L. Struening and Marcia Guttentag (eds.), *Handbook of Evaluation Research.* Beverly Hills, Calif.: Sage Publications, 1975.

Dunn, Dennis, J., et al. *Placement Services in the Vocational Rehabilitation Program.* Menomonie, Wis.: Research and Training Center, Stout Vocational Rehabilitation Institute, University of Wisconsin-Stout, December 1974.

Eber, H. W. "Multivariate Analysis of a Vocational Rehabilitation System." *Multi Behavioral Research Monograph* 66-1, 1966.

Florida Division of Vocational Rehabilitation. *Florida Difficulty Index in Achieving Rehabilitation.* Tallahassee, Fla.: 1973.

Gibson, D. L., et al. *Manual for the Minnesota Satisfactoriness Scales.* Minnesota Studies in Vocational Rehabilitation XXVII, Bulletin 53. Minneapolis, Minn.: University of Minnesota, 1970.

Glaser, E. M. "Knowledge Transfer and Institutional Change," *Professional Psychology* 4, 1973: 434–444.

Goodyear, Don L., and Bitter, James A. "Goal Attainment Scaling as a Program Evaluation Measure in Rehabilitation," *Journal of Applied Rehabilitation Counseling* 5(1), Spring 1974: 19–26.

Hawryluk, Alex. "Rehabilitation Gain: A Better Indicator Needed," *Journal of Rehabilitation* 38(5), September–October 1972: 22–25.

Hefferin, Elizabeth A., and Katz, Alfred H. "Issues and Orientations in the Evaluation of Rehabilitation Programs: A Review Article, Part I," *Rehabilitation Literature* 32(3), March 1971: 66–74, 95.

———. "Issues and Orientations in the Evaluation of Rehabilitation Programs: A Review Article, Part II," *Rehabilitation Literature* 32(4), April 1971: 98–107, 113.

Human Interaction Research Institute. *Putting Knowledge to Use: A Distillation of the Literature Regarding Knowledge Transfer and Change.* Los Angeles: 1976.

Kay, Harold B. *Program Product and Priorities.* (Unpublished paper), 1977.

Kunce, Joseph T., et al. *Rehabilitation in the Concrete Jungle.* Research Series No. 3. Columbia, Mo.: Regional Rehabilitation Research Institute, University of Missouri, 1969.

Kunce, Joseph T., and Miller, Douglas E. "Simplified Prediction: A Follow-Up Study," *Journal of Counseling Psychology* 19(6), November 1972: 505–508.

Miller, Leonard A., and Barillas, Mario G. "Using Weighted 26-Closures as a More Adequate Measure of Counselor and Agency Effort in Rehabilitation," *Rehabilitation Counseling Bulletin* XI, December 1967: 117–121.

Moriarity, Joseph B. "Issues in Evaluating Vocational Rehabilitation," *Professional Psychology* 8(4), November 1977:27–31.

Muthard, John E. (ed.). *Training Guides in Caseload Management for Vocational Rehabilitation Staff.* Washington, D.C.: Vocational Rehabilitation Administration, 1965.

Muthard, John E., and Miller, Leonard A. *The Criteria Problem in Rehabilitation Counseling.* Iowa City: College of Education, University of Iowa, 1966.

———. *The Rehabilitation Counselor Rating Scale.* Studies in Rehabilitation Counselor

Training, No. 6. Joint Liaison Committee of the Council of State Administrators of Vocational Rehabilitation and the Rehabilitation Counselor Educators, 1968.

Noble, John H., Jr. "Actuarial System for Weighting Case Closures," *Social and Rehabilitation Record* 14(5), 1973: 34–37.

Reagles, Kenneth W., and Butler, Alfred S. "The Human Service Scale: A New Measure for Evaluation," *Journal of Rehabilitation* 42(3), May–June 1976: 34–38.

Reagles, Kenneth W., Wright, George N., and Butler, Alfred J. *A Scale of Rehabilitation Gain for Clients of an Expanded Vocational Rehabilitation Program.* Wisconsin Studies in Vocational Rehabilitation, Monograph XIII, Series 2. Madison: Wisconsin Regional Rehabilitation Research Institute, 1970.

Research Utilization Laboratory, Jewish Vocational Service. *Goal Attainment Scaling Manual.* RUL #5. (RSA Grant No. 22-P-577-6.) Chicago: September 1976.

———. *Lab Notes,* Special Issue, January 1977.

Rubin, Stanford E. *Analysis of Rehabilitation Counselor Sub Role Behavior: Development of a Rehabilitation Counseling Interview Sub Role Behavior Scale.* Fayetteville, Ark.: Arkansas Rehabilitation Research and Training Center, University of Arkansas/Arkansas Rehabilitation Services, 1973.

Rubin, Stanford E. (ed.). *Studies on the Evaluation of State Vocational Rehabilitation Agency Programs.* Fayetteville, Ark.: Arkansas Rehabilitation Services, 1975.

Rubin, Stanford E., and Reagles, Kenneth W. "Assessment of Counselor Performance." In: Brian Bolton (ed.), *Handbook of Measurement and Evaluation in Rehabilitation.* Baltimore: University Park Press, 1976.

Schneiderman, L. *Ohio State University: Plan for Evaluating the PA/VR Franklin County Expansion Grants Project.* SRS Project Grant 25-P-65-439/5-01. Columbus, Ohio: Ohio State University, 1972.

Sermon, Duane. *The Difficulty Index—An Expanded Measure of Counselor Performance.* Research Monograph No. 1. St. Paul, Minn.: Minnesota Division of Vocational Rehabilitation, March 1972.

Serot, D. E. *Indices of Cost, Output and Productivity for Use in Evaluating Rehabilitation Service Programs.* Working Paper No. 187/RS013. Berkeley, Calif.: Institute of Urban and Regional Development, University of California, 1972.

Seventh Institute on Rehabilitation Services. *Recommended Standards for Closure of Cases.* Information Memorandum RSA-IM-71-24. Washington, D.C.: U.S. Department of Health, Education and Welfare, Social and Rehabilitation Service, Rehabilitation Services Administration, 1969.

Silver, D. L. "A Look at Evaluation of Vocational Rehabilitation Counselor Performance," *Journal of Rehabilitation* 35, November–December 1969: 13–14.

Tenth Institute on Rehabilitation Services. *Program Evaluation—A Beginning Statement.* Washington, D.C.: U.S. Department of Health, Education and Welfare, Social and Rehabilitation Service, Rehabilitation Services Administration, 1972.

U.S. Department of Health, Education and Welfare, Rehabilitation Services Administration. "Criteria for Closing Case Records." In: *Rehabilitation Services Manual.* (Draft 1549.01-1549.03) Washington, D.C.: 1971.

———. *Vocational Rehabilitation Manual.* Washington, D.C.: Social and Rehabilitation Service, 1971.

Vash, C. *The Ghost in the Counseling Office or Living Up to Professional Role Expectations (Especially When You're Not Exactly Sure What They Are).* (Unpublished paper), 1978.

Vialle, Harold D. *Operations Research Program in the Oklahoma Vocational Rehabilitation Agency.* Report of Grant No. RD-946. Oklahoma City: Oklahoma Vocational Rehabilitation Agency, 1968.

Wallis, Janice H., and Bozarth, Jerold D. "The Development and Evaluation of Weighted DVR Case Closures," *Rehabilitation Research and Practice Review* 2(3), Summer 1971: 55–60.

Walls, Richard T., and Tseng, M. S. "Measurement of Client Outcomes in Rehabilitation." In: Brian F. Bolton (ed.), *Handbook of Measurement and Evaluation in Rehabilitation.* Baltimore: University Park Press, 1976.

Weisinger, Marvin. "Overview of Outcome Measures." In: Isabel P. Robinault and Marvin Weisinger (eds.), *Program Planning and Evaluation for Vocational Rehabilitation.* New York: ICD Rehabilitation and Research Center, September 1975.

Weisinger, Marvin, Robinault, Isabel P., and Bennett, Eleanor C. (eds.). *Program Evaluation: Selected Readings.* New York: ICD Rehabilitation and Research Center, 1975.

Weiss, D. *Manual for the Minnesota Satisfaction Scale.* Minnesota Studies in Vocational Rehabilitation XXII, Bulletin 45. Minneapolis, Minn.: University of Minnesota, 1967.

Westerheide, William J., and Lenhart, Lowell. *Case Difficulty and Client Change: A Review of the Literature.* Monograph 1. (ERIC Report ED 099 719.) Oklahoma City: Department of Institutions, Social and Rehabilitation Services, 1972.

Westerheide, William J., Lenhart, Lowell, and Miller, Clinton M. , III. "Case Difficulty: Summary." In: Marvin Weisinger, Isabel P. Robinault and Eleanor C. Bennett (eds.), *Program Evaluation: Selected Readings.* New York: ICD Rehabilitation and Research Center, 1975.

Wheeler, D. *The Measure of Job Relatedness for Job Occupational Evaluation.* (ERIC Report ED 053 318.) St. Paul, Minn.: Minnesota Research Coordinating Unit in Occupational Education, 1971.

Zadny, Jerry J., and James, Leslie F. *Another View on Placement: State of the Art 1976.* Studies in Placement Monograph No. 1. Regional Rehabilitation Research Institute. Portland: School of Social Work, Portland State University, March 1976.

9
Independent Living*

SUSAN STODDARD, M.C.P.
With a Foreword by Edward V. Roberts

Traditionally the term independent living *has been used to refer to the aids to daily living, the wheelchairs, arm braces, specially designed housing, etc., that allowed severely disabled persons to care somewhat for their own survival needs.*

When those active in the disabled movement today use the term, they are referring to the ability of the severely disabled person to actively and generally share in the joys and responsibilities of community life. They are referring to the social services that we all take for granted but that may be denied the disabled person because of architectural and/or attitudinal barriers. Independent living services are an important part of comprehensive rehabilitation for the severely disabled.

"Independent Living" explains the concepts as developed in the consumer movement and provides an up-to-date report of the major developments in independent living service delivery models. It is intended to inform vocational rehabilitation administrators, counselors, and planning personnel about the major issues in independent living, and the importance of this opportunity for consumers.

The chapter reviews pertinent legislative history and current issues and discusses estimates of the target population. Major models of independent living services in the United States are also presented. Because expansion of these services to all physically disabled individuals will require a substantial commitment of government resources, economic benefits of independent living are presented in a discussion of its costs and benefits.

*This chapter is based on a mongraph of the same title that appeared as one of a series called "Emerging Issues in Rehabilitation," published by the Institute for Research Utilization (Washington, D.C., 1977) with funding support by the Rehabilitation Services Administration. The author wishes to thank the following individuals who contributed to the preparation of the earlier monograph: Mr. Edward Roberts, Ms. Joan Leon, Ms. Judy Senkevitch, Mr. Bruce Schmidt, Dr. Frederick Fay, Mr. Lex Frieden, Mr. Don Galloway, Ms. Judy Heumann, Dr. Herbert Liebowitz, Dr. Elizabeth Pan, Dr. Thomas Backer, Dr. Carolyn Vash, Dr. Herbert Dorken, Mr. Bertrum Griffis and Dr. Frederick Collignon.

INTRODUCTION

Independent living for persons with severe physical disability is an important rehabilitation concept in the 1980s. The concept is new and constantly developing. It is not surprising, then, that the definition of independent living is unclear to many.

A useful perspective about independent living is provided in the following statement by Edward V. Roberts, Director of the California Department of Rehabilitation.

> In its broadest implications the independent living movement is the civil rights movement of millions of Americans with disabilities. It is the wave of protest against segregation and discrimination and an affirmation of the right and ability of disabled persons to share fully in the responsibilities and joys of our society.
>
> The movement's strength comes from the fact that it represents all people with special needs—the aged, the physically disabled, the developmentally disabled, and the mentally ill. At no time was this more apparent than during the Section 504 demonstrations in April 1977. At that time, people of all different disabilities joined hands and demanded their full human and civil rights as equal Americans. This demonstration capped a series of efforts by the general public and legislators to achieve laws and guidelines that would open the doors to education, employment, housing, transportation, and recreation for people with special needs.
>
> Medical and rehabilitation technology has made tremendous advances in the last few decades, and we are now able to help persons with even the most severe disabilities to the point of independence. The problem we now face is how to make changes in our environment so that these persons can complete the rehabilitation process and become actively participating and valued members of our communities.
>
> The independent living movement has made all of us aware of our society's underdevelopment and the scarcity of resources available for people with special needs. As I learned from personal experience as a post-polio respiratory quadriplegic, a disability is a conditon that can usually be stabilized and assimilated into one's self-image, but a handicap is a conditon that is created by the service gaps and architectural and attitudinal barriers in society. It's the handicap that is so limiting. We can, by focusing our efforts on the development of society's capability to accommodate and sustain people with special needs, cause that handicap to disappear. It's important to realize that disability can happen to anyone and that there are literally hundreds of thousands of people in this country who, because of age, disability, or other factors are now denied the chance to lead a full and active life because of the underdevelopment of our communities and social service systems.
>
> I believe that the basic premise of the independent living movement is that everyone has potential to live more independently. Our experience

shows that even the most severely and profoundly disabled individuals can be independent—they may need all kinds of help—but that they can be in control of their lives.

Today, our vocational rehabilitation system addresses only a part of the overall need of the individual and serves those most easy to rehabilitate. As we attempt to carry out the mandate of the Rehabilitation Act of 1973, which requires state rehabilitation agencies to serve people with severe disabilities as a first priority, we are becoming increasingly aware of the gaps that exist in our programs and the lack of community services. We are realizing that our programs tend to systematically reject the people with the greatest needs. Many people with severe disabilities need extensive independent living and pre-vocational services in order to be helped by our vocational programs and once they complete our programs, they continue to need independent living services to varying degrees for the rest of their lives. For the most part these services do not exist in our communities. This review focuses on independent living services and the new self-help programs that have emerged to provide these services, and advocacy for people with severe disabilities. It also discusses the importance of these organizations to our rehabilitation system and the continuing improvement of the system's ability to serve people with even the most severe disabilities.

The largest and best known of the independent living programs is the Center for Independent Living (CIL) in Berkeley, which in its six years of operation has had a major effect on the accessibility and responsiveness of the Bay Area community and the ability of that community's residents to live more independently. CIL was started by a group of people with severe disabilities who came from an experiential base and felt a strong dissatisfaction with the institutional network that society had set up to help them. I was one of the founding members. One of the keys to CIL's success was that our dissatisfaction with the existing level of services was shared by many people in the helping professions, government and the general public, and that those who were receptive to CIL's ideas and goals lent their support in terms of energy, commitment and dollars to the development of CIL's programs. As a result of this support we were able to develop an innovative concept into an important link in our medical/rehabilitation system.

Organizations such as CIL fill a major gap in our medical/rehabilitation network. Their focus is on integration and the services needed to move people into the mainstream. Independent living programs deal with the quality of life people lead in the communities; they are service and training centers, but primarily they are advocates working to develop a public awareness of the needs and capabilities of people with severe disabilities, as well as an awareness within the disabled individual of his potential for a life of greater participation and involvement.

In California, the State Department of Rehabilitation has in the past . . . used its new Innovation and Expansion (I&E) Grant capability to stimulate the development of independent living programs throughout the state. Currently there are fourteen of these organizations in California, nine of which were started by I&E grants. We regard these programs as essential compo-

> nents in the network of community-based services. The programs help clients move toward vocational goals and are valuable resources in developing in employers, helping professionals, and the general public a greater awareness of the employment and independent living potential of all people with disabilities. We anticipate that these programs will help the department reach out to the many people who have been excluded from Department of Rehabilitation programs for reasons of severity of disability, and that they will function as important resources for supportive services, counseling, prevocational and vocational training throughout the rehabilitation process.
>
> California is not the only state that has done this. State rehabilitation agencies in Michigan, Massachusetts and others have also begun to facilitate development of independent living programs in their communities. This trend has gone hand in hand with the growing conviction of state rehabilitation agencies that they can and should serve a wider range of clients—including those people who, for many reasons, do not have an employment goal, but who can be helped significantly toward greater independence and integration. It is significant that at a recent meeting of the Council of State Administrators of Vocational Rehabilitation (CSAVR), 88% of the state directors felt that independent living services should be a part of state rehabilitation programs. A few years ago only a few state directors felt that way. . . . Making independent living a reality for people with severe disabilities is not the sole responsibility of rehabilitation. It's a responsibility shared by all government programs, the general public, business and industry, and private service agencies. We need to work together to build a complementary social system in this country, one that makes it possible for people with special needs to live as equal citizens.[1]

When those active in the disabled movement use the term *independent living,* they are referring to their ability to participate actively in society—to work, have a home, raise a family, and generally share in the joys and responsibilities of community life. They are referring to the human services necessary to reduce barriers to such community participation. Independent living is an integral part of the rehabilitation process for the severely disabled, an essential component of a program that hopes to help people with severe disabilities achieve their personal and vocational objectives. This new definition of independent living has developed from three previous independent living concepts that in themselves provided partial and limited solutions for the individual with a severe disability.

Three Partial Concepts of Independent Living

Physical Modification (Aids to Daily Living)

First is the traditional concept of independent living services as aids to daily living—the wheelchairs, orthopedic devices, special equipment, and housing modifications that permit people with severe physical disabilities to care, somewhat, for their own survival needs. The focus of this concept is on modification of the physical environment to make activities of daily living more feasible. Concern with such needs is the basis for some important new programs established with the title "independent living." For example, the U.S. Department of Housing and Urban Development (HUD) has established a new Office of Independent Living with a concern for special housing. The focus on physical modification is a crucial but still only partial answer to the needs of individuals with severe disabilities.

Independent Living Rehabilitation (ILR)

A second concept of independent living developed in drafts of vocational rehabilitation bills. Vocational rehabilitation services are available to handicapped individuals for whom vocational objectives are feasible. Many have argued that a separate program could provide services without respect to vocational objectives. In other words, this assumed a clear distinction between individuals in need of independent living services (vocationally "nonfeasible") and those for whom vocational goals are feasible. By definition, this concept of independent living as distinct from vocationally oriented services may preclude vocational goals for the individual with severe disability.

Consumer Rights

A third concept developing at the same time focused on attitudes and on the rights of people with disabilities. It includes consumers and professionals, advocating change in general attitudes and provision of the services that individuals with disabilities need in order to take part in community life. While the first two concepts are essentially programatic in nature, the third has not been restricted to any one program or service system but has advocated an integrated service system focused on the services needed to help people be independent. The concept enhances the belief that people with disabilities have the right to services that enable them to be equal and independent members of the community.

Comprehensive Definition

The development of a comprehensive definition of independent living has been recent and is still going on. The ideas from these three previous models are complementary, although each in itself is incomplete. The independent living movement has provided impetus for changes in programmatic approaches to independent living.

Housing

For example, the concept of housing for the disabled is changing in HUD from large, segregated and institutional housing projects to a range of housing alternatives that provide varying degrees of services and control depending on needs of residents. There is a new commitment to the least restrictive and most integrative environments, compatible with the goals of the independent living movement.

Rehabilitation

Since the Rehabilitation Act of 1973 called for priority to the individuals with most severe handicaps, vocational rehabilitation professionals are more aware that independent living services are often needed by individuals with severe disability in connection with the vocational rehabilitation process, and may be needed before, during, and after "rehabilitation." Independent living services may be necessary in order to compensate for the fact that many severely disabled individuals have not gained skills needed to be independent or had the opportunity to develop motivation toward vocational goals. Vocational rehabilitation counselors are finding that independent living need not be a parallel and separate system but can complement vocational rehabilitation objectives.

Independent Living Organizations

While the independent living movement has brought about some changes in how major programs view service need, the emphasis has not been on government agencies as exclusive providers of independent living services. Alternative, consumer-run organizations ("centers for independent living") have developed coordinate and complement services provided by government. These centers, which will be described in detail below, are organizations based on the new meaning of independent living that has developed, combining physical modification services, rehabilitation, and consumer rights into a comprehensive network of service for the person with a severe disability. The goal is a network that provides a continuum of services from the onset of disability at whatever age throughout the person's lifetime.

The focus in this model is on the individual rather than the program. In this context, vocational education and vocational rehabilitation services may be utilized by the individual as he or she gains the ability to benefit from them and develops the self-direction needed to choose a life goal. Figure 1, illustrates the relationship between the individual with a disability, the family, established service systems such as state rehabilitation agencies, and the many distinct "independent living" services that make up the comprehensive rehabilitation package. The

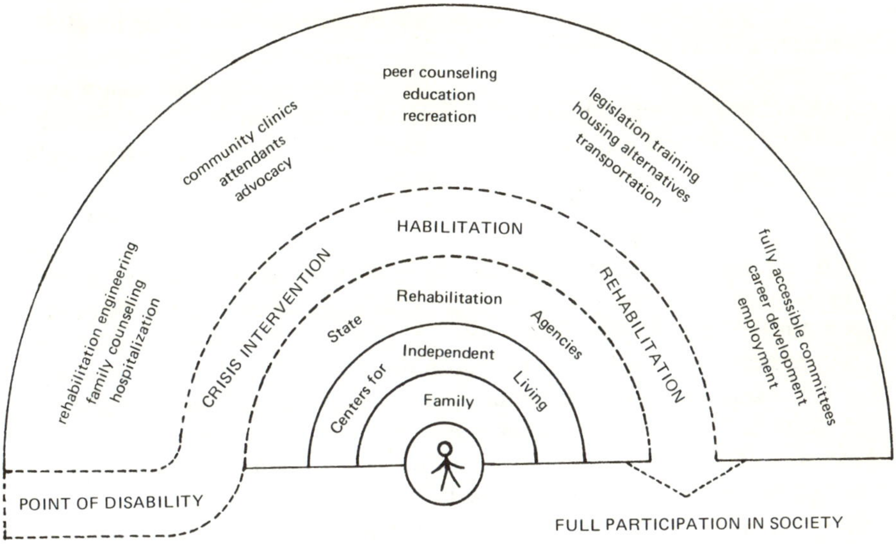

FIGURE 1

diagram was created in 1975 by Ed Roberts and the staff from CIL, Berkeley, working with Dr. Herb Liebowitz of RSA, Region IX, for the Conference on Independent Living held in Berkeley, through RSA funding, in 1975.

The continuum is made up of a complementary network of services provided both publicly and privately. The services needed at the time of crisis intervention (diagnosis or onset) include family counseling, medical care, and rehabilitation engineering (equipment and prostheses). This *crisis intervention period* usually is defined as the time the individual is undergoing major medical care leading to the treatment and the stabilization of health. As the individual gains the ability to leave a hospital environment, a second period called *habilitation* begins. This is the period during which primary emphasis is on personal adjustment to disability and on increasing independence and self-reliance.

During habilitation, appropriate housing alternatives are critical. Historically, a great many people with severe disabilities moved from hospital environments to nursing homes and other care institutions. There are now new alternatives that facilitate the development of independence and a positive self-image (Cole and Frieden, 1977).

It is during this period that the independent living centers can play a critical role through the provision of life-support services and peer counseling, and also when vocational rehabilitation programs may begin to support the career development of the individual. The length of time necessary for the habilitation phase depends on the individual and on the community environment. Clients in independent living programs have achieved habilitation in less than a year, while previously, without independent living programs and services, the process might have taken five years—if habilitation was achieved at all.

The next stage is defined as *rehabilitation,* the period of development of a definite life style and career objective, which could range from homemaker, part-time and intermittent employment, to full-time employment in the primary labor market. The work aspect of the continuum is critically important because it is only through work and other productive activities that an individual really becomes a part of the mainstream, a valued member of the community. Therefore, to the extent that an individual chooses and can attain a vocational objective, these objectives are an integral part of the independent living process.

Figure 1 shows an end to the individual's process as "point of full participation." This does not necessarily mean the end of independent living services. Such services as attendant care and peer counseling may always be important as support services for the independent person with severe disability.

In summary, *independent living* has six basic elements:

- *Focus on the individual* with disability, and maximization of that individual's opportunity for participation in society.
- *Provision of the services* needed by that individual, either through established service organizations or through independent living centers that integrate public and private services available in the community and provide other services not available elsewhere.
- *Focus on choice* for the individual, on alternative ways that housing and service needs might be met.
- *Integration* of an individual's need for support services and achievement of habilitation or a living situation that works, with life goals such as vocational and educational objectives.
- Provision of both *"crisis" or intervention services* related to the onset of disability and *ongoing services* that support stabilization and individual development during and after rehabilitation.
- *Advocacy* of the rights of individuals with disability.

Scope and Purpose

The sections of this chapter cover a number of important issues and programs related to the provision of independent living services.

The next section, "Independent Living and Federal Rehabilitation Legislation," reviews attempts to introduce independent living as a component of vocational rehabilitation services, illustrating a number of planning issues that still confront policy makers.

The following section discusses the problem of "Defining the Target Population" inconsistencies in the use of definitional terms.

Following this is a description of "Alternative Delivery Strategies" for independent living services. The centers for independent living that have emerged throughout the country provide, for the disabled, linkages with services and funding upon which they depend in order to live in the community. Several major dimensions of these programs are identified. In addition, several examples of independent living service models are reviewed.

Next are reviews of two important programs in which alternatives for organization and delivery of independent living services are being systematically evaluated.

The next section reviews analytical and theoretical work to date on estimating the costs and benefits of independent living. Traditional economic justification of vocational rehabilitation services for the disabled has rested on the program's focus on gainful employment. Even if the legislative mandate were to be expanded to permit independent living closures, difficulty in defining independent living gain presents a major obstacle in economic analysis.

The conclusion reemphasizes the main programmatic features of the consumer model of independent living and outlines major policy questions and the agenda for exploration of new alternatives.

Following the conclusion is a "Checklist for Developing Independent Living Projects" prepared for the BCIL report.

INDEPENDENT LIVING AND FEDERAL REHABILITATION LEGISLATION[2]

The legislative history of vocational rehabilitation program funding shows congressional concern for independent living as a part of vocational rehabilitation legislative process dating back to 1959. This brief review of attempts to introduce independent living as a component of vocational rehabilitation services illustrates a number of planning issues that currently confront the policy maker:

- What are the service needs related to independent living?
- Who should be served?
- How should an independent living program be administered?
- How should independent living rehabilitation relate to vocational rehabilitation?
- How much would an independent living program cost?

1959–1971

Vocational rehabilitation legislation dates back as far as 1920, when the original Smith-Fess Act, Public Law 66–236, authorized training, counseling, and placement services for the physically handicapped, related to vocational goals. However, it was not until 1959 that independent living rehabilitation services were proposed in Congress. In that year, two bills, HR 361 and HR 5416, contained titles relating to "independent living rehabilitation services." Emphasis in this early bill, however, was on reduction of the public burden by reducing a disabled person's need for an attendant and increasing "ability of independent living."

Bills of similar spirit were introduced in 1961 containing titles on "Independent Living Rehabilitation Services." These called for a cooperative arrangement between the state agencies to provide independent living and those ancillary social services needed for independent living. The intent was to establish a separate program for independent living. The authors, primarily the National Rehabilitation Association (NRA), indicated that due to lack of administrative experience in the area of independent living, two programs should exist. "This arrangement will assure that attention given to the new program will not detract from emphasis on vocational rehabilitation" (Urban Institute, 1975, p. 7).

The administration opposed these provisions. Indecision on the part of the Department of Health, Education and Welfare (HEW) in designating who was to administer the provision—public health, rehabilitation, or social services—has been cited as the ultimate cause of failure (Urban Institute, 1975, p. 8). Even though "independent living rehabilitation" legislation failed, a number of programmatic gains affecting the ability of disabled individuals to obtain services and dollars and to make changes in the environment were achieved in rehabilitation, mass transit, Social Security, and Medicare legislation during this period. Money for attendants and for health care became more available to the disabled through other state and federal social programs. And in 1972, rehabilitation bills greatly expanding the concept of independent living services to the severely disabled were written.

1972

In 1972 HR 8395—written as a new act to replace the Vocational Rehabilitation Act (scheduled to expire June 30, 1972)—outlined a considerably expanded mandate for vocational rehabilitation, including comprehensive services to the severely handicapped. *Severely handicapped* were defined as: (1) having a physical or mental disability so serious that it limited substantially the ability to function in the family and community as one without such a serious disability may be expected to function; and (2) who, with the assistance of comprehensive rehabilitation services, can reasonably be expected to improve substantially the ability to live independently and function normally in the family and community (Barrett, 1975, Addendum, p. 5).[3]

Senate hearings considered a number of bills on the handicapped, including HR 8395 as reported out of the House committee. Emphasis on the severely handicapped gained momentum in the Senate subcommittee hearings. Not only were supplementary funds approved to provide comprehensive rehabilitation services for the severely handicapped without vocational objectives, but priority service to the severely handicapped was provided in the basic vocational rehabilitation program as well.

HR 8395 was reported out of conference on October 11, 1972, with no dissenting votes. Senator Alan Cranston, as Chairman of the conference committee, stated, "the crucial thrust of the conference report Title I program is to eliminate the creaming and shift the focus to harder cases in order to serve individuals with more severe handicaps."

Definitions in the bill are of particular interest. *Comprehensive rehabilitation services* meant vocational rehabilitation services and any other goods or services provided under the act that will make a substantial contribution in helping handicapped individuals to improve their ability to live independently or function normally with their family and community (Barrett, 1975, p. 13).

Handicapped individual meant any individual who: (1) has a physical or mental disability which for such individual constitutes or results in a substantial handicap to employment; and (2) can reasonably be expected to benefit from vocational rehabilitation services or comprehensive rehabilitation services.

Rehabilitation, for purposes of Title II of the bill, meant the goal of achieving, through the provision of comprehensive rehabilitation services, substantial improvement in the ability to live independently or function normally with the family or community on the part of the handicapped individual who was not capable of achieving a vocational goal at the present time (Barrett, 1975, p. 15).

The report on HR 8395 was agreed to unanimously by the Senate and House and presented for approval on October 14, 1972. President Nixon announced his pocket veto on October 27, 1972. President Nixon's Memorandum of Disapproval stated, in part:

> This measure would seriously jeopardize the goals of the vocational rehabilitation program and is another example of congressional fiscal irresponsibility. Its provisions would divert this program from its basic vocational objectives into activitives that have no vocational element whatsoever or are essentially medical in character. In addition, it would proliferate a host of narrow categorical programs which duplicate and overlap existing authorities and programs. Such provisions serve only to dilute the resources of the vocational rehabilitation program and impair its continued valuable achievements in restoring deserving American citizens to meaningful employment (Urban Institute, 1975, p. 9).

The vetoed bill was reconsidered by the 93rd Congress and while some changes were made, the independent living provisions were retained. Again President Nixon vetoed the bill (in this case, Section 7).

The Rehabilitation Act of 1973

Veto of HR 8395 resulted in a continuation of the existing Vocational Rehabilitation Act through July 1973 at 1972 funding levels. In 1973, failing at the second attempt to override the presidential veto, the House and Senate developed a compromise bill. It dropped the provisions for the new independent living comprehensive service program, but did mandate priority of service in the basic vocational rehabilitation service program to the severely disabled and included authorization for a major study of the comprehensive needs of the severely disabled (Section 130).[4]

Other sections of the Rehabilitation Act of 1973 that pertain especially to the goals of community integration and independent living are Sections 501, 502, 503, and 504, which call for affirmative action programs for employment of the disabled in the federal government and firms contracting with the government; provision of barrier-free work areas in such firms; removal of architectural and transportation barriers to the handicapped; creation of the Architectural and Transportation Barriers Compliance Board; and nondiscrimination on the basis of handicap for programs and activities receiving or benefiting from federal financial assistance (*Federal Register,* Wednesday, May 4, 1977, part IV).

1974 to the Present

In 1974 the Vocational Rehabilitation Act was amended. Of particular interest in these amendments was the authorization of a White House Conference on the Handicapped and a broader definition of *handicapped individual* to focus on substantial limitations of an individual's functioning in one or more major life activities rather than on handicap to employment, vocational objectives, or potential benefits from vocational rehabilitation services.

Since the amendments of 1974, there has been no major vocational rehabilitation legislation pertinent to independent living definitions or expansions of vocational rehabilitation scope of services to cover independent living services. There have been other major laws that have directly affected independent living capabilities. Among them:

- Education for all Handicapped Children Act of 1975 (Public Law 94–142), which calls for a sharply increased federal commitment to ensure that all handicapped children receive full and appropriate educational services.
- Developmentally Disabled Assistance and Bill of Rights Act (Public Law 94–103).
- Supplemental Security Income (SSI) amendments (among them, Public Law 94–566, Public Law 94–365, Public Law 94–569, and Public Law 94–585) extending SSI benefits to aged, blind, and disabled recipients in publicly operated community residences and a new assistance program for SSI-eligible children.
- National Housing Act Amendments of 1975 (Public Law 94–173), Title I, which includes provisions for the removal of barriers, hazards, and inconvenient features of housing for handicapped people.

In addition to these new laws, an Office of Independent Living was established in HUD in June 1977. Secretary Patricia Harris announced the creation of the office at the White House Conference and stated that the overall objectives of the office are to promote the creation of independent living centers across the country and to make more and better housing available to the handicapped.

President Jimmy Carter in late 1978 signed into law Public Law 95–602. Among other things, the law provides for independent living rehabilitation. The law requires state rehabilitation agencies to submit state plans for independent living to the Commissioner of the Rehabilitation Services Administration. These state plans will present a three-year proposal describing the services to be provided, present assurances of compliance with accessibility legislation, provide assurances that individual written rehabilitation programs will be developed for each client, and in other ways assure that the services will be comprehensive in scope and available to those who qualify. *These plans must* "provide assurances that handicapped individuals shall have a substantial role in developing the State plan."

A review of all major legislation benefiting the handicapped is compiled biannually by the Office for Handicapped Individuals (OHI), HEW (1974, 1975–76). For more detailed information about legislation pertaining to the handicapped, the reader is referred to these OHI summaries or to the legislation itself.

DEFINING THE TARGET POPULATION

It is the severely disabled for whom independent living services are so critical and for whom the programs discussed in this chapter have been designed. Yet, there are numerous definitional issues that have impeded policy planning and program development.

Definition of Terms

Most authors on independent living policies have adopted the following definitions of *disability, impairment, severity,* and *handicap:*

- *Impairment*—a physiological or anatomical loss or other abnormality or both.
- *Disability*—the limitation on an individual's capacity to perform some key life function caused by an impairment.
- *Handicap*—the limitation imposed by a disability on an individual's ability to carry on his or her usual activities.
- *Severity*—the degree of impairment, disability, or handicap; at the worst degree of severity, the above three terms are virtually synonymous.

These terms are used in this chapter and are consistent with materials from the Comprehensive Needs Study (Urban Institute, 1975), the HEW audit study of vocational rehabilitation services (Barrett, 1975), and others.

Measures of Severity

In mandating priority for the *severely handicapped*, the 1975 Rehabilitation Act called for a definition useful for eligibility decisions and for recording type of caseload. The present system is limited to an indication on a list of diagnostic categories which automatically or with qualification mean severely disabled, including all Social Security Disability Insurance (SSDI) beneficiaries and all blind and disabled SSI recipients as severe cases, and allows for other cases on the basis of functional limitation factors and the requirement of multiple vocational service over an extended time. In general, those doing substantive work in assessing how to implement policy regarding severe cases opt for emphasis on handicap, or the limitation imposed by a disability interacting with other variables to prevent carrying out activities. A comprehensive review of alternative approaches to the definition of severity was prepared by Beverly DeGraaf (Berkeley Planning Associates [BPA], January 1977).

Current definitional work within vocational rehabilitation centers on vocational goals. As DeGraaf points out, another debate in the field addressed by Congress in its deliberations prior to the passage of the 1973 law and by the literature is whether priority to severe cases should go to those for whom the only true goal might be some degree of independent living rather than employment. The Comprehensive Needs Study (Urban Institute, 1975) advocates opening up vocational rehabilitation to nonwork-related services, and many studies suggest definitional schemes for classifying severity which include independent living in the disability scale.

Estimates of the Target Population

What is the number of individuals potentially eligible for independent living services? The policy concern is obvious. What must the program coverage be? Except for the institutionalized population, which is readily counted, the severely disabled have not been accurately estimated in any census. One difficulty, of course, is the definitional issue mentioned above. The key reference on this topic is the fourth chapter of the Urban Institute's Comprehensive Needs Study report, "Estimates of the Severely Disabled Population Not in Institutions." The Urban Institute's estimates are for the noninstitutionalized, eighteen to sixty-four years of age, and were based on the methods of the Survey of Disabled Adults (SDA) of the Social Security Administration. The following definitions were used:

- *Most Severely Disabled*—those individuals who reported that their health kept them from working at all and who were either not in the labor force during the year prior to the survey or had become permanently disabled during that year.
- *Severely Disabled*—those individuals with a health condition which allowed them to work but only occasionally or irregularly. This group also includes those persons who had said that their health prevented them from working but who did not satisfy the other criteria necessary to be considered most severely disabled.
- *Partially Disabled*—those individuals who were able to work regularly but had a health condition which limited the amount or kind of work (including housework) they could do.

Using existing surveys and these definitions, the Urban Institute estimated the working-age noninstitutionalized population of severely disabled and most severely disabled in 1975 as shown in Table 1.

For the institutionalized, the Urban Institute estimate was 1,786,876, or 93.3 percent of the total population in institutions (Urban Institute, 1975, p. 87, Table 5–2).

These estimates from the Comprehensive Needs Study indicate the numbers of individuals who are potential clients for independent living services. The actual numbers are dependent upon the particular descriptions of "severity" and "need" used.

TABLE 1
Estimates of Noninstitutionalized Disabled Population, Aged 18 to 64, for July 1, 1975

	Number in Thousands	*Percent*
Total U.S. population	124,800	100.0
Total disabled population	23,300	18.7
Most severely disabled	4,200	3.4
Severely disabled	3,900	3.1
Partially disabled	15,200	12.2

Source: Urban Institute, 1975, p. 72, Table 4–4

Many of the severely disabled individuals have been "invisible," living isolated lives in institutions or at home, with little integration into the mainstream of society. In recent years, some of these individuals have organized and begun to form consumer organizations and self-help groups, and to lobby for programs that would improve their abilities to live full active lives in the community. The next section discusses some of the alternative forms for community-based delivery of services that have emerged through the efforts of the severely disabled themselves.

ALTERNATIVE DELIVERY STRATEGIES: MODELS FOR DELIVERY OF INDEPENDENT LIVING SERVICES

The independent living centers that have emerged throughout the country provide, for the disabled, the linkages with services and funding upon which they depend in order to live in the community. "Independent living" means freedom from isolation or from the institution; it means the ability to choose where to live and how; it means the individual's ability to obtain the services necessary to carry out activities of daily living that the nondisabled often take for granted.

Several sources provide a comprehensive overview of the range of service needs considered in independent living programs. The Comprehensive Needs Study report (Urban Institute, 1975) includes the results of surveys conducted on the service needs of individuals closed from service by vocational rehabilitation for reasons of severity, and also of individuals contacted through Comprehensive Medical Rehabilitation Centers (CMRC's). Laurie (1977) provides a review of "guidelines and experiences in independent living" which includes a discussion of many of the service systems. Everett and Collignon (1975) analyze the cost and policy considerations of major service needs for improving the capacity for independent living. The *BCIL Report* (Fay et al., 1977) contains a checklist of relevant services (included as a section of this chapter).

Each severely disabled individual has unique service needs and requirements for independent living goals. No one service prescription or housing situation will be the answer for everyone in an independent living program. Rather, the independent living movement has stressed individual *choice* of alternatives for each service.

One problem the independent living movement has faced is the existence of *gaps* in existing service systems and the lack of alternatives from which to choose. The Comprehensive Needs Study reviewed the many programs within HEW that provide services and financial assistance to the handicapped. The writers of the Comprehensive Needs Study found that the programs serving the severely handicapped are inequitable, contain severe gaps in services, suffer from inadequate control, and are operated with insufficient knowledge and resources (Urban Institute, 1975). Similar problems in children's service were found by the Rand Corporation in its study *Improving Services to Handicapped Children* (Brewer, 1974). The Comprehensive Needs Study report cites a major shortcoming in the design of programs for the disabled in the preoccupation with the medical aspect, "with emphasis on the *dis* rather than the *ability,* and a lack of attention to the social aspects."

In response to this disorganized and incomplete service delivery condition nationwide, there have been a variety of alternative service delivery models developed privately in nonprofit corporations and with local, state, and national governmental assistance and seed monies, to explore alternatives for delivery of independent living services and for making independent living in the community a possibility for the severely handicapped.

As we have discussed in the introduction, these organizations, or centers for independent living, provide a wide range of services, which may include:

> Activities of daily living, Architectural barriers/barrier free design, Attendant services, Chore services, Coalition development communications, Community organization, Consumer affairs information, Economic support services, Educational liaison, Employment services, Equipment repair, Home health aide, Homemaker, Housing development and adaptation, Independent living training, Information services, Legal services, Lobbying, Life support services, Medical services, Mobility skills, Outreach and recruitment, Personal care assistants (recruitment, selection, training), Public relations, Education, Recreation, Rehabilitation services, Sex education, Social services/State agency liaison, Transportation, Vocational liaison (Fay et al., 1977, p. 2).

This section discusses several of these alternative systems that have developed across the country. These programs exemplify what is happening in independent living. They provide laboratories for the demonstration of alternative approaches and visibility for the disabled in their continuing campaign for more independent living services.

Common to these programs is an emphasis on peer support and advocacy of the rights of persons with disabilities. Some of the major dimensions of difference among these programs are as follows:

• *Residential versus nonresidential setting*—Independent living may mean living in the community, in nonsegregated housing, or in specially adapted housing projects. Sometimes these housing units have been funded through HUD. These residential alternatives do not imply institutionalization but rather specialized housing. In many cases, the housing programs are integrated with service delivery.

• *Direct services versus referral to community services*—In some instances, services are provided directly by the organizations, and many include transportation, peer counseling, and wheelchair repair. Most services are provided by referral to important financial services and counseling programs, such as vocational rehabilitation and SSI.

• *Population served*—The organization may serve one disability group or severity level such as the blind, the deaf, or the spinal cord disabled, or may serve many disability groups. Some organizations may maintain traditional separation by disability. The trend, however, is to organize around commonly shared service needs.

• *Professional base versus consumer base*—In some organizational models, emphasis may be on professional service workers, such as counselors, medical workers, and therapists. In other organizations, there may be a consumer approach to service delivery with perhaps a "peer counselor" approach.

• *Vocational versus nonvocational emphasis*—Independent living services were traditionally viewed in vocational rehabilitation as other than vocational. However, many independent living achievements can relate directly to vocational goals. Organizations may vary in the extent to which their overall program, and individual service components, are related to vocational goals of the severely disabled.

• *Transitional versus ongoing services*—Another basic difference in the design of these organizations is the goal of providing transitional services (say, from onset of disability until some independent living skill is achieved) or permanent sustaining services (keeping continual contact with the client, providing ongoing services in referral, counseling, and support).

We will review several examples of independent living service models which have achieved national prominence because of their success in helping people with severe disabilities live more independently. These examples illustrate some of the basic ways that programs in independent living vary. Perhaps the major distinction in organizing the delivery of independent living support services is whether or not the service center is residential—that is, whether program participants live in the community or in housing provided by or in the center. Therefore, the following descriptions are arranged according to nonresidential and residential models.

Nonresidential

Center for Independent Living (CIL),
Berkeley, California

It has been stated by Laurie in *Housing and Home Services for the Disabled* (Laurie, 1977) that CIL in Berkeley is "the most effective self-help service program in the United States." There is no doubt that Berkeley's CIL is innovative and relatively comprehensive in its approach to independent living.

CIL serves approximately 3,500 persons in the San Francisco Bay Area and represents a broad coalition of disabilities, including spinal cord injury, post-polio, severe cerebral palsy, muscular dystrophy, multiple sclerosis, Fredericks ataxia, blind, deaf, multiply disabled, and the elderly.

The organization's goal is total integration of people with severe disabilities into community life, or *mainstreaming.* To this end, CIL provides basic services, such as family counseling, personal counseling, mobility training, attendant referrals and training, wheelchair repair, self-care counseling, preventive health care, transportation, job development services, referral to important social service agencies, and programs including vocational rehabilitation, and community advocacy. These and other CIL services are designed to stabilize the environment of an individual with severe disability, thereby minimizing the handicapping aspects of disability and helping the person to gain equal opportunity.

In its advocacy work on the local, state, and federal levels, CIL is actively involved in the efforts to remove architectural and attitudinal barriers and to gain equal rights for all people with disabilities. In its own community its advocacy efforts have been extraordinarily successful, and Berkeley is considered the most accessible community in the country.

CIL is not a residential center. Persons who use CIL's services or work for CIL live in houses and apartments throughout the community. The organization does offer a referral service of available accessible housing and provides housing renovation assistance to improve accessibility for clients.

In addition to these services, CIL considers itself a training institution for people with disabilities; every job is a training job leading, hopefully, to employment in the primary labor market. Currently, CIL employs 105 persons, half of whom are severely disabled. There are training programs in computer programing and paralegal services, and a university degree program coordinated with Antioch College/West. Many people with disabilities work as volunteers within the organization. All major executive offices, and the majority of executive board seats, are held by severely disabled individuals.

Under grants and special funding from various sources, CIL has developed a number of special projects. Significant funding includes an I&E grant from the California Department of Rehabilitation to design a strong and versatile electric wheelchair, a research and demonstration (R&D) grant from RSA, HEW, to demonstrate the effectiveness of CIL's peer counseling model for providing independent living services to the severely disabled (a part of the Comprehensive Needs Study), and a contract from the Veterans Administration (VA) to test reliability and acceptability of equipment provided by VA for the disabled.

In summary, CIL is a consumer operated service organization geared toward making support services in the community available to the disabled. Its services are both directly and indirectly provided. It utilizes community services whenever possible and aims at maximizing independence of the handicapped individuals via integration into the mainstream of the community. Other independent living programs in California have been modeled after CIL.

Residential

Most independent living models provide at least some direct residential services. As Lex Frieden points out in his paper "Independent Living Arrangements," "residence programs may be compared on two fundamental dimensions. These are dwelling type and life support service style. Dwelling types range from single family dwellings to dormitories. Life support service styles range from informal arrangements to highly organized programs . . . Those independent living arrangements which involve large groups in multiresident dwellings and employ many attendants in an organized program are more institutionalized than those arrangements which involve a single individual in a single family dwelling who depends on a neighbor to provide his care" (Frieden, 1975, p. 3).

New Options, Houston, Texas
(Cole, Holden, and Frieden, 1976)

In June 1976, the Texas Institute for Rehabilitation and Research (TIRR) in Houston began a model transitional living program, New Options, designed to foster the integration of severely physically handicapped individuals into their communities. Goals of integration may include the establishment of an independent living situation, involvement in educational and vocational opportunities, active social participation in the mainstream of society, the enhancement of important personal skills, and the medical stabilization required to maintain independent living gains. TIRR continues to support the program, which has received additional funding from RSA through an R&D grant.

Three years of experience with a previous R&D residential project, the Cooperative Living project, provided valuable background information in the design of the New Options program. Forty severely disabled young adults have lived in the Cooperative Living project since it opened in January 1972. Cooperative Living provided a first opportunity to begin involvement in advocacy, education, vocational training, or employment. Almost all of the Cooperative Living residents made important gains in independence during their stay in the project. The program removed many constraints that existed in residents' former living environments but contained no elements of structured transitional programing. Gains in independence thus occurred largely as a result of residents' own efforts over an average fifteen-month stay.

In New Options, a planned and structured program, incorporates many of the features fostering independence that operated implicitly in the earlier program, but is designed carefully to provide more information and experience and to enable participants to acquire important independent living skills in a much shorter period of time. Due to the structure, detailed studies can be made of controlled and directed transitional processes that in the Cooperative Living project were left largely to chance.

The New Options project is housed in TIRR's Maximum Independence Center, a dormitory-style building. Each project participant has a private room. The professional staff organizes group activities, and in addition, each of the staff is involved in goal setting and problem solving with participants on a one-to-one basis. The purpose of this counseling is to help individuals learn to solve problems on their own. In addition to the professional staff, a number of active handicapped persons from the community lead program activities.

A series of ten training modules are in place to show participants the range of options available in living arrangements, education/vocational training and employment, transportation, performance of physical tasks, meeting medical needs, and sexual relationships; and to help people develop new skills in managing financial affairs, managing attendants and budgeting energy, developing social skills and assertiveness, and goal setting and problem solving.

An important element of New Options, in addition to the program content, is the experience of living for six weeks in a dormitory-type setting with a nonprofessional attendant staff. Many participants have never been away from the personal care of family members or a nursing staff, and learning to manage attendants and direction of their own care is crucial to independent living.

Boston Center for Independent Living (BCIL) (Fay et al., 1977)

BCIL had its roots not only in the anger of disabled individuals "incarcerated" in public and private institutions but also in the frustration of rehabilitation professionals who found the noninstitutional community inaccessible to clients and patients following rehabilitation. All three co-founders had firsthand knowledge of the complexity of integrating persons with severe disabilities into the larger community. Paul J. Corcoran, M.D., now RT-7 Project Director, contributed his knowledge of medically acceptable alternative living situations and links to university support. Frederick A. Fay, Ph.D., now RT-7 Research and Training Director and a quadriplegic psychologist, brought energy and enthusiasm from firsthand knowledge of other centers for independent living. Rehabilitation counselor Bob McHugh, with his intimate knowledge of the state Vocational Rehabilitation system, was a link to avenues of cooperation and funding between agencies and the idea. Their goal was a base of operations—a program rather than a facility—for disabled individuals to bridge the gap between total dependence on an institution and independent living. The BCIL founders envisioned a consumer-run self-help community integrated with the able-bodied where severely disabled persons could develop independent living skills.

In September 1974, the first resident rolled into modified quarters in Boston University's theology building and BCIL was underway. In the three years since its founding, BCIL and the roughly fifty individuals who have participated in its program have demonstrated that independent living is a realistic and preferred goal for many severely disabled persons.

Today BCIL is a small, nonprofit corporation coordinating three separate phases of independence that have evolved over the years:

1. *Transitional living.* Providing the first basic steps in training for social and physical skills, transitional living began in modified dormitories at Boston University. As BCIL attracted disabled persons not necessarily interested in a full-time education this concept was expanded, and in March 1977 the first residents moved into a second transitional facility in Brookline Village, an apartment complex in a Boston suburb.

2. *Cluster housing.* For those who have mastered the skills of independent living, cluster housing offers greater independence. Located in East Boston, this is an apartment building with several apartments modified for handicapped persons, with a pool of personal care assistants and a night-time attendant.

3. *Independent living.* As facilities and funding for attendants became available in the greater Boston area, individuals began moving to accessible apartments, usually shared with a personal care assistant, where they now live as students and professionals.

Atlantis

Atlantis Community, Inc., Denver, Colorado, a private nonprofit program, was born out of actions taken by a group of disabled persons dissatisfied with traditional nursing home programs. This group joined forces with various organizations for the disabled—the Denver Chapter of the National Paraplegia Foundation, United Cerebral Palsy Association, Muscular Dystrophy Association, Vantage House Youth Wing Council, Young Disabled Adults from Life Center, Mobility Among the Disabled, Multiple Sclerosis Society, the Denver Community Design Center, and the Mayor's Commission on the Disabled.

The Atlantis housing service originally consisted of leasing seven first-floor apartments from the Denver Housing Authority. Now it offers a variety of residential living arrangements to the severely disabled. According to the project booklet, the goal of the community will be to "provide needed services while respecting the individual residents' freedom and privacy." Some of these needed services are provided directly by Atlantis, such as attendant care, transportation, housing, social activities, and counseling. Others are provided indirectly, such as medical care (via referral) and transportation by the Regional Transportation District, which has adapted some buses with special apparatus.

The project is financed by a variety of means. In the past, grants have been won from various federal agencies, such as the Denver Housing Authority. United Way has also contributed grant money in the past to help with attendant care.

The Atlantis Community serves severely disabled persons in the Boulder/Denver areas of Colorado. Many members of this project take an active political interest in all levels of government. The program's strategy is directed toward integration into society's mainstream, maximizing traditional avenues of approach, and implementing new ones when possible.

Campus Living

Campus programs have been tremendously important to the independent living movement. It wasn't until the University of California at Berkeley Cowell Hospital project, sponsored by the California Department of Rehabilitation, opened in 1962 that quadriplegic students were able to attend a university. Since that time, disabled students and others have convinced universities of the necessity of removing architectural barriers that impeded mobility on campus. Their success on campus has also affected nearby communities, which slowly have become more accessible for all disabled people. The same has been true of attitudinal barriers. As disabled students became more visible on campuses and in communities and succeeded educationally and socially, they broke down many of the attitudinal barriers of the general public toward all disabled.

Many of the service delivery programs discussed earlier had their roots in a campus-based program for disabled students. CIL grew out of the Physically Disabled Students Program (PDSP) at the University of California, Berkeley, and BCIL started its first program at Boston University.

The first campus-based program began operation in the early 1950s at the University of Illinois (Laurie, 1977, p. 147). This program has grown and continues to provide services.

UIREP and the Rehabilitation Education Center make it possible for qualified individuals with severe, permanent physical disabilities to pursue higher education and to benefit from all related experiences which are so much a part of college education and common to all students. The comprehensive approach of the program includes offering barrier-free access, both in its immediate setting and to all aspects of campus life. There are currently 150 students in wheelchairs totally integrated on the campus who live primarily in 28 large barrier-free dormitories. This program is an arm of the University and is headed by Dr. Timothy Nugent.

Tanbrier House at the University of Illinois serves several quadriplegics or severely handicapped persons. Tanbrier House is basically a consumer-run organization with nonprofessional attendant care. In Tanbrier, the various duties such as hiring and firing staff, bookkeeping, and ordering of food are shared by the residents.

These programs are examples of organizational models that have been emerging in the United States in the last few years. There are many other examples that could have been cited, and other alternatives to be explored. Additional information on programs such as these can be found in Laurie (1977), which includes an extensive review of independent living arrangements and transitional projects. *The BCIL Report* (Fay et al., 1977), Cole and Frieden (1977), Fay (1974), and the Comprehensive Needs Study report (Urban Institute, 1975) are also relevant references.

These emerging organizational strategies for the delivery of independent living services are very significant. They represent a variety of models that have been developed in response to the obvious need for the support services that will allow the severely disabled to live in the community and free of institutional walls. In many cases, these organizations have emerged as grass-roots organizations, in storefront offices, and have survived day-to-day and week-to-week on hope and on impermanent and sometimes fickle funding sources. That they have survived, and that new organizations continue to develop based on these pioneering models or expressing new organizational forms, attests to the real need for the services and the growing pressure for independence.

SYSTEMATIC EVALUATION OF ALTERNATIVES: SECTION 130, AND INNOVATION AND EXPANSION APPROACHES

In addition to these community alternatives for service delivery, there are a growing number of demonstration programs, "experiments" in various strategies for offering independent living services. Notable are the six "Section 130" demonstration programs funded as a part of the Comprehensive Needs Study (Urban Institute, 1976), and a commitment of vocational rehabilitation I&E grants monies to exploration of independent living options. Such I&E programs have been initiated by state rehabilitation agencies in California, Michigan and Massachusetts.

Section 130 Demonstration Projects

The Rehabilitation Act of 1973 authorized the Comprehensive Needs Study. This study addressed a number of the issues raised in the legislative process; however, some issues which could not be addressed were:

- Does Rehabilitation know how to serve the most severely handicapped?
- What organizational arrangements seem most efficient and effective for an ILR program?
- What other programs and services can support an independent living thrust?
- What services, especially what new services, may be required? Who should provide them?
- What manpower will be required and at what level can caseloads be handled?
- What are the approximate outcomes for given levels of expenditure? What are the costs for different types of outcomes?

- What limits should be placed on who is served (are there persons too severely handicapped to benefit even from ILR)?
- What are the objectives for an ILR Program for which reasonable accountability can be maintained?

Due to resource limitations not all of these issues could be included in the demonstration strategy. Six projects out of twenty-two applications were funded:

- One consumer-based model (CIL, Berkeley)
- Two models in CMRC's (University of Washington, New York State)
- Three models using the state vocational rehabilitation agency as the sole focus of responsibility for ILR (Utah, Texas Blind, Illinois)

The status and role of the projects as summarized in the Urban Institute's *First Year Report* (July 1976) on these projects are:

- Each project in the series illuminates more than one issue, some with greater emphasis than others.
- Each project highlights a possible service delivery model for establishment of an independent living program.
- Each project will demonstrate its ability to organize and meet objectives of an ILR-type program for persons not usually served in a state vocational rehabilitation program.
- Each project will describe experiences with other programs.
- Each project will be developing services not usually in the vocational rehabilitation program, illuminating general aspects of rehabilitation service technology.
- Each project will be developing information on cost and personnel implications.

Consumer-based Model: CIL, Berkeley, California

One of the six demonstration programs selected as part of the Comprehensive Needs Study is a demonstration of the effectiveness of the peer counseling approach to service delivery used at CIL, Berkeley, California. Peer counselors, who are themselves disabled individuals, work with severely disabled clients to assist them in learning independence skills and obtaining basic survival services and resources which can then enable the client to live independently in the community. In the CIL perspective, the rehabilitation system is seen as a network of public and private agencies in which several serious gaps exist. The peer counselor serves three important functions. First and most important, the peer counselor provides a role model, that of a disabled person (two of the four counselors are in wheelchairs, one a quadriplegic), working in an organization in a professional role and living an independent life. Secondly, the peer counselor provides training in a range of independent living skills. Thirdly, the peer counselor serves as the client's link to the services that are available either through CIL, the Department of Rehabilitation, or other resources and organizations in the community. The principal objectives of this project are to show that a consumer-based organization can deliver services which may not otherwise be provided to severely disabled persons and to facilitate independent living for these individuals within the community as well as to provide assistance in vocational exploration and job placement. Of the six projects originally funded under Section 130, this is the only project housed in a community-based consumer organization.

Comprehensive Medical Rehabilitation Center (CMRC) Projects

Because the more severely disabled are more likely to have a higher proportion of medical needs, one possible approach to the delivery of independent living services is through CMRC's. Two such projects are included in the Section 130 demonstrations. (Urban Institute, July 1976).

University of Washington Department of Rehabilitation Medicine, Seattle. This demonstration is conducting comprehensive evaluations of the rehabilitation needs of persons with severely handicapping conditions and organizing state agency activities as well as community resources to provide increased services and care to the handicapped. The Urban Institute lists the specific procedures to be used in this demonstration as follows:

1. Interviewing the severely handicapped to determine their medical, housing, transportation, educational, vocational, economic and other rehabilitation needs.
2. Recommendation of appropriate rehabilitation services, based on interviews and further information gathered from evaluations of client status. For example, if medical help is indicated during the interview, medical examination by appropriate specialists would be recommended.
3. Since vocational training and counseling are frequently needed, two types of evaluation may be used: administration of interest, aptitude, and achievement tests, and on-the-job observation.

Also, with the client's permission, observations of the work situation are performed. Assistance is provided, if needed, in job interviewing skills, resume preparation, and job seeking techniques by a vocational counselor.

4. To evaluate the helpfulness of rehabilitation services, interviews and evaluation are administered after services are provided. Services continue as long as there is need for them (pp. 3–4).

New York State Agency and the Institute for Rehabilitation Medicine (IRM). The focus of this project is the coordination of the CMRC with other rehabilitation facilities and other programs through the state rehabilitation agency itself. This tests both the coordination and case management aspects of a potential independent living program. While the Seattle project is designed as if the independent living program were assigned to medical centers alone, the New York project is designed as if a state rehabilitation agency were responsible but must work with the CMRC resource.

The basic structure of this demonstration is as follows:

> A state agency counselor is stationed with the IRM staff which includes a physician, public health nurse, social worker, physical therapist and other specialists as required. Clients will be primarily those with neuro-muscular diseases such as muscular dystrophy. Individuals go through a complete rehabilitation medicine workup, and receive medical services and equipment as appropriate, usually on an outpatient basis. Rehabilitation will be carried out with focus on the individual's home, family and work situation. Counseling in emotional adjustment to these progressive diseases, use of aids-to-daily-living, housing and transportation modification, and family counseling are included in project focus. (Urban Institute, July 1976)

State Agency Projects

An alternative way of administering independent living services is through the state agency responsible for the basic vocational rehabilitation program. That is, if the bill containing independent living provisions had not been vetoed in 1972, how might the state program be handling independent living services? (pp. 5–6)

Utah State Vocational Rehabilitation Agency. The project that Utah State proposed for demonstration is aimed at provision of specialized and timely programs to include a full range of comprehensive rehabilitation services for a limited number of very severely disabled and handicapped people.

The purpose is not to serve active state vocational rehabilitation cases but rather to operate parallel to the vocational rehabilitation program, borrowing useful models such as the client-counselor model and innovating when necessary. During the project demonstration period, the project is developing and implementing a practical system for identifying and assessing the total needs of the most severely handicapped.

The client population for this project includes individuals whose rehabilitation cases have been closed due to severity of disability—those with catastrophic disabilities including central nervous system dysfunction, multiple orthopedic or muscular loss, muscular dystrophy, multiple sclerosis, cerebral palsy, epilepsy, severe cardiovascular conditions, severe kidney disease, severe rheumatoid arthritis, deaf, blind, and other severe neurological or orthopedic loss or disability.

The project provides services that are not routinely available to all rehabilitation clients, such as assistance in mobility, communication, social activities, and those activities necessary to maintain and restore general life functions. Vocational goals may be achieved, but clients are expected to gain in their ability to become more self-sufficient.

Texas Blind Agency. The individuals served by the Texas Blind Agency in its demonstration project are blind and with one or more of the following secondary disabilities: chronically mentally ill, central nervous system dysfunction, multiple orthopedic disability, severe developmental disabilities, severe cardiac disorder, chronic pulmonary disease, and/or severe auditory impairment.

This project provides a comprehensive milieu of services to test the feasibility of rehabilitation services for these individuals, who, because of multiple handicaps, are traditionally restricted from vocational rehabilitation due to severity of disability. The purpose is to determine the individual needs, develop a program to meet these needs, and provide training in independent living.

The method used focuses on a team approach combined with assessments of the individual client's need. Rehabilitation professionals are available to work with every client to meet his or her individual needs. The project utilizes three areas of expertise developed in the Texas Commission for the Blind:

- Vocational rehabilitation services to the blind multiply handicapped, as exemplified by Sunrise, which serves blind profoundly or severely retarded institutionalized young persons.
- A long-established commitment to involve all available community resources.
- The team approach, which has been utilized by the Texas Blind Agency in its basic program. The project expects to demonstrate

that the provision of concentrated individualized services can help clients achieve a functional level of independent living, and in some cases reentry into the traditional vocational rehabilitation process.

Illinois State Vocational Rehabilitation. The Illinois Vocational Rehabilitation agency proposed the implementation of two-way interactive cable television to individuals with the most severe handicaps who are either homebound or confined to long-term care facilities. A pilot project was planned in Peoria, Illinois, to provide services and training to people in a range of living situations. Planned services included instruction to family members in physical therapy; instruction in activities of daily living; and training for semi-skilled and high-skilled jobs such as insurance claims adjustment, microfilming, and data entry processes. The project was discontinued due to implementation difficulties.

Innovation and Expansion Projects

Vocational rehabilitation I&E funds are being used currently to explore independent living strategies. There is potential for more development through I&E. In California, the State Department of Vocational Rehabilitation in June 1976 made grants totaling $645,115 in I&E funds "to establish and maintain community-based and consumer managed centers for the provision of the vocational and independent living services." The I&E grants only partially fund these programs, which are also seeking support from individuals, corporations, local government, and foundations in their geographic area.

In awarding these grants, the California Department of Rehabilitation was attempting to replicate the effectiveness of CIL in Berkeley, California, but recognized that the new groups would vary considerably in both organization and services delivered due to the particular characteristics of their geographic location. These centers were established in nine communities with a broad geographical spread. The groups applying for these funds also varied: three student-affiliated groups; two existing nonstudent disabled organizations; one comprehensive rehabilitation facility; and two groups of severely disabled individuals who formed for the purpose of the grant. From October 1976 to June 1977, 1,615 clients were served by the nine projects. The Table 2 shows the location, number of clients, services provided, and admission criteria for each project.

These projects provide direct (i.e., counseling, transportation) and indirect (i.e., community services for transportation, medical care, etc.)

TABLE 2
Numbers and Types of Clients Served and Services Provided at Independent Living Projects in California (Innovation and Expansion) (California State Department of Rehabilitation)

City Where Project Located	*Number of Clients Served 10/1/76–6/30/77*	*Services Provided*	*Admission Criteria*
Fresno	N/R	1. Establish a center for physically handicapped. 2. Provide peer counseling and advisory services. 3. Assist in obtaining qualified attendant care. 4. Information library and newsletter. 5. Promote public awareness and sensitivity to needs of handicapped. 6. Coordinate agency services that affect disabled people. 7. Recruit and utilize volunteers to help operate the center.	Need for services
Mt. Diablo	131	1. Provide supportive services for the severely disabled to enable them to function as heads of households, attend school, seek and retain employment, perform volunteer services, and undertake most other activities as any other able-bodied person. 2. Advocacy for the disabled population to existing organizations and institutions. 3. Intend to offer counseling and advisory services, physical assistance, mobility services, housing information and training, and centralized information regarding other services and resources.	Individual's need for services (physical, emotional, financial, social and educational needs will be considered).
Sacramento	80	1. Establish center for service delivery. 2. Outreach to disabled individuals previously overlooked. 3. Compile registers of attendants, readers, interpreters, drivers, accessible housing, sources for equipment. 4. Establish services for personal maintenance (attendant care, counseling, advocacy).	Any individual who is unable to accomplish a given personal objective due to limitations imposed by some physical, sensory, or communications disability.

TABLE 2 Continued

City Where Project Located	*Number of Clients Served 10/1/76–6/30/77*	*Services Provided*	*Admission Criteria*
Sacramento (continued)		5. Mobility (specialized transportation, mobile repair service). 6. Newsletter, publications library.	
San Diego	227	1. Advocacy for clients to various community agencies. 2. Information and referral: maintaining central resource library, laws and codes, legislative information, accessible shopping, doctors, housing; maintaining reader, interpreter, attendant lists. 3. Mobility services with purchase of a van. 4. Counseling by both peer and nondisabled for vocational, sexual, interpersonal problems, and assertiveness training.	As above
San Francisco	215	1. Along with San Francisco Chapter of CAPH, they have undertaken jointly to establish a self-help center with ultimate goal of integration of San Francisco residents with physical disabilities into the full life of the community. 2. Services will include attendant referral and assistance, independent living skills training, peer counseling, financial counseling and assistance, housing and architectural accessibility, assistance in job placement. 3. Intend to extend and supplement the programs of Berkeley CIL in their respective areas. They will also exchange information of serving disabled and of successful advocacy with other organizations and institutions.	Any person with a physical disability who feels a need for the services offered. Preference will be given to those persons residing in the City and County of San Francisco.
Santa Rosa	203	1. Roster of attendants. 2. Advocacy for recognition of attendants (wages, skill training). 3. Wheelchair and equipment repair and service.	Dependent upon need.

TABLE 2 Continued

City Where Project Located	Number of Clients Served 10/1/76–6/30/77	Services Provided	Admission Criteria
Santa Rosa (continued)		4. Liaison with low-cost housing managers and officials. 5. Information and referral services and library. 6. Advocacy and Ombudsman service with systems and agencies affecting handicapped people. 7. Communications network between handicapped people within the county.	
Van Nuys	72	1. Outreach for severely disabled. 2. Financial counseling. 3. Recruitment and screening of attendants/homemakers; maintaining lists for referral. 4. Inspection of apartments and housing for suitability of use by disabled clients. Inspect and offer consultation on new construction. 5. Refer disabled clients to appropriate agencies for services. 6. Publish monthly newsletter. 7. Provide 24-hour answering service. 8. Maintain speaker's bureau to speak on problems of handicapped before public agencies, private groups, in hospitals. 9. Provide counseling service.	Anyone asking for services in person, in writing, or on the telephone.
Watts	564	1. Peer counseling, individual family and group counseling. Drop-in rap sessions. 2. Pre-vocational counseling. 3. Financial aid counseling. 4. Referral services for attendants/homemakers, readers for the blind, interpreters for the deaf, service people to do minor modifications; referral to proper agencies, listing of accessible housing. 5. Reference library will catalog journals, books, and articles relevant to the needs of the disabled.	Any physically disabled adult may apply.

TABLE 2 Continued

City Where Project Located	*Number of Clients Served 10/1/76–6/30/77*	*Services Provided*	*Admission Criteria*
Watts (continued)		6. Equipment Loan Bank; donated "sickroom" equipment will be stored and available for loan. 7. Attendant recruitment service and management course. Attendants will be recruited and screened. 8. Self-help health program; a lecture series on preventive medicine for the disabled. 9. Low-vision aides will be provided for partially-sighted. 10. TTY terminal and limited interpreter time will be provided for the deaf. 11. A wheelchair-accessible van will be bought for transportation. 12. Surveys conducted for lists of accessible housing.	
Los Angeles	123	1. Outreach to identify, serve, and refer disabled clients to appropriate agencies. 2. Provide crisis intervention services by hot-line counseling and/or in-home counseling. 3. Provide counseling services to overcome problems of disabled in socialization, family relations, sexual adjustment, and spiritual adjustment. 4. Provide activities of daily independent living skills to families of disabled. 5. Provide advocacy and referral services. 6. Provide special interest workshops to the disabled. 7. Develop a goal attainment scaling model appropriate for use with the minority disabled.	A person must be disabled and live in, or be a student at, a school, college, or university located within the target area.
Summary, all projects	1,615		Need for services offered; sometimes residence criteria on addition

Source: California Department of Rehabilitation.

services. However, each of the nine projects may emphasize or not include whatever services it so desires. For example, one project emphasizes a medical supplies service, while others emphasize housing, homemaker chores, and attendant services. These nine centers are, as far as line functions go, autonomous, reporting only to the Department of Rehabilitation quarterly on budgetary matters.

Currently there are plans for RSA funding of a systematic evaluation of the California I&E experience.

The state of Michigan and Massachusetts have also allocated I&E funds for development of independent living services.

While these programs do represent increasing government commitment to exploring the potential of independent living service delivery, there remain basic questions about the costs of such services if provided throughout the nation. The Section 130 projects, now well into their third year, routinely collect cost information and should provide meaningful program planning data. In addition to evaluation of program impact and demonstration of a program's ability to serve severely disabled clients and to fill gaps existing currently in rehabilitation services, the Section 130 projects and the many other independent living programs in the country can provide needed information on the costs of coordinating or directly delivering independent living services.

COSTS AND BENEFITS OF INDEPENDENT LIVING

Traditional economic justification of vocational rehabilitation services for the disabled has rested on the program's focus on gainful employment. As we have seen, the vocational mandate in rehabilitation services has persisted despite legislative attempts since 1959 to extend rehabilitation benefits to persons for whom no vocational objective is obvious. This vocational emphasis brings with it an eligibility requirement that clients be "feasible"—that is, potentially employable. Those individuals disabled to the degree that their participation in the labor force is considered "infeasible" are refused services.

With the 1973 change in mandate to serve, as a priority, the severely disabled, there has been some experience in the system with economic costs associated with such services. But because of the formative nature of independent living concepts and programs, the economics of independent living is still an emerging field. Traditional economic analysis of vocational rehabilitation stresses gainful employment, reflecting vocational rehabilitation's legislative mandate. Even if the legislative mandate is expanded to permit independent living closures, difficulties in defining independent living gain and its dollar values present a major obstacle in economic analysis. Such analysis is critical. As Berkowitz et al. point out (White House Conference, *Awareness Papers,* 1977):

> Clearly chances of handicapped individuals achieving their goals are enhanced if they can establish that expenditures made on their behalf are justified and thus provide the basis for continued and expanded efforts on their behalf (p. 234).

Most benefit-cost ratios computed for the basic program in vocational rehabilitation show a substantial return to society for investment in services. Conservative estimates indicate a benefit-cost ratio of 5 to 1. Berkowitz (White House Conference, *Awareness Papers,* p. 234) agrees with the conservative figure, but cites ratios as high as 70:1. These benefits are based on earnings of rehabilitated clients. In considering a program of independent living, outcomes other than gainful employment may be included. A conclusive benefit-cost analysis has not been done. But policy makers and analysts have expressed concern about the costs of such programs.

Costs

Cost is a major policy issue. The Comprehensive Needs Study developed cost estimates by considering a program to serve only the eighteen-to-sixty-four age group of 68,000 individuals closed for severity by vocational rehabilitation in 1972. With *modest assumptions* of care needs—two round trips per week by taxi, one hour a day for an attendant, one hour per week for a home health aid, one meal per day brought to the home, four hours of counseling per year, and, for 10 percent of the individuals $1,000 in college tuition—the total estimated cost per year was $115,100,000 (Turem, 1976).

An internal RSA memo on "Independent Living," dated July 1977, cites this cost estimate in discussing current policy and costs of programs. It is important to realize how conservative the figure of $115.1 million really is, in considering provision of independent living services to the population in need. The Urban Institute emphasized that these costs are associated with modest assumptions of care needs of only 68,000 individuals. In fact, the costs indicated are those associated with maintaining an independent life style with a relatively low level of services (for instance, the estimate assumed one hour of attendant care per day; many individuals with severe disability require attendant care for five or more hours per day). These are unit costs for a low level of service use, not total estimates for a program that provided CIL-type services across the country.

To give some idea of the difference in scale between the Urban Institute estimate and the likely real social costs of such services, some benchmark statistics from the State of California Homemaker/Chore services will be helpful. The Homemaker/Chore program, as has been mentioned, pays for attendant care and has provided, in California, the attendant system that makes independent living possible for many in the state. In 1976–1977, this program spent $115 million dollars, serving 72,000. Fully 65 percent of the population served were elderly, 30 percent disabled, and 5 percent blind. Approximately 9 percent of all served were severely disabled, needing twenty hours per week of Homemaker/Chore services. In 1977–1978 projected expenditures were $140 million. Estimates from Homemaker/Chore services indicate that the severely disabled individuals served in 1976–1977 used 32 percent of the funds, or $36 million dollars.[5] These figures should indicate how conservative the Comprehensive Needs Study estimates really were. The figures indicate *not* the level of resources needed for independent living but merely for some support services.

Some of the more specific reports prepared as a part of the Comprehensive Needs Study do provide more detail of the sort needed for a more comprehensive cost estimate. For example, Everett and Collignon (1975) conducted an extensive study entitled *Cost and Policy Considerations in Improving the Capacity for Independent Living of the Most Severely Handicapped.* In this study the authors have presented estimates of independent living needs and the costs and benefits of implementing the following programs for independent living needs of individuals most severely handicapped: transportation, relocation, architectural barriers and housing, medical care, employment, and other consumption activities. As a part of the Comprehensive Needs Study, this study analyzes the costs and some of the impacts of the various alternative services mentioned above and the approaches for meeting the needs of the most severely handicapped.

In a related study, *Cost Analysis of Alternative Transportation Systems for the Handicapped,* by Jones (1975), various ways of improving the mobility of the 7,600,000 persons in the United States who suffer from chronic mobility limitations are looked at primarily with consideration of the impact and cost of each alternative. The alternatives discussed are: curb modification, wheelchairs, modified automobiles and vans, fixed-route transit system, demand-responsive systems, and mobility counseling. With specific regard for independent living this paper states that "the non-economic social benefits accruing to over 3 million unemployable handicapped persons provide compelling reasons for implementation of a national program" (p. 62). The paper concludes that a national mobility-improvement program should include curb modification, door-to-door transportation service, the phasing-in of the "transbus," limited subsidies for modified automobiles and vans, and the provision of power wheelchairs and mobility counseling to those persons needing them. The analysis indicates that such a program would return substantial social and economic benefits, including a $6.4 billion increase in the earnings of the handicapped.

The paper also concludes that adapting existing subways and buses, and building accessibility into new subway systems, are not cost-effective solutions to the mobility problems of the handicapped.

Looking at costs from another point of view, Frieden, in a paper titled "Independent Living Arrangements for the Severely Disabled" (1975), speaks of housing for the disabled not solely as housing but an entire "life support system." According to Frieden, the suitability of the housing determines the independency or dependency of its occupants. The author presents a philosophic and pragmatic approach to independent living which includes an everyday cost breakdown of living expenses, such as attendance fees and scheduling, food expenses, and transportation costs. The author compares the costs and benefits in quasi-economic terms for multiresidences (i.e., occupied by more than one individual) versus living alone. As might be expected, costs are higher in single-unit dwellings as compared to multiresidences. Benefits in this study are basically seen as intangibles: freedom, privacy, social interaction, and self management, whereas costs are measured in dollars.

Benefits

Frieden's paper points out a central problem in the economic analysis of independent living programs: the measurement of "intangible" or no-dollar benefits associated with a disabled person's gain—in self-esteem, in choice.

Estimation of an Individual's Nonincome Gains

The *Valuation of Homemaker Services* (Loshin and Collignon, 1975) illustrates that services not traditionally included in the economic arena can indeed be given a dollar value. Estimation attempts in this study have included opportunity cost estimation of women who are homemakers and, alternatively, the replacement cost estimation of homemakers. The findings of this study offer recommendations for methods of calculating accurate replacement cost estimates.

Another relevant study, contracted by RSA, is being conducted as a part of the development and refinement of vocational rehabilitation program evaluation standards (BPA, 1977). This work includes consideration of standards for measuring nonvocational or independent living outcomes. The work builds on a previous study of nonvocational outcome measurement conducted for the California Department of Rehabilitation (Schmidt, 1976).

Attempts to measure benefits of other than gainful employment represent an important step in the economic analysis of independent living. It is important to consider that from a social cost point of view independent living programs may create a net social gain due to:

Reduction of costs of institutionalization. Many argue that, in fact, it costs more to maintain an individual in an institution than to provide the services and dollars that the same person needs to live independently (Laurie, 1977).

Support for gainful employment. Many severely disabled individuals, when given adequate equipment and services, are a part of the active work force. Countless others want such an opportunity. The benefits and costs of the gainfully employed severely disabled should be reviewed more carefully. Studies conducted with Washington and Michigan State Vocational Rehabilitation data showed that severely disabled individuals are not more difficult to rehabilitate for employment than other vocational rehabilitation clients, although closure is more costly (Collignon, Dodson, and Skaburskis, 1975).

Much work remains to be done on the economics of independent living. Economic justification of investment in independent living programs is an important policy concern. But we should be equally aware of the importance to the disabled person of the choices and the independence that the nondisabled take for granted. Some of the intangibles associated with self-esteem and independent living gain will never be a part of a benefit-cost calculation, but they are centrally important in the lives of the individuals with severe disability.

CONCLUSION

The Rehabilitation Act of 1973 provided the basis, within vocational rehabilitation, to investigate extension of independent living services to the severely disabled. A number of notable events provide landmarks in the rapid change in independent living from an idea to a more and more clearly defined expression of need for services, legislation, and resources. These landmarks in the articulation and development of independent living include:

- The Comprehensive Needs Study and its five ongoing demonstration projects, based in hospitals, state vocational rehabilitation programs, and in a consumer-run organization.

• The first national Conference on Independent Living, sponsored by RSA and held at the Claremont Hotel in Berkeley, California, in October 1975. The newly emerging concept of independent living clashed with more traditional, maintenance-based concepts in this conference.

• The inclusion of independent living topics in important national rehabilitation planning conferences. For instance, at the 1977 National Conference of the Council of State Administrators of Vocational Rehabilitation (CSAVR), an entire afternoon agenda was devoted to discussion of independent living and where, governmentally, an independent living program might be housed.

• The increasing interest in exploring independent living alternatives, as in the recent allocation of state I&E dollars to the development of independent living programs, and the evaluation of the program's ability to deliver needed services and to integrate independent living services with the vocational rehabilitation basic program.

• Development of new professions, such as peer counseling, in which disabled individuals counsel other disabled individuals on activities of daily living, disability experience, and provide role models for independent living.

• The inclusion, in the White House Conference on the Handicapped, of papers on housing and service needs for independent living and the economics of disability.

• The recent opening, within HUD, of an Office of Independent Living.

• The recent successful mobilization of disabled people nationally, in San Francisco, California, and then Washington, D.C., to force the long-delayed implementation of Section 504 of the Rehabilitation Act of 1973.

• RSA funding of a second national Independent Living Conference, held in 1978 in Texas.

While these are all indicators of rapid advances in independent living, there is still much to be done. More alternatives should be explored. The existing centers for independent living have begun to develop intervention strategies and support systems. There are many arrangements and programs that should be tried. Among them are:

- Research on the appropriate outcome measures of independent living rehabilitation.

- Exploration of the relationship of aspects of independent living programs, such as peer counseling, to the vocational rehabilitation basic program.

- Investigation of new strategies for intervention.
- Data and analysis of the costs of providing independent living services.
- Longitudinal information on the benefits of independent living services.
- Clarification of the major definitional issues impeding implementation of independent living legislation.
- More investigation as to the organizational structures most effective and efficient in the provision of independent living services, through an expanded program of experiments and demonstration projects.

While many of these questions remain unanswered, the evidence seems to indicate that centers for independent living, following the definition described in these pages, provide the most viable and dynamic answer to consumer choice and participation.

Following is a checklist, developed by Frederick Fay, which outlines many of the major parameters and issues which must be dealt with in establishing an independent living program. Some consumers have criticized the checklist as being too simplistic to serve as a guide in actually establishing such a program. However, it is considered a very good overview to acquaint the reader with the types of considerations which must be confronted.

CHECKLIST FOR DEVELOPING INDEPENDENT LIVING PROJECTS[6]

I. Review literature on other centers for independent living.

II. Develop nucleus of committed people who are willing to work.

A. Develop selection criteria for board, officers, and advisory committee (consumer majority? provider support? abilities? disability representation? interest? commitment? fiscal management skills?).
B. Determine initial officers (President, Clerk, Treasurer . . .).
C. Identify and involve potential members for Board of Directors and Advisory Committees.
   1. Representatives of key consumer constituencies (National Paraplegia Foundation, National Association of the Physically Handicapped, National Association of the Deaf, Paralyzed Veterans of America, American

Council of the Blind, Disabled in Action, and/or other consumer organizations).

2. Representatives of provider organizations (State Departments of Vocational Rehabilitation, Medicaid, Social Services, Regional Rehabilitation Research and Training Center, state or local housing authorities, area rehabilitation facilities, Easter Seal Society, and/or other service providers).

III. Discuss and agree on the center for independent living's program philosophy, purposes and target population.

A. Develop written preliminary program description.
B. Interest and involve broad base of support.

IV. Select and develop an appropriate organization structure for carrying out the center's purposes.

A. Review state and federal laws on incorporation and tax status of organizations (e.g., 501(c)3 vs. 501(c)4).
B. Prepare the center's articles of incorporation and by-laws. Some of the areas by-laws should cover are:
   1. name of the organization
   2. principal office location
   3. applicable definitions
   4. fiscal issues
   5. purposes of the organization
   6. leadership responsibilities
   7. membership responsibilities
   8. process for calling meetings
   9. process for board and/or membership nominations, elections, voting, resignations, suspension and removal
   10. authority to enter into financial agreements
   11. personal liability
   12. process for amending by-laws
C Submit organizational papers to appropriate authorities for incorporation, tax status, and employee identification number.
D. Affiliate with state coalition or national organization.

V. Establish short and long term goals and objectives for the center (one, three and five year plans).

A. Determine what services other organizations in the area provide adequately.
B. Determine which services the center will advocate for and which it will provide itself:

Activities of daily living, Architectural barriers/barrier free design, Attendant services, Chore services, Coalition development communications, Community organization, Consumer affairs information, Economic support services, Educational liaison, Employment services, Equipment repair, Home health aide (Fiscal conduit services), Homemaker, Housing development and adaptation, Independent living training, Information services, Legal services, Lobbying, Life support services, Medical services, Mobility skills, Outreach and Recruitment, Personal care assistants (recruitment, selection, training), Public relations/education, Recreation, Rehabilitation services, Sex education, Social services/State agency liaison, Transportation, Vocational liaison.

C. Determine funding sources for each high priority service objective; to pay for program services, develop fundable proposals and contracts with private foundations and public agencies. Some of the many options to consider include:
    1. individuals
    2. private sector (foundations, civic groups)
    3. State Vocational Rehabilitation Agency
    4. State Housing Finance Agency
    5. City Housing Authority
    6. Department of Community Affairs
    7. Department of Housing and Urban Development
    8. Rehabilitation Services Administration
    9. Veteran's Administration
    10. Department of Public Health
    11. Bureau of Developmental Disabilities
    12. Department of Labor-Comprehensive Employment Training Act
    13. CETA (10)
    14. Department of Public Welfare
        a. Medicaid (Title XIX)
        b. Social Services (Title XX)
    15. Rehabilitation Research and Training Centers
    16. Department of Health, Education and Welfare

D. Secure adequate start-up funds.

VI. Develop a comprehensive written program plan to meet the center's advocacy and service objectives. This plan should include a description for proposed implementation describing:

A. Priority activities to be undertaken.
B. Persons responsible for carrying out activities (board, committees, executive directors, staff volunteers).
C. Methods used in carrying out activities.
D. Location of implementation of activities.
E. Anticipated time duration of activities.

VII. Draw up a budget for the center's comprehensive program plan and organizational operating costs. Make cost projections for the long term plans (three and five year plans).

VIII. Develop and implement a management system to administer the center's plan. Systems to provide accountability should be *in writing* and should include:

A. Program Content
   1. internal record keeping system (data collection) on program utilization
   2. a process to prepare external program reports at appropriate times
   3. calculations of specific program costs
   4. evaluation processes to measure program effectiveness and growth
   5. standards for quality service
   6. written program descriptions
   7. an operational planning process
   8. geographical scope of program

B. Program Participant
   1. confidentiality protection
   2. standard means to periodically review client policies
   3. program eligibility criteria
   4. standardized forms
   5. efficient application admission and graduation procedures
   6. measures of performance
   7. objectives of participation

C. Fiscal Controls
   1. accounting procedures with back-up information on cash receipts, cash disbursements, payroll, closing procedures, budgets, etc.
   2. use of standard report forms
   3. annual audit by certified persons
   4. a control system for making and receiving payments
   5. a plan to correct deficiencies
   6. a plan to seek continuing financial support (grant, fee for services, etc.)

D. Facility Operations
   1. appropriate site location
   2. costs to occupy
   3. signed lease
   4. office procedures regarding correspondence, hours, absences
   5. inventory of all equipment
   6. building safety and appropriate insurance

E. Personnel Policies
   1. hiring practices
   2. benefits plan
   3. assurance of compliance with federal and state laws
   4. job descriptions

5. job evaluations
6. appropriate supportive equipment
7. staff training
8. system to measure job performance
9. staff reporting
10. salary and pension plans

IX. Develop an assessment system to measure progress toward objectives.

A. Review at least annually.
B. Prepare an annual report.

X. Select effective staff.

NOTES

[1]From Mr. Roberts' Foreward to the monograph *Independent Living* in the "Emerging Issues in Rehabilitation" series, Washington, D.C., 1977.

[2]This legislative review draws heavily from the reviews included in the *Report of the Comprehensive Service Needs Study* (The Urban Institute, 1975) and in Barrett (1975).

[3]A detailed review of the legislative history of the ill-fated 1972 bill, as well as the 1973 act, can be found in Linda Barrett, *Legislative Review,* Berkeley Planning Associates, September 1975.

[4]Included in this Comprehensive Needs Study are six demonstration projects, which are reviewed later in this chapter.

[5]Mike Perine, California Department of Health, Sacramento, CA.

[6]Frederick Fay et al. *The BCIL Report,* ed. Peter Reich. Boston: Regional Medical Rehabilitation Research and Training Center No. 7, Tufts, July 1977.

REFERENCES

American Society of Landscape Architects Foundation. *Barrier Free Site Design.* Washington, D.C.: U.S. Government Printing Office, 1974.

Arneson, Kathleen. "Residential Choices and the Handicapped," *American Rehabilitation* 2(1); September–October, 1976: 25–29.

Baker, M., Fischetti, M. A., Williams, L. A., and Young, E. M. *State and Local Efforts to Eliminate Architectural Barriers to the Handicapped.* Washington, D.C.: National League of Cities, Department of Urban Studies, 1974.

Barrett, Linda W. *Legislative Review of the Specific Provisions for Priority to Individuals with Most Severe Handicaps and the Individualized Written Rehabilitation Program.* Berkeley Planning Associates, September 1975.

Berkeley Planning Associates (BPA). *Vocational Rehabilitation Program Evaluation Standards: A Critique of the State of the Art.* RSA Contract #105–76–4116. January 7, 1977.

Brewer, Garry D., and Kakalik, James S. *Improving Services to Handicapped Children, Summary and Recommendations.* R-1401-HEW. Santa Monica, Calif.: Rand, May 1974.

Center for Independent Living, Berkeley, California. *Report of the State of the Art Conference, Center for Independent Living, October 21–23, 1975.* RSA Grant 45-P-45484/9–01.

Cole, J. A., and Frieden, Lex. *Transitional Living: A Program Fostering Community Integration of Severely Physically Handicapped Persons.* Houston: Texas Institute for Rehabilitation and Research, June 1977. Interim Report on RSA Project Grant #13P57889/6–01 (RT 4).

Cole, J. A., Holden, B. L., and Frieden, Lex M. *The New Options Project: A Live-In Program to Foster Social Adaptive Skills.* Paper presented at scientific sessions of 53rd Annual Session of the American Congress of Rehabilitation Medicine and the 38th Annual Assembly of the American Academy of Physical Medicine and Rehabilitation, San Diego, November 7–12, 1976.

Collignon, Frederick C., Dodson, Richard, and Skaburskis, Andrejs. *An Evaluation of the Costs and Effectiveness of Vocational Rehabilitation Service Strategies for Individuals Most Severely Handicapped, (IMSH).* Berkeley: Berkeley Planning Associates, May 1975. Subcontract to the Urban Institute, Comprehensive Needs Study HEW-SRS-74-54-3.

Council of State Administrators of Vocational Rehabilitation (CSAVR). "Independent Living Rehabilitation Survey Results" *CSAVR Memorandum* CSA77–40, August 4, 1977.

"Eliminating Barriers," *American Rehabilitation* 1(2), November–December, 1975, 32.

Everett, Todd H., and Collignon, Frederick. *Cost and Policy Considerations in Improving the Capacity for Independent Living of the Most Severely Handicapped.* Berkeley: Berkeley Planning Associates, May 1975.

Farber, Douglas A. *Housing and Related Services for Exceptional Persons: A Source Book.* Monticello, Ill.: Council for Planning Libraries, 1973.

Fay, Frederick. *Housing Alternatives for Individuals with Spinal Cord Injury.* Boston: Tufts Rehabilitation Research and Training Center, 1974.

Fay, Frederick, et al. *The BCIL Report,* ed. Peter Reich. Boston: Regional Medical Rehabilitation Research and Training Center No. 7, Tufts, July 1977.

Fink, Charlotte, Manus, Muriel R., and Manus, Gerald I. *Housing for Disabled Persons: Annotated Bibliography.* New York: United Cerebral Palsy Association, 1975.

Frieden, Lex. "Independent Living Arrangements for the Severely Disabled," *Report on the State of the Art Conference, Center for Independent Living, October 21–23, 1975.* RSA Grant 45-P-45484/9-01.

George Washington University. Rehabilitation Research and Training Center. *Development of Modern Vocational Objectives For Severely Disabled Homebound Persons: Remote Computer Programming, Microfilm Equipment Operations, and Data Entry Processes.* Washington, D.C.: 1974.

Jones, F. Ron. *Cost Analysis of Alternative Transportation Systems for the Handicapped.* Working paper No. 256. Berkeley: Institute of Urban and Regional Development, University of California, 1975.

Lassen, Peter L. *Barrier Free Design: A Selected Bibliography.* Washington, D.C.: Paralyzed Veterans of America, Inc., 1973.

Laurie, Gini. *Housing and Home Service for the Disabled: Guidelines and Experiences in Independent Living.* New York: Harper & Row, 1977.

Lewis, Sylvia. "The Disabled Are Tired of Being Pushed Around," *Planning* 43(6), July 1977:9–13.

Loshin, Ronald S., and Collignon, Frederick C. *Discussion and Survey of Benefit Cost Studies of Vocational Rehabilitation.* Berkeley: Berkeley Planning Associates, 1975, Subcontract to The Urban Institute, Contract No. HEW-SRS-74-54-3.

Motlock, W. M. *Mobility for Spinal Cord Impaired Patients.* Presented at Conference on Mobility for Spinal Cord Impaired People, National Academy of Science, held at Rancho De Los Amigos, Downey, California, February 1974.

Nau, Louis Y., and Turem, Jerry S. "The Comprehensive Needs Study," *American Rehabilitation* 1(2), March–April 1975: 9–12.

Overby, Charles M. "Will Technology Change Work Living Patterns?" *Journal of Rehabilitation* 39(6), November–December 1973: 18–19, 41.

Rehab Inc. *An Analytical Appraisal of the Definition of Severe Handicap: A Final Report.* 1976. Project sponsored by RSA, HEW.

Schmidt, Bruce L. *An Alternative Approach to Assessing Client and Social Benefits Resulting From Services Provided by the California Department of Rehabilitation.* A working paper written for the California Department of Rehabilitation, 830 K St., Sacramento, California, 1976.

"Transportation for the Disabled: What is the Government Doing? When? Where? With What?" *Accent on Living* 20(1), Summer 1975: 40–42.

"Travel," *Rehabilitation Gazette* 17; 1974: 2–11.

Turem, Jerry S., "Testimony Prepared for the Subcommittee on Handicapped, Committee on Labor and Public Welfare, United States Senate." Washington, D.C.: The Urban Institute, March 21, 1976.

Turem, Jerry S., and Nau, Louis Y. "Comprehensive Needs Study, Part II," *American Rehabilitation* 1(4), March–April 1976: 6–9.

U.S. Architectural and Transportation Barriers Compliance Board. *Freedom of Choice: Report to the President and to the Congress on Housing Needs of Handicapped Individuals.* 2 vols. Washington, D.C.: 1975.

U.S. Department of Health, Education and Welfare, Office for Handicapped Individuals. *A Summary of Selected Legislation Relating to the Handicapped, 1975–76.* Washington, D.C.: May 1977.

U.S. Department of Health, Education and Welfare, Rehabilitation Services Administration. *Rehabilitation Services Manual.* Washington, D.C.: October 15, 1975.

U.S. Department of Transportation. *Transportation for the Handicapped: Selected References.* Bibliographic List No. 8. Washington, D.C.: 1975.

The Urban Institute. *Report of the Comprehensive Service Needs Study.* Washington, D.C.: Rehabilitation Services Administration, June 1975. Contract #HEW 100-74-0309.

The Urban Institute. *First Year Report on Section 130 Demonstration Projects.* Washington, D.C.: July 1976.

Van Vechten, Doris, and Pless, I. Barry. "Housing and Transportation: Twin Barriers to Independence," *Rehabilitation Literature* 37(7), July 1976: 202–207, 221.

The White House Conference on Handicapped Individuals, *Delegate Workbook. Workshop VII, Special Concerns (1) Severely Disabled: Service Delivery; Housing.* Washington, D.C.: May 22–27, 1977.

The White House Conference on Handicapped Individuals. *Volume One: Awareness Papers.* Washington, D.C.: May 23–30, 1977.

10
Consumer Involvement in Rehabilitation

FRANK BOWE, PH.D.
FREDERICK A. FAY, PH.D.
JANET A. MINCH, M.A.

The purpose of this chapter is threefold: (1) to review the recent history of the consumer involvement in rehabilitation of disabled persons through the 1970s; (2) to describe the current state-of the-art in terms of research studies and model programs; and (3) to identify issues and trends relevant to future consumer involvement growth. The reader will gain an understanding of the scope of consumer involvement programs and how they are defined. Federal legislative requirements and guidelines for incorporating consumer involvement in vocational rehabilitation systems are detailed in the history section. Specific examples of models currently being implemented by state vocational rehabilitation agencies and consumer organizations are described in the section on participation roles. Future issues and trends are briefly identified at the end of the chapter.

The chapter aims to inform vocational rehabilitation agency administrators, rehabilitation counselors, disabled individuals, and representatives of persons interested in rehabilitation in understanding consumer involvement. This orientation will assist individuals in using the current state-of-the-art to resolve current and future issues. In particular, policy decision makers within the rehabilitation system should find the information useful.

> Government must be kept open. If we intend to rebuild confidence in the government process itself, policy must be shaped through the participation of Congress and the American people.[1]
>
> —Jimmy Carter

Consumer involvement in rehabilitation is a process of participation between disabled consumers and the organizations which represent them, and providers of services and/or policy makers on issues which ultimately affect the recipients of these services. A few popular terms for consumer involvement are *citizen participation, community partic-*

ipation, or *client involvement.* One might associate with these terms a wide number of organized programs whose purpose is to intentionally and systematically promote communication between the providers and the users of services. The overriding purpose for the development of consumer involvement processes is to advance the effectiveness of rehabilitation services in enabling disabled individuals to live and work independently. To that end, processes for consumer participation provide opportunities for individuals and organizations that are interested in rehabilitation to influence the decisions and the decision makers who provide the services that ultimately affect the consumers. The basic purpose of consumer involvement programs in policy development in vocational rehabilitation as defined in federal guidelines is

> . . . to give the people for whom the programs are designed full opportunity to participate in policy formulation and initial planning to assure that "their" programs are relevant to their needs and responsive to their priorities. This concept fits us well as a society for it is one form of participation of the governed in their government.[2]

WHO ARE THE CONSUMERS?

In its most narrow sense, the word *consumer* describes an individual who directly secures a service or a commodity and is thus a client of rehabilitation services. In a broad sense, the term has been used to include people who are affected directly or indirectly by actions of vocational rehabilitation agencies, such as parents and/or guardians of mentally ill or retarded individuals; former, current, and future clients of vocational rehabilitation agencies; representatives of organizations composed of disabled persons, as well as individuals who by choice do not identify themselves as disabled or do not belong to groups but qualify as disabled. In addition, in a broad sense *consumers* refers to persons who represent the interests of disabled persons, sometimes referred to as *advocates.*

Consumers or persons who directly use or benefit from a commodity or service have a level of understanding that, if utilized, can improve the effectiveness of rehabilitation services. To do this, disabled persons have recognized and developed opportunities through individual and collective action. Recently, persons from different disability groups have become more organized, speaking with one voice on cross-cutting issues. Such organizing has occurred at several levels. The American Coalition of Citizens with Disabilities, an umbrella group of organizations concerned with different special interest areas at the national level, has defined a method to work together on issues of common concern described in the book *Coalition Building* (Bowe et al., 1978). Founded in 1974, its membership includes groups such as Paralyzed Veterans of America, the American Council of the Blind, the National Association of the Deaf, and the National Spinal Cord Injury Foundation, and others.

On the state level, many different types of organizations exist. Recent years have seen the growth of statewide coalitions in Florida, Ohio, Texas, Massachusetts, and other states. These groups are joined together for action on common issues. Many groups have formed around one disability and sometimes relate to a national group. Some examples of these groups are state chapters of the Association for Retarded Citizens, United Cerebral Palsy Associations, Association for the Deaf, and the Federation of the Blind. These groups are usually established as nonprofit organizations and devote time to program and advocacy services. Finally, through funding from the federal Rehabilitation Services Administration, Developmental Disabilities Councils have been established in each state to work in planning and advocacy for developmentally disabled persons. The councils have consumers as part of their membership and are active in statewide issues.

Self-help groups and consumer-based organizations at state and local areas have emerged over the last several years to provide information, support, and advocacy within their membership as well as a broader community. The most visible type of organization representing this area are the Centers for Independent Living that have organized and grown over the last several years. Established informally or as nonprofit organizations, these groups provide services in a variety of areas (legal, housing, peer counseling, transportation, and so on).

A BRIEF HISTORY

Inherent in the fundamentals of a democratic society are many methods for affecting decision making: voting rights, filing legislation, public hearing processes, and others. Depending upon the status of particular concerns, various processes may be incorporated. Sherry Arnstein describes a theoretical model of citizen participation entitled "A Ladder of Citizen Participation" (Arnstein, 1969). At the bottom of the ladder are nonparticipation roles, described by the author as therapy and manipulation techniques; in the middle, an area of "tokenism" that is chiefly a one-way communication of consumers giving information but having no authority; and at the top of the ladder, areas of "consumer power" where some control and/or decision-making authority is in the hands of consumers. If one adapts Arnstein's theory to the vocational rehabilitation system, different types of organized patterns for consumer involvement would be reflected. At the bottom of the ladder, in the area of "nonparticipation," one will find opportunities for consumers to express their concerns as a means for venting frustrations but without administrative expectation of policy impact. On the manipulation rung, administrators use consumers as public relations devices to promote their own ends. "Rubber stamp committees" is the name often given to this area.

Through the various degrees of "tokenism," a number of approaches are incorporated in the vocational rehabilitation system. Newsletters, public hearing processes, or memoranda are means of informing consumers about activities of the administration. Use of disabled persons as consultants is sometimes included in preparing annual reports and state plans. Consumers sometimes feel these methods are tokenistic, especially when the material and issues presented is complex and/or not clearly presented, thus limiting their input. Some persons feel they lack sufficient background experience to provide input quickly and appropriately.

"Consumer power" might best be typified by consumer organizations that establish and run independent living programs or informational services or provide other services. Here, the consumers have taken on the responsibility for the provision of rehabilitation services encompassing authority and accountability.

Most social programs such as welfare, housing, and health care, to name only a few, have incorporated various approaches for citizen participation. "Today virtually all programs in which Federally appropriated funds are used require citizen access to the decision-making process."[3]

Within the vocational rehabilitation system, the scope of consumer involvement is broad and participation roles are diversified. Consumer involvement as previously defined would include counselor-client interaction around a required communication process of the Individualized Written Rehabilitation Plan (IWRP). The statutory provisions in Section 102 of the Rehabilitation Act of 1973 describing the IWRP emphasize the client's participation, rights, and remedies, and are specific objectives and measurements of achievement. This one-to-one communication system is one highly personalized form or method to ensure the participation of the client in a dialogue with the agency.

At another level, a statewide advisory board composed of elected representatives from organizations of disabled persons who recommend and review policies of a state rehabilitation agency has potential impact on the whole service delivery system. The advisory board approach is more likely to affect policy issues than specific individual service issues.

Cooperation and open communication appear to be important and essential components of consumer involvement programs. Remmes stressed the importance of positive interaction and openness to dispel what he called the "cold war" between providers and consumers (Remmes, 1972, 1974). Rehabilitation Services Administration Commissioner A. S. Adams (1976) later identified the need for each party to understand the others' perspectives in obtaining the cooperation necessary to implement an effective consumer involvement program. Gaining insight into consumers' needs and evaluating the effectiveness of methods and approaches helps to influence the way in which rehabilitation programs are run (Thursz, 1969).

Benefits to consumer involvement were cited in a federal document (*Rehabilitation Services Administration Manual,* 1975) as:

- increased awareness of client needs;
- realistic insights as to how various aspects of the state vocational rehabilitation program are functioning and how they might be improved;
- establishment of better working relationships between the agency and clients, providers and other individuals and organizations active in rehabilitation in the state;
- better information sharing and clearer understanding of the state agency's mission, goals and objectives;
- increased and more effective advocacy for the state agency's programs and its program needs;
- and the establishment of a mechanism to permit continuous external feedback from all segments of the population on current and proposed operations and plans.[4]

Others have recognized the advantages of consumer involvement to both providers and recipients (Adams, 1976; Bartels, 1972; Drake, 1973; Fay, 1978; Howe et al., 1979; Institute on Rehabilitation Issues, 1975; Minch and Spaniol, 1978; Thursz, 1969).

RELATIONSHIP TO OTHER SOCIAL MOVEMENTS

A broad perspective on the relationship between consumer involvement in rehabilitation to other social movements is presented by Gerben DeJong (1978). DeJong's paper provides an analysis of how the movement for independent living has taken shape at a time when other complementary social movements were developing. These movements include civil rights, consumerism, self-help, demedicalization, and mainstreaming. As DeJong observes, "The civil rights movement of the 1960's has had an impact far beyond the racial minorities it sought to benefit."[5] Other interest groups became more aware of both their rights and of how to achieve them. Disabled citizens observed the philosophy and strategies of the blacks, other minorities, and women during the 1960s and became more active in demanding civil rights for themselves.

A key event that catalyzed disabled leaders from different disability backgrounds was the National Citizens Conference on Rehabilitation of Disabled and Disadvantaged (NCCRDD) in 1969. The NCCRDD brought together the leadership of many organizations of different disability groups, as well as minority leaders from the black, Chicano, and other communities. The Planning Committee for the Conference determined that one of the top five priorities for conference attention was the topic "Consumer Involvement in Rehabilitation." Thursz documented the state of the art with respect to consumer involvement and rehabilitation in 1969 as a background paper for that conference. In fact, the paper had very little to say, directly, with respect to consumer involvement in rehabilitation; it spoke more to other movements and the history of consumerism in general.

During the 1960s and, more intensively, the early 1970s, disabled consumer activists pressured Congress to include amendments to the rehabilitation legislation that would assure affirmative action programs and put an end to discrimination. Title V of the Rehabilitation Act of 1973, which was passed with considerable support by disabled people, includes provisions for affirmative action programs for the employment of disabled persons within the federal government (Section 501) and by organizations contracting with the federal government (Section 503). Section 502 created the Architectural and Transportation Barriers Compliance Board. Probably the most significant section for disabled people is Section 504, which bans discrimination on the basis of handicap in any program or activity receiving federal financial assistance.

The civil rights movement has had an effect not only on the securing of certain rights (e.g., Title V, the "civil rights act" for disabled citizens) but also on the manner in which these rights have been secured. When more traditional strategies have been exhausted, disabled persons have employed other techniques of social protest such as demonstrations and sit-ins. The Rehabilitation Act Amendments of 1974, which established the White House Conference and clarified the civil rights provisions—as well as the Rehabilitation Act Amendments of 1978, which established independent living and strengthened further the civil rights provisions within the law—were all passed, in part, as a result of street demonstrations by disabled citizens throughout the country.

The civil rights provision itself, Section 504, while passed in 1973, was not implemented through regulation until 1977. Section 504 includes a strong requirement for consumer involvement: As recipients of federal funds develop transition plans for compliance in barrier removal, they are required to involve disabled persons in the process. Demonstrations coordinated by disabled citizens throughout the country put the pressure on the administration to finally promulgate those implementing regulations.

CONSUMERISM

As DeJong (1978) points out, "The parameters of the consumer movement are hard to define. It is a movement that affects nearly all social classes and groups. The movement is most personified by Ralph Nader but also includes public interest lawyers representing various disadvantaged groups. The movement embraces both the person who devotedly reads *Consumer Reports* and the person who campaigns for new consumer protection legislation. . . ."[6] DeJong observes that the rise in consumer sovereignty is challenging professional dominence in rehabilitation policy making. As observed earlier, the IWRP required joint involvement by the client and the counselor in developing the rehabilitation plan. Independent living centers have developed with strong consumer involvement on both the policy-making boards of directors and on the staff (Fay et al., 1976). The substantial involvement by disabled persons in management and implementation of the independent living centers, where disabled people frequently have majority control, is based in part on the assumption that disabled individuals, with several years of disability experience, are frequently better aware of the needs of disabled people and better informed about government benefits than able-bodied professionals in the rehabilitation delivery system.

Section 101 (A) 18 of the Rehabilitation Act of 1973 requires consumer involvement at the policy level. The policy consultation required of the state or local agency specifies that it must "take into account, in connection with matters of general policy arising in the administration of the plan, the views of individuals and groups thereof who are recipients of vocational rehabilitation services, or, in appropriate cases their parents or guardians working in the field of vocational rehabilitation and providers of rehabilitation services."[7] This provision provided a thrust, along with pressure by consumers and their representatives, for RSA to thoroughly revise its chapter on what is now called "Policy Development Consultation." Before turning to the details of "Chapter 25," as it has come to be known by consumers interested in influencing their state agency's policies, it's worthwhile to trace briefly other social movements that have influenced the development of consumer involvement.

SELF-HELP

As DeJong points out in describing the self-help movement, it "embraces a large variety of groups: from the Female Improvement Society to Alcoholics Anonymous. There now appears to be a self-help group for almost every conceivable human condition or problem—alcoholism, drugs, gambling, death, homosexuality, child abuse, women's health, old age, sex, neighborhood crime, cigarette smoking, child birth, and of prime interest here, physical disability."[8]

For disabled citizens, two major self-help developments have provided the impetus for a greater voice by disabled people in rehabilitation decision making. First, centers for independent living have developed in Massachusetts, Texas, California, Michigan, and many other states as vehicles for both advocacy and service delivery. The independent living centers provide services such as peer counseling and advocacy that are not provided by the established vocational rehabilitation agencies. The second major vehicle for self-help activities is the coalition. The best-known example of this is the American Coalition of Citizens with Disabilities. It was formed in 1974 by leaders of different "individual disability self-help groups" who saw a need for a united force by disabled persons, whether blind, deaf, spinal cord injured, or whatever, on common concerns such as attitudinal barriers and discrimination. The coalition brings together under one umbrella organization the leadership not only of national self-help disability groups but also state coalitions and state and local organizations of citizens with disabilities. Self-help groups give disabled people the opportunity to exercise control over their own lives and the services they use.

Several other social movements have had an impact on the growing interest of disabled people to be involved in rehabilitation decision making. "Demedicalization," for example, is a trend which challenges the medical profession in certain spheres of human life. Once a physically disabled person is medically stabilized, the day-to-day management of the disability is primarily a personal rather than a medical matter. A continued medical presence in the lives of disabled persons fosters dependency and is thus in conflict with rehabilitation goals.

Several other trends, including the self-care movement described above, as well as the movements described by terms like *deinstitutionalization, normalization,* and *mainstreaming,* are related to the issue of consumer involvement in the decisions that affect one's life. DeJong concludes that there are three major assumptions or propositions that cut across all of the major movements discussed above:

> *Consumer Sovereignty*—disabled persons (consumers), not professionals, are the best judges of their own interests; they should ultimately determine how services are organized on their behalf.
> *Self-Reliance*—disabled persons must rely primarily on their own resources and ingenuity to acquire the rights and benefits to which they are entitled.
> *Political and Economic Rights*—disabled persons are entitled to freely pursue their interests in various political and economic arenas.[9]

CHAPTER 25

In a very real sense "Chapter 25," the *Rehabilitation Services Manual* chapter on policy development consultation, is the key to the future of consumer involvement and rehabilitation. The chapter provides vocational rehabilitation agencies and consumers with guidelines for the involvement of disabled persons in a formal program for receiving and considering the views of recipients of Vocational Rehabilitation services. The Chapter 25 cover letter from then RSA Commissioner A. S. Adams states the expectation that each state agency would immediately take steps to formulate in writing its policy development consultation program and have that program in operation no later than December 25, 1975.

In passing the Rehabilitation Act of 1973, Congress incorporated the concept of "consumer participation" into the RSA service delivery system, just as it had into several other federal programs in recent years. In the past, state Vocational Rehabilitation agencies had to varying degrees involved consumers in some of their activities. However, as is observed in Chapter 25, "for all state VR agencies, therefore, involving clients, service providers and others in policy development and administration will not be a new experience. What will be new, probably for all States, will be extending the breadth and depth of their participation. Hence, every State agency will, in all likelihood, need to go far beyond present practices to meet the requirements of the Rehabilitation Act and the Regulations as set forth in Manual Section 525.02."[10]

Chapter 25 requires each state Vocational Rehabilitation agency to assess its current position with respect to consumer involvement and to develop a program which in scope, degree, and continuity of client, provider, and other person participation meets the requirements of the act and regulations (*Rehabilitation Services Administration Manual,* 1975). The chapter also calls for a written description of each state's program for consumer involvement that would be made available to the public. Neither Congress nor the Rehabilitation Services Administration prescribed one particular approach to consumer involvement in state agency policy formulation, but Chapter 25 does present broad principles which the state agencies must consider in structuring their programs for policy development consultation by disabled persons.

Chapter 25 documents the program benefits of consumer involvement as well as different models for securing consumer input; functional consultation areas; composition of advisory groups and selection of members; and responsibilities of state agencies and consumer representatives. The guidelines indicate several program areas for policy development consultation where views and recommendations of consumers are helpful:

- Program evaluation
- Program planning and development
- Legislative proposals and budgets
- Assessment of physical accessibility
- Proposing research
- Assistance in studies and surveys
- Interpretation of agency policies and program services
- In-service training and staff development
- White House Conference activities
- Securing and utilizing local community resources
- Implementation of Rehabilitation Act Amendments
- Establishment of centers for independent living

Consumer involvement program models take a variety of forms. The examples identified in this chapter are obtained through research studies undertaken at Tufts Research and Training program. Often consumers and agency personnel are utilized in more than one method at a time. In fact, there is no one perfect way to implement a consumer involvement program. Diversified forms of involvement enhance the ability to include a wide variety of consumers and to interact with various levels of administration. Such interaction may take place in various administrative functions, such as agency planning processes (budget and program), staff development (hiring, reviewing, or training), or facility utilization (accessibility considerations). Other program models might focus specifically on service provision. Here, consumers participate in active roles as "providers" of basic and auxiliary rehabilitation services, such as counseling or information sharing.

Policy areas may include reviewing standardized forms and manuals, identifying gaps in service delivery, or recommending changes to better meet service needs of disabled persons. Issues such as accessible housing, transportation, and adaptive equipment often emerge in discussions focusing on the agency's position and directions.

State Vocational Rehabilitation agencies note the area of program evaluation as the most frequently utilized for gathering information from consumers (Howe et al., 1979). Client satisfaction studies are one of the most common examples of this model. Questionnaires are routinely mailed to clients whose cases have been closed in order to assess service delivery systems. Separate federal program standards require evaluation in this area. In California, comprehensive program studies are undertaken (such as the recent one for the Orientation Center for the Blind) that use substantial information contributed by disabled persons (Howe et al., 1979). Opinion and assessment surveys have been utilized as well.

The statewide Consumer Advisory Board in Arkansas, consisting of twenty persons (ten of whom are disabled) who represent the eight service regions of the state, has assisted the agency in establishing a deaf service program. As a priority program issue for the committee, they provided leadership and support in improving services to the state's deaf population.

Many states (e.g., Arkansas, Texas, California, Minnesota, and Massachusetts) indicate that advisory groups and consumers review the agency's annual state plan and program budget information prior to submission to RSA. Some states indicate the use of consumers on an ad hoc basis in planning discussions. Massachusetts uses consumers as paid consultants to review program plans.

Independent living is a new area for most state Vocational Rehabilitation programs. As the planning and implementation of these services proceed, particularly where community-based independent living centers with disabled persons on the board and staff will be a prime vehicle for delivering independent living rehabilitation services, it is critical to involve consumers. This approach has proven effective in states like California, Massachusetts and Michigan, where Innovation and Expansion (I&E) grants have been awarded to consumer organizations for developing such centers. As states move from planning to implementation, consumer review of proposed projects and centers can assure "peer" review. The Rehabilitation Act Amendments of 1978 require that grant applicants for independent living centers "provide assurances that handicapped individuals will be substantially involved in policy direction and management of such center and will be employed by such center."[11]

Consumer assistance in developing legislative proposals and budgets is exemplified by consumer success in addressing the problems of economic disincentives in two states. In California, successful lobbying for state funds has enabled severely disabled persons who return to work to retain their medical coverage. A current California effort would provide state funding to continue the independent living programs once their I&E grants run out. In Massachusetts, a coalition of consumers and providers got state legislation passed to enable a new employee with a severe physical disability to retain his or her personal care assistance (attendant care), at gradually reduced support levels, up to an income of $18,000.

An innovative telecommunications system is under development in Oklahoma to provide a means of dialogue between consumers and the Vocational Rehabilitation agency throughout the state on policy issues. The sophisticated television talk-back equipment brings instant contact and response when persons are separated geographically.

Another communication device, a statewide toll-free telephone WATS line or "hotline," provides an opportunity for consumers to call with questions and provide information. The Illinois Division of Vocational Rehabilitation has provided extensive service in this area through a program entitled "DIAL." Equipped with a telecommunications typewriter (TTY) for use by deaf persons, the service provides and receives information about programs, services, and organizations of and for handicapped persons. Close documentation assists the staff in defining gaps in available services and in recommending changes through position papers. Newsletters and brochures are other methods used to communicate information.

Individual policy consultants are hired through a consumer involvement program in Massachusetts funded with I&E grant money. This program enables the Vocational Rehabilitation commission to utilize services of consumer consultants on a request basis. Some areas in which consultants have been used include: hiring new staff, reviewing grant proposals, developing and reviewing policy areas, developing affirmative action plans, and assessing facility accessibility.

Several studies have been undertaken by consumers on a paid fee basis to determine accessibility (California, Massachusetts), and many more indicate unpaid use of consumers. Consumers have participated in key roles in workshops, seminars, and informal training, as well in educating individuals about mobility barriers and their removal. They were actively involved in a workshop developed through the Oregon Vocational Rehabilitation Division for architects and engineers on barrier-free design. A panel of disabled persons, representing many different aspects of mobility difficulties, discussed environmental access and accessibility issues (Bowe et al., 1978).

The Governor of Illinois recently established a Technical Advisory Committee on Coordination of State Handicapped Services among state human service agency directors who provide services to the handicapped. They, in turn, appointed a citizen committee to hold statewide hearings to identify major issues within the handicapped community.

In Texas, a significant number of rehabilitation staff regularly attend consumer organization meetings. Through this process, staff persons learn firsthand about needs within the consumer community at large. Workshops have been held in some states to provide intensive training in service areas such as independent living.

Consumer trainers may provide specific information to particular disability groups (e.g., how to obtain interpreter services for a deaf client). Frequently, consumer groups fill some of the gaps left by the Vocational Rehabilitation service delivery system and can provide training to counselors on how to interface with "self-help service providers." Knowledge of consumer group information, referral and follow-up services, meetings, newsletters, hotlines, and client assistance and advocacy efforts can be a valuable resource for counselors new to independent living rehabilitation. Consumer involvement in staff development may include helping to select and evaluate counselors who provide independent living services.

RESEARCH STUDIES

Consumer involvement programs have been in existence in various forms for several years. However, very little research or evaluation has been undertaken in this area. In 1975 the Arkansas Rehabilitation Research and Training Center coordinated a study group in consumer involvement chaired by Young M. Orsburn of the Arkansas Rehabilitation Services (Institute on Rehabilitation Issues, 1975). For two days in San Antonio, Texas, approximately sixty people from all parts of the country convened to discuss consumer involvement and to finalize a document that might serve as a guide for future studies and action in consumer involvement. The report, entitled *Consumer Involvement: Rehabilitation Issues,* is one of the few documents available that explore the major issues, implementation considerations, and training needs in consumer involvement in vocational rehabilitation.

Tufts Research and Training Center (Boston) developed a core research area in 1976 to explore the area of consumer involvement. This core area was developed in response to studies that included the participation of the Massachusetts Council of Organizations of the Handicapped. Through that program effort, Tufts Research and Training Center cooperated in financing a study on consumer advocacy. The project focused on developing leadership capabilities within the disabled consumer community but also detailed the level of activism and organized ability of various consumer organizations in working with those systems that affect their lives.

The consumer involvement core area has two basic goals. One is "to explore the role of the consumers themselves as a force in advancing the effectiveness of the rehabilitation system"; the other is "to explore methods for meaningful involvement of consumer organizations in the planning, delivery and evaluation of medical, vocational, environmental and independent living rehabilitation services."[12] Through several other Tufts projects, model or pilot approaches to facilitating the participation of disabled persons in service programs were explored. Specific references for these programmatic aspects are explained in three 1978 reports: *Access to Science, A Management Training for Severely Physically Disabled Individuals,* and *Vocational Rehabilitation: Consumers as Citizens.*

In late 1977, Tufts developed a research study to survey the state-of-the-art of consumer involvement in Vocational Rehabilitation agencies. The perceptions of 81 Vocational Rehabilitation agency personnel have been compared with response from 343 disabled consumers. This state-of-the-art study identified the methods of communication between consumers and their state Vocational Rehabilitation agencies, the extent to which these methods are employed nationwide, the specific aspects of each state agency's operation in which consumers actually participated, and how well both consumers and state Vocational Rehabilitation agencies were meeting their responsibilities as defined in Chapter 25 of the *Rehabilitation Services Manual.* Objectives of the study also included the identification of the training and technical assistance areas most desired, how consumer involvement activities benefit state Vocational Rehabilitation agencies and disabled persons, and the perceptions of the level of effectiveness of policy consultation by consumer advisers.

The findings indicate that 50 percent of the states' Vocational

Rehabilitation agencies surveyed have a written plan for consumer involvement. Many states only describe a portion of consumer involvement activities in these formalized plans. Agencies serving the blind were more likely (63 percent) than were general agencies serving both blind and general clients (36 percent) to have a written plan (Howe et al., 1979). Many essential aspects of a consumer involvement plan, such as methods utilized for communication, methods used by agencies to ensure that recommendations are heard, and payment mechanism for financial reimbursement, are not incorporated. The data support the conclusion that several different methods (i.e., advisory boards, ad hoc consultants, public hearings, conferences or meetings, and questionnaires) are used by state Vocational Rehabilitation agencies, with the advisory committees being the most frequent.

Comparing areas of consumer involvement practices, the survey indicates that communication between vocational rehabilitation agencies and consumers is not clear. For example, consumers are not often aware of written information, methods of consumer representation, or follow-up methods to notify consumers of the status of recommendations.

The policy area where consumer involvement occurs most frequently was reported as program evaluation; it occurs least frequently in training Vocational Rehabilitation staff. Several other functional consultation areas were rated, such as program planning and development, assistance in developing legislative proposals and budgets, and interpreting agency programs to the public. All these areas were reported as used throughout the country to varying degrees. At least 50 percent of the vocational rehabilitation agencies nationwide used consumers in areas of program evaluation, planning and development, studies about handicapped individuals, and special facilities and programs for the handicapped. Consumers felt they assisted most in the affirmative action area and in the development of special facilities and programs.

Agency personnel perceive consumers consistently in all areas as effective in carrying out consumer involvement responsibilities. Most effective was their willingness to work constructively. Consumers perceived wide variations in evaluating their effectiveness in different areas. Dealing with problems as issues and not in a personal or vindictive manner was perceived by consumers as their most effective area. Overall, they felt least effective about keeping their constituency informed (Howe et al., 1979). Both groups support the belief that the strongest program benefit from consumer involvement is the increased awareness of client needs. Technical assistance and training, particularly in leadership, communication, and policy skills, are perceived as helpful and needed.

The Consumer Involvement Core Area at Tufts Research and Training Center received an I&E grant in 1976 from the Massachusetts Rehabilitation Commission to explore the feasibility of several consumer involvement models. The program goal is to demonstrate and evaluate several different approaches to consumer involvement in vocational rehabilitation in Massachusetts. The models include development of local advisory councils, policy review teams, individual consultation by disabled persons on hiring, program development, and grants review. Areas where consumers provided services were via information centers, peer counseling, and a newsletter on rehabilitation information. Six major areas developed through a nominal group process defined priority project outcome areas to be measured. These are:

1. Attitude change
2. Consumer awareness of State Rehabilitation Agency
3. Independent living
4. Consumer-state rehabilitation communication
5. Improving state rehabilitation agency services to clients
6. Organizational development

During the first program year, complementary questionnaires were distributed to state Vocational Rehabilitation agency personnel and disabled consumers who participated in the program. The following year, the same questionnaire, with additional questions designed to assess policy development, was again distributed to program participants (both Vocational Rehabilitation personnel and disabled consumers).

The first-year results show that both agency and consumers "express attitudes [that] were similar and tended to be positive towards the consumer involvement program. Consumers did appear to feel more strongly about having a role in agency decision making, knowing more about how the agency is spending its money and knowing more about how the state agency is organized."[13]

The second-year follow-up evaluation study reinforces the consistent theme of the importance and value of consumer involvement activities. The important factor is that consumer and agency staff at all levels engage in structured, long-term, participative problem solving (Minch and Spaniol, 1978). Consumers generally feel a stronger need for involvement in policy issues. A large and diversified number of policy matters were identified. The participation processes "generated personal enthusiasm where it had been lacking. This included a better understanding of the problem of other people and a greater awareness of handicapped people."[14]

Another research study that has looked at the extent and effectiveness of consumer involvement in vocational rehabilitation was conducted by the American Coalition of Citizens with Disabilities (ACCD) in 1978. This group provided evidence that policy-related involvement is beginning to occur five years after enactment of the law.

The ACCD surveyed forty-two state directors and their top policy aides in summer 1978 (Bowe, 1979; Varela, 1978). The six questions asked formed three areas of inquiry. First, the coalition sought to determine which techniques of communicating with members of the consumer population were used, how frequently each was applied, and how effective each appeared to be. Second, the agency officials were questioned about the quality of consumer input in each of twelve areas of agency activity. And third, they were asked about means of improving consumer involvement in policy making.

Many of the answers were surprising, both to the coalition and to rehabilitation professionals. While almost all agencies surveyed used a broad range of techniques of consumer participation, the highest-rated was employment of disabled consultants. Meetings between agency representatives and consumer-organization officials were the most frequently reported avenues of consumer input and the second highest rated. Advisory bodies, telephone contacts, and questionnaires were also used but were not as highly rated in effectiveness.

Consumers were perceived by the agency administrators as most helpful in assessing accessibility of facilities, recruitment of disabled employees, legislative and budgetary proposal preparation, independent living, and evaluation of agency program services. The respondents were particularly pleased with the input of disabled people who had been chosen by their peers or jointly by the agency and consumer groups; less satisfactory was the advice of disabled persons selected by the agency alone.

Asked to rank-order approaches to improving consumer involvement, the officials chose a central office liaison with consumer groups as the most likely to succeed. Other choices, in descending order of preference, were: election of advisory-group members by organizations of disabled people; conferences on how to influence rehabilitation programming and organize groups effectively; newsletters for consumers; and training in leadership for consumer representatives.

ISSUES AND FUTURE TRENDS

The White House Conference on Handicapped Individuals *Implementation Plan* provides insight into future trends regarding consumer involvement. The conference itself would not have occurred but for the activism of disabled persons. On October 29, 1974, President Gerald Ford vetoed the Rehabilitation Act Amendments of 1974, which provided for the convening of the conference. Demonstrations and lobbying by disabled persons throughout the country contributed to Congress's override of the veto. The delegates to the White House Conference in 1977 represented probably the most comprehensive gathering of disabled citizens and others to develop policy recommendations regarding programs affecting disabled persons.

The legislation that developed the White House Conference included a policy from Congress that the federal government would work jointly with the states and with local citizens to develop recommendations and plans for action to solve the many problems of persons with handicaps. The amendments also established a National Planning and Advisory Council. The council was mandated to include a majority of "individuals with handicaps appointed to represent all individuals with handicaps" and "parents of individuals with disabilities appointed to represent all such parents and individuals" (Rehabilitation Act Amendments of 1974). The state conferences that led up to the National White House Conference included similar consumer involvement activities.

In 1978, President Jimmy Carter stated his administration's commitment to consumer involvement at the White House Conference when he said, "I am committed to the proposition that disabled people deserve to control and shape their own lives. I am committed to ensuring that our disabled citizens have the rights and opportunity to function independently and creatively in our society, rather than be segregated from it."[15]

The letter from Hank Viscardi, Conference Chairperson, to President Carter transmitting the conference's Implementation Plan, highlighted a few major recommendations. The first of these dealt with consumer involvement in federal decision making.

The conference delegates expressed their desire for a clearly defined public policy throughout federal and state governments. Viscardi, and through him the delegates, called for involvement of "individuals with handicaps, their parents or guardians and organizations representing their interests in all decision making bodies impacting upon their lives as individual citizens. Representation by the handicapped consumer on these bodies shall not be less than one half of the total group constituted."[16]

The second major recommendation touched on the areas in which it was considered essential for the administration and Congress to recognize the unique and distinct needs of individuals who are handicapped. These major initiatives included "welfare reform, tax reform, health insurance, labor and economic reform, and social security programs. Immediate action should be taken to appoint handicapped consumers, as well as their parents/guardians and organizations representing them, to all committees established to deal with these issues at the appropriate administrative levels."[17]

The "major findings" section of the Implementation Plan provided more details on the consumer involvement recommendations of the White House Conference. The plan presents the recommendation of the White House Conference that handicapped individuals and their parents and/or guardians must be represented at the highest level of policy setting and decision making:

> It is recommended that the President identify and designate an individual within his Office at the Domestic Council level to coordinate policies and administration activities affecting handicapped individuals and their families. To recommend that an individual with this responsibility be placed within the Office of the President is to recognize that the concerns of persons with disabilities cross-cut many Departments, including Justice, Transportation, Housing and Urban Development, Labor and Commerce as well as the Department of Health, Education, and Welfare.
>
> An administrative net shall be developed at the Department level with each Secretary or Department head appointing a Special Assistant to provide coordination and follow-through in every agency. Priority should be given to individuals with disabilities in filling these positions.
>
> A National Planning Council or National Commission on Handicapped Individuals is recommended which should contain more than the collective power of a number of lesser committees and councils currently in existence. More than half of the individuals on this consolidated, powerful body should be persons with disabilities with an additional twenty five per cent parents and guardians of individuals with disabilities. Due consideration should be given to membership of non-whites with representation from concerned racial/ethnic minority organizations. This body should have a well-defined legislative mandate and adequate funding to allow the Commission to play a meaningful role in National government.[18]

The Implementation Plan called for similar councils at the state level to assure ongoing grass-roots involvement. The plan then spelled out some of the key elements of what in many ways is a national plan for consumer involvement in disability policy decision making:

> Persons with disabilities and parents or guardians must have a voice in decisions that affect their lives. This means full voting membership on boards and committees at that policy-setting level. While the nature of advisory committees makes them important to decision making, actual participation on the decision making board is a more important and appropriate role. The lack of visibility suffered by persons without significant economic or political influence means that government and the private sector must seek out individuals for these positions. Major initiatives of the Administration and the Congress in areas of human services such as welfare reform, health care delivery, National health insurance, White House conferences, employment training and placement are among areas which demand participation of individuals with disabilities. Funding to provide for ordinary and extraordinary expense should be made available in order to enable individuals—regardless of economic status—to serve in such decision-making capacities. Funding should also be made available for training of persons with disabilities, parents, guardians and advocates in communication skills, leadership and organization to enable them to effectively represent themselves and participate in a meaningful way.[19]

Of the 420 action items that were included in the Implementation Plan, well over 60 related to "Consumer Involvement." This pervasive interest by disabled leaders in the decision-making end of federal and state government that affects the lives of disabled individuals is quite apparent.

Several of the issues raised in the above quotation have been identified in other documents as critical to the successful involvement of consumers in the decisions that affect their lives. The Rand report *Citizen Organizations: Increasing Client Control Over Services* focuses on the ability of such organizations to achieve simultaneously the Department of Health, Education and Welfare goals of devolving power, reducing alienation, and improving program effectiveness (Yin et al., 1973). Its major conclusions are that certain organizational characteristics serve to devolve power more effectively than others: "In particular, characteristics such as the citizen organization having its own staff, having the power to investigate grievances and to influence substantially the formation and execution of service budgets, having an elected citizen membership and having an umbrella-like organizational structure all are associated with the ability of a citizen organization to exert its own influence and control."[20]

Both the White House Conference recommendations and the Rand report highlight several issues that will determine the future of consumer involvement in rehabilitation. Perhaps the best way to state the issues is in the form of questions. The resolution of these issues, or the answers to these questions, will ultimately determine the extent to which consumers are involved in the rehabilitation service delivery system. The issues or questions are:

1. Is there a *commitment* from the top management of the agency to involve disabled individuals in the planning, delivery, and evaluation of rehabilitation services?
2. How *extensively* does this commitment from the top permeate the agency's policies, programs, and activities.
3. How *substantial* is the consumer *representation* in the decision-making process (e.g. tokenism vs. consumer involvement and/or control)?
4. Is the commitment to consumer participation backed up by a *well-defined mandate* and *adequate funding* to allow consumers to play a meaningful role in the agency?
5. Is *training* available for persons with disabilities to develop advocacy, communication, leadership, and organizational skills to enable them to effectively represent themselves and participate in a meaningful way?

IMPLICATIONS

The ACCD and Tufts research surveys are virtually the only major studies of consumer involvement in rehabilitation to have yielded valid and reliable information. Other findings tend to confirm those of the ACCD survey, indicating that consumer involvement was sought, at least to some extent, on a broad range of agency issues and activities. That the area is so little studied illustrates the newness of the concept and the field's tendency to regard it as peripheral rather than central to the "real" business of rehabilitation. Yet consumer participation is inherent in the very nature of rehabilitation: it is not only that disabled people know what they need and want; the essence of a rehabilitated individual is one who has come to understand the self and the rehabilitation process well enough to appreciate the relationship of the two and to design a sequence of activities that will bring both the individual and other disabled people to their optimum level of development. These surveys provide the first concrete evidence that the field is beginning to understand this fact. Now that a start has been made, improvements appear indicated in three key areas:

• *Communication.* Perhaps the most startling finding of the Tufts survey was the disparity between agency and consumer respondents on the extent and effectiveness of consumer involvement. It is evident that disabled people and rehabilitation officials will have to meet, exchange data, and plan together so that the two groups will better understand and appreciate each other. Bowe, Jacobi, and Wiseman (1978) have outlined a model by which consumers may communicate in a common and coherent voice that will be heard by rehabilitation administrators. This or some other approach will clearly be needed to bridge the information gap Tufts has discovered.

• *Election of Consumer Advisors.* The ACCD survey presented strong evidence that only consumers who have been selected by, and are accountable to, their peers will initiate a two-way consultation process such that both the agency and the disabled population will benefit from the advisory group approach to consumer participation. Consumers chosen by the agency are often not known to clients and potential clients, or, if known, are not known to be serving as advisors. Similarly, these persons have little or no responsibility to the agency clients. Accordingly, they may easily be seen as, or become, Uncle Toms. An alternative to consumer election of advisors is agency selection from a list of consumer-chosen designees.

• *Broadening Areas of Involvement.* Both the Tufts and the ACCD surveys identified a wide array of agency activities in which consumer involvement was reported. However, both studies also revealed a definite emphasis upon the more narrow kinds of participation (e.g., accessibility surveys, recruitment of disabled employees, client-service evaluation) and a corresponding neglect of broader and higher-order involvement (e.g., training of agency personnel, assistance in identifying research and evaluation targets, overall agency goals and objectives). The Tufts survey revealed one possible reason for the slant: current and former clients predominatd among consumer advisors. The findings of the two surveys suggest, however, that consumers have much more to offer than is now being tapped by the agencies. Solicitation of consumer input in research and training appears most likely to prove successful.

CONCLUSIONS

Based on the rapid growth of the consumer movement, as reflected in the development of national and state coalitions of disabled citizens, as well as the receptivity of federal and state rehabilitation agency staff to consumer participation, it seems quite likely that consumerism and rehabilitation will expand from sporadic tokenism to meaningful consumer involvement throughout the entire rehabilitation service delivery system.

Consumer participation in rehabilitation may perhaps best be described as a participation process still in its infancy. Only half of the state agencies report having written plans describing how the advice of disabled people and their advocates will be sought and used in determining agency policy and procedures. Similarly, a majority of disabled people remain unaware of agency policies on consumer involvement. The opportunities for significant advances are thus bright, particularly if each party approaches the process with an open, cooperative spirit. The possibilities are still flexible, the rules not yet rigid. But the time to act is now.

NOTES

[1]Community Services Administration. *Citizen Participation. Rapido Press,* San Jose, Calif., January 1978, inside front cover.

[2]*Rehabilitation Services Administration Manual.* Program Regulation Guide, Chapter 25, Section 525.03. Washington, D.C., October 15, 1975.

[3]Community Services Administration. Introduction, *Citizen Participation. Rapido Press,* San Jose, Calif., January 1978.

[4]*Rehabilitation Services Administration Manual,* Chapter 25, Section 525.04–525.05. Washington, D.C., 1975.

[5]Gerben DeJong. *The Movement for Independent Living: Origins, Ideology, and Implications For Disability Research.* Tufts Rehabilitation Institute, Tufts-New England Medical Center, Boston, Mass., November 17, 1978, p. 20.

[6]Ibid., p. 22.

[7]Rehabilitation Act of 1973, U.S. Government Printing Office, Washington, D.C., Section 101 (A) 18.

[8]DeJong, *The Movement for Independent Living,* p. 23.

[9]Ibid., p. 34.

[10]*Rehabilitation Services Administration Manual,* Chapter 25, Section 525.02.

[11]*Rehabilitation Act Amendments of 1978.* Washington, D.C., U.S. Government Printing Office, March 10 and 14, 1978.

[12]Paul J. Corcoran, *Annual Progress Report, 1977.* Tufts Research and Training Center, Tufts-New England Medical Center, Boston, Mass., p. 223.

[13]Janet Minch, and LeRoy Spaniol,. *Involving Disabled Consumers in Vocational Rehabilitation.* Tufts-New England Medical Center, Boston, Mass., 1978, p. 53.

[14]Janet Minch, and LeRoy Spaniol,. *Involving Disabled Consumers In Vocational Rehabilitation: An Evaluation Report of the Second Year,* Boston, Mass., Tufts-New England Medical Center, January 1979.

[15]The White House Conference on Handicapped Individuals, Volume Three: *Implementation Plan,* Washington D.C., U.S. Government Printing Office, June 1978, p. 9.

[16]Ibid., p. iv.

[17]Ibid., p. iv.

[18]Ibid., p. 9.

[19]Ibid., p. 10.

[20]Robert K. Yin, William A. Lucas, Peter L. Szanton, and J. Andrew Spindler. *Citizen Organizations: Increasing Client Control Over Services,* Santa Monica, Calif., April 1973, p. vii.

REFERENCES

Adams, A. S. "Rehabilitation Consumerism: Confrontation or Communication and Cooperation?" *Journal of Rehabilitation,* 42:23–25, 29, January–February 1976.

Arnstein, S. R. "A Ladder of Citizen Participation." *American Institute of Planners Journal,* 35:216–224, July 1969.

Back, Kurt, W., and Taylor, Rebecca C. "Self-Help Groups: Tool or Symbol." *Journal of Applied Behavioral Science,* 12 (July–August–September 1976):295–309.

Bartels, E. C. "Consumer Involvement in the Rehabilitation Process." (Unpublished paper, 1972).

Bowe, F. "Approaches to Consumer Involvement." *American Rehabilitation.* Washington, D.C.: Rehabilitation Services Administration, H.E.W., March–April 1979.

Bowe, F., Jacobi, J., and Wiseman, L. *Coalition Building.* Washington, D.C.: American Coalition of Citizens with Disabilities, Inc., 1978.

Carlucci, John, and Fellenz, Peter. *A Final Report: Feasibility Study Of A Management Training Program For Severely Physically Disabled Individuals.* Boston, Mass: Tufts Research and Training Center, Tufts-New England Medical Center, October 1978.

Community Services Administration. *Citizen Participation.* San Jose, Calif.: *Rapido Press,* 1978.

Corcoran, Paul J., *Annual Progress Report, 1977.* Boston, Mass.: Tufts Research and Training Center, Tufts-New England Medical Center, 1978.

Corcoran, Paul J., Fay, Fred, and DeJong, Gerben. *Integration of Independent Living Into the Total Rehabilitation Process.* Boston, Mass.: Tufts Research and Training Center, Tufts-New England Medical Center, 1978.

DeJong, Gerben. "The Movement for Independent Living: Origins, Ideology, and Implications for Disability Research" (Monograph). Boston, Mass.: Tufts Rehabilitation Institute, Tufts-New England Medical Center, 1978.

Drake, J. "Minnesota's Consumer Advisory Project." *Rehabilitation Record,* 14(2):25–27, March–April 1973.

Fay, Fred, Bartels, Elmer, Corcoran, Paul, and McHugh, Robert. *The BCIL Report.* Washington, D.C.: Health, Education and Welfare, Office of Human Development, Rehabilitation Services Administration, 1976.

Fay, Fred, Fortunato-Schwandt, Wayne, Minch, Janet, Redden, Martha, and Schein, Andrea. *Access To Science.* Boston, Mass.: Tufts Research and Training Center, Tufts-New England Medical Center, October 1978.

Howe, Susan, Minch, Janet, Fay, Fred, and Goldberg, Richard. *Consumer Involvement in Vocational Rehabilitation: State of the Art Study.* Boston, Mass.: Tufts Research and Training Center, Tufts-New England Medical Center, 1979.

Hurwitz, Nathan. "The Origin of the Peer Self-Help Psychotherapy Group Movement." *The Journal of Applied Behavioral Science,* 12, 283–294, (July–August–September 1976).

Institute on Rehabilitation Issues. *Consumer Involvement: Rehabilitation Issues.* Arkansas Rehabilitation Research and Training Center: June 1975.

Minch, Janet, and Spaniol, LeRoy. *Involving Disabled Consumers in Vocational Rehabilitation.* Boston, Mass.: Tufts Research and Training Center, Tufts-New England Medical Center, 1978.

Minch, Janet, and Spaniol, LeRoy. *Involving Disabled Consumers in Vocational Rehabilitation: An Evaluation Report of the Second Year.* (forthcoming report).

Nelson, John. *Evaluation Report, Vocational Rehabilitation: Consumers As Citizens.* Boston, Mass.: Tufts Research and Training Center, Tufts-New England Medical Center, September 1978.

Rehabilitation Act of 1973, Public Law 93–112. Washington, D.C.: U.S. Government Printing Office, September 26, 1973.

Rehabilitation Services Administration Manual. Program Regulation Guide, Chapter 25, (RSA-PRG-76-7). Washington, D.C., October 15, 1975.

Remmes, H. S. "Consumer Involvement in Rehabilitation." *Rehabilitation Record,* 13(4): 33–35, January 1972.

Remmes, H. S. "Consumer Feedback: Tiny Tim is Dead!" *Rehabilitation Literature,* 35(10):298–300, June 1974.

Thursz, D. *Consumer Involvement in Rehabilitation.* U.S. Department of Health, Education and Welfare, Social and Rehabilitation Service, Washington, D.C., 1969.

Varela, R. *Self-Help Groups in Rehabilitation.* Washington, D.C.: American Coalition of Citizens with Disabilities, Inc., 1978.

The White House Conference on Handicapped Individuals. Volume Three: *Implementation Plan.* Washington, D.C., U.S. Government Printing Office, June 1978.

Withorn, Ann. *To Serve the People: An Inquiry into the Success of Service Delivery as a Social Movement Strategy* (Unpublished dissertation, Brandeis University, 1977).

U.S. Congress. Senate. *Rehabilitation Act Amendments of 1978.* 95th Cong., 2nd sess. Washington, D.C.: U. S. Government Printing Office, 1978.

Yin, Robert K., Lucas, William A., Szanton, Peter L., and Spindler, Andrew J. *Citizen Organizations: Increasing Client Control Over Services.* Santa Monica, Calif., April 1973.

11
The Psychological, Social, and Vocational Adjustment to Spinal Cord Injury*

ROBERTA B. TRIESCHMANN, PH.D.

There is growing recognition that the psychological, social, and vocational aspects are important to the rehabilitation of persons with spinal injury, yet these aspects have not received sufficient emphasis in the rehabilitation process. Dr. Roberta B. Trieschmann summarizes the research on this topic and outlines the implications of these findings for those concerned with the rehabilitation of the spinal cord injured. She describes the major inadequacies of some of the research that has been conducted to date and suggests an alternative focus for research of the future: the development and testing of treatment strategies to assist every disabled person to achieve some success in life rather than a search for winners and losers.

INTRODUCTION

The incidence of spinal cord injury is greatest among males who are in their late teens and twenties. Thus, at the peak of their physical and emotional vigor, these young men face a loss of the ability to ambulate, a loss of sensation over those parts of the body below the level of the injury, a loss of bladder and bowel control, and an altered ability to participate in the physical aspects of sexual relationships. Men in their mid-thirties to mid-forties comprise another group who sustain spinal injuries frequently. Females account for approximately 20 percent of the spinal injury population.

In the past, rehabilitation efforts have been focused upon activities of daily living, mobility training, and vocational education and training.

*The research which provides the basis for this chapter was supported in part by a research grant from the Rehabilitation Services Administration, DHEW, Grant No. 13-P-59011/9-01.

However, both professionals and persons with spinal injury have been increasingly concerned that, to be successful, rehabilitation should include attention to the psychological and social parameters of the disability and should emphasize psychosocial integration into the community as a goal of rehabilitation. As a result of this concern, the Rehabilitation Services Administration sponsored a research project to evaluate the information available in the literature regarding the psychological, social, and vocational adjustment to spinal injury so that a comprehensive research program could be planned for the future to increase our knowledge in this area (Trieschmann, 1978).

This chapter will point out that there are significant gaps in our knowledge about the adjustment process to spinal injury. Unfortunately, much of the research to date has focused on the intrinsic characteristics of the injured person which lead to successful adjustment rather than on person-environment units. In essence, such research seeks to predict the successful candidates for rehabilitation and to screen out the failures. For example, research has identified a preinjury history of vocational accomplishment as predictive of employment but has ignored the financial disincentives to productivity. Thus, a study of the critical environmental influences on the behavior of the person with spinal injury can potentially lead to the development of intervention strategies to assist more injured persons to achieve a successful and rewarding life following onset of a disability. Topics to be reviewed in this chapter include the psychological factors associated with spinal injury, the social implications of the disability, factors associated with productivity, sexuality, the impact of the treatment environment, and intervention strategies which will produce behavior change. Emphasis will be placed on the identification of what we know and do not know about the adjustment to spinal cord injury. Suggestions for future research will also be given.

PSYCHOLOGICAL FACTORS ASSOCIATED WITH SPINAL INJURY

A recent exhaustive review of the literature on the psychological, social, and vocational adjustment to spinal cord injury reveals that there are significant gaps in our knowledge about the process of adjustment (Trieschmann, 1978). This lack of knowledge is rather shameful, especially when viewed in light of clinical evidence that there is a high suicide rate in this population. Although there are no direct studies of suicide among these with spinal cord injury, some inferences can be drawn from morbidity studies in the literature. Such studies suggest that 12 to 46 percent of the deaths of persons with spinal injury who survive the acute stage of treatment may involve self-neglect or self-destructive behaviors. Most of these deaths occur within five years of injury. Consequently, it appears that our psychological rehabilitation efforts have not been very successful up to now. In the future, we must explore the processes of adjustment and rehabilitation to identify appropriate behavioral goals for each individual and effective intervention strategies to accomplish these goals.

Emotional Factors

Little information about the immediate consequences of spinal injury has been reliably demonstrated. There has been widespread speculation that the early weeks, perhaps months, involve a state of psychological shock in which the person actively denies what has happened, but there are no data which substantiate this notion. An alternative hypothesis proposes that any clouding of the sensorium during the acute stage results from a combination of circumstances, such as anesthesia from surgery, medication for pain, sensory deprivation, and sleep disruption, rather than denial. Consistent with this hypothesis, it has been reported that a large percentage of patients actively desire information about their injury within two weeks of onset (Braakman, Orbaan, and Dishoeck, 1976).

The literature is full of articles which purport to describe the stages of adjustment to spinal injury, and the same unsubstantiated ideas are repeated like a litany. For example, the stage theory of adjustment proposes that the immediate reaction to disability is denial, followed by profound depression (Kerr and Thompson, 1972). This theory proposes that people must go through these stages and mourn their loss in order to become adjusted to the disability. It is feared that the adjustment process will not be complete until the person has experienced depression and truly mourned.

However, the data tend to suggest the opposite (Bourestrom and Howard, 1965; Dinardo, 1971; Goldiamond, 1973; Kalb, 1971; Klas, 1970; Lawson, 1976; and Taylor, 1967). Recent research suggests that those who are least depressed tend to function better during rehabilitation and following discharge. Those who do become significantly depressed may do far worse after discharge. There is no evidence to substantiate the stage theory of adjustment, and on the average, only mild depression during the second or third week has been noted in these studies.

The research which documents the emotional reaction to spinal injury has been complicated by the finding that spinal injury itself may reduce the experience of emotional feelings because of disruption of the autonomic nervous system (Hohmann, 1966). The higher the level of the lesion, the greater the reduction in experienced emotional feelings. Patients report, however, that they often act "as if" they were feeling emotional, because it is expected of them by those around them, and they get attention for their requests. Consequently, in studying the emotional reaction to spinal injury, the use of multiple levels of measurement, including a biochemical measure, and several direct behavioral measures of emotion may circumvent this "as if" phenomenon. Most research in the past has used staff ratings of the person's emotional behavior as the criterion measure, this type of measurement being most susceptible to distortion by the "as if" phenomenon. Longitudinal research seems to be the more effective way of reliably determining the fluctuating role of emotions in the adjustment process, rather than cross-sectional research, as has been the case up to now.

Motivational Factors

Motivation has been considered the key to the rehabilitation process. If the patient is "motivated," it is believed that success in ensured. Ordinarily, motivation has been viewed as a drive within the individual to get better; in actuality, however, it is often equated with overt cooperation with the rehabilitation staff and their decisions. Using this concept of motivation, the emphasis in the literature has been on the identification of those with motivation and on the attempt to screen out those with a motivational deficit (Fordyce, 1975). No one has identified a remedy for a deficit in motivation using this approach, and psychotherapy apparently has proved unsuccessful in this regard (Diamond, Weiss, and Grynbaum, 1968).

However, if motivation is viewed in terms of those rewards and satisfactions in the environment for which the person will work, motivation becomes external to the person and is capable of being influenced by rearranging the environmental rewards. There is much evidence that this approach works. "Unmotivated" patients can change their behavior through use of behavior therapy techniques, which gives credibility to this view of motivation (Malament, Dunn, and Davis, 1975; Sand, Fordyce, and Fowler, 1973; Trotter and Inman, 1968).

Locus of control appears related to the concept of motivation, and it may become a critical issue in working with the disabled person. *Locus of control* is defined as the degree of belief that one's behavior controls the rewards of the world. Persons with an *external* locus of control believe in fate, luck, chance, and powerful others, and those with an *internal* locus of control believe that their own behavior controls their rewards. Externals tend to become more depressed following spinal injury and to do less well after discharge (Dinardo, 1971). Internals tend to show less depression and to function much better following discharge. Furthermore, externals may be more susceptible to the experience of learned helplessness (Seligman, 1975). The onset of spinal injury may be one of the most extreme examples of helplessness in the natural environment, and if some persons are susceptible to learning that they are helpless to control the rewards of the world, they may function very poorly in the rehabilitation center and after discharge. Thus, it appears that the behavioral view of motivation and the concepts of locus of control and learned helplessness may provide keys to the improved functioning of a large percentage of persons with spinal injury.

Body Image and Pain

Body image, as a psychodynamically defined personality variable, has not been demonstrated to relate to the adjustment to disability. However, body image as a sensory response to parts of one's body has been shown to be disrupted in a large percentage of persons with spinal injury soon after onset (Bors, 1951; Conomy, 1973). The perception of the body in positions other than the one visually noted is the most common experience. However, these body image distortions tend to disappear in a large proportion of persons within several months of injury.

Pain is a frequent experience immediately after the injury, but it tends to disappear within several weeks unless there is extensive surgery which produces scarring or unless the person is not managed well psychologically in the early stages of injury (Burke, 1973). Furthermore, Burke suggests that persons who have not received proper psychological management may have more pain complaints than those who have received proper care. The correlation between the incidence of pain complaints and a prior history of alcohol or drug abuse is suspected but not proven.

Personality Factors

There is no evidence of a unitary spinal cord injury personality. In fact, there is considerable evidence to suggest that the population of persons with spinal injury is a heterogeneous one. Very few persons exhibit significant psychopathology after the spinal injury unless they had a preinjury history of hospitalization for depression or suicide attempts, or some other evidence of severe psychological maladjustment (Hohmann, 1975). Hohmann also notes that psychotic persons who sustain a spinal injury may show a remission of the psychotic symptoms until pressured to leave the hospital and resume functioning in the outside world.

The research into the factors associated with adjustment to spinal injury reveals that youth, a warm and loving family background, financial resources, a history of accepting responsibility for educational and vocational plans, an internal locus of control, the presence of interpersonal support, creativity in problem solving, having many goals, and having goals in the accomplishment versus physical function area are associated with success in rehabilitation (Goldberg and Freed, 1976; Kemp and Vash, 1971; Kerr and Thompson, 1972; Swenson, 1976). We have already noted that much of the research has focused exclusively on features of the person. In addition, such research activity tends to identify the successes so that we screen out the failures. However, this assumes that all responsibility for success depends on the intrinsic characteristics of the person, and suggestions are not usually given as to how to deal with the failures. This limited approach may be too costly if we consider the death rate from self-neglect as one indication of the problem.

Psychological Testing

The use of psychological tests to predict outcome has been the focus of little research. However, in cases in which they have been used, they have not accounted for much of the variance in behavior. The Minnesota Multiphasic Personality Inventory (MMPI) has been used to assess the immediate emotional response to spinal injury; only mild depression has been found, in contrast to the massive psychological distress which had been predicted (Bourestom and Howard, 1965; Fordyce, 1964; Taylor, 1967). However, these studies contain the implicit assumption of homogeneity of the population with spinal injury—and this assumption is probably erroneous. Rather, the population seems to be a very heterogeneous one and may be composed of several distinct groups. Therefore, the averaging of psychological test data for the entire group before determining the nature of the population may produce misleading results. Furthermore, the MMPI has been found to contain items which a person with spinal injury would have to answer in the deviant direction, not because of psychological problems but because of the spinal injury (Taylor, 1967, 1970). This inflates the profiles spuriously unless a correction is made for these items.

There is no data which relates the results of intelligence or projective tests to outcome. However, there is some evidence to suggest that tests of creativity and problem-solving ability may relate to outcome (Kemp and Vash, 1971). Therefore, it is recommended that psychological test data be considered only one of many kinds of measurements of behavior. Greater emphasis should be given to the direct observation of behavior in our evaluation and research activity.

SOCIAL IMPLICATIONS OF THE DISABILITY

While emphasis in rehabilitation has traditionally been focused on the physical parameters of the disability, the social implications may be devastating and should receive equal attention in rehabilitation programs. The concept of difference is learned at an early age, as is the concept of physical attractiveness, and we learn to evaluate people on these two dimensions (Berscheid and Walster, 1974). Thus, persons with a spinal injury may devalue themselves according to these internalized standards and know, too, that others will devalue them accordingly. As a result, they tend to withdraw from social situations after discharge from the rehabilitation center (Cogswell, 1968). Through a process of self-socialization, they learn to cope with the world to some degree, but the degree of skill they achieve in managing social situations varies greatly. Thus, it appears that a key to a successful outcome after spinal injury is the variety of social skills which the injured person possesses (Dunn, 1977; Dunn, Van Horn, and Herman, 1977; Romano, 1976). Therefore, a major emphasis for the future must be the development of techniques to teach social skills to disabled persons and research to identify which technique is best suited to which behavioral goal.

Demographic Factors

Demographic variables may be quite influential on function following spinal injury. There is some evidence that, on the average, the younger person adjusts somewhat better than the older person (Kerr and Thompson, 1972), and the age range of twenty to thirty-five may have the greatest variability in ultimate functioning (Wilcox and Stauffer, 1972). Within this latter age group, some adjust splendidly and others do poorly. There is no evidence that severity of disability per se influences adjustment to disability. Rather, person and environment characteristics play a more important role in determining outcome. We have no evidence on the influence of duration of disability, although it may take two to four years to learn to live with the disability with some degree of comfort and satisfaction (Kerr and Thompson, 1972).

Sex of the individual may be a variable in ultimate response to spinal injury. However, we have no evidence on the difference between men and women in adjusting to the disability, since most of the research to date has been based on men. Socioeconomic status has been implicated as a factor in one study (Kalb, 1971), but we do not know enough about its role at this point. Socioeconomic status and culture may have very powerful influences on adjustment to spinal injury, since these environmental variables are correlated with the injured person's resources and with expectations regarding behavior. Both of these issues may enhance or interfere with the rehabilitation process. We do not know the effect of urban versus rural residence on spinal injury. Thus, research is needed to document the influence of demographic variables on adjustment to spinal injury.

Family Factors

Disability can have a great impact on the family, but we have little data to document the types of problems and the intervention strategies that are most effective as remedial devices. Statistics on marriage and divorce among U.S. veterans suggest that approximately 26 percent of preinjury and postinjury marriages end in divorce, in comparison to a 33 percent divorce rate for able-bodied persons nationally and 50 percent in California, the residence of most of the research subjects (El Ghatit and Hanson, 1975, 1976). However, we have no data on the civilian spinal injury population, who may not have the same financial security as many veterans. Thus, there is concern that this data may not be representative of the entire population of persons with spinal injury.

Recreational Factors

Recreation has often been viewed as entertainment rather than a therapeutic activity. However, it appears that active participation in a sport may have physical and psychosocial benefits, but this is an issue which deserves to be studied. Since recreation of some kind is an important part of everyone's life, a person with a disability needs to learn new leisure-time activities if the preinjury ones are no longer available. The effects of active participation in sports and other recreational activity should be studied in terms of productivity and in terms of the death rate.

FACTORS ASSOCIATED WITH PRODUCTIVITY

Traditionally, there has been an emphasis on full-time employment as the outcome of rehabilitation efforts. However, employment may not be an appropriate goal for everyone, and there are obstacles within the system which prevent everyone who desires a job from becoming employed. Therefore, it seems more reasonable to consider one of our goals to be productivity, which includes educational and avocational activities, group membership, and family and community participation, in addition to employment.

The data suggest that persons with paraplegia are somewhat more likely to obtain employment than persons with quadriplegia (Brown and Chanin, 1974; Dvonch, Kaplan, Grynbaum, and Rusk, 1965; Felton and Litman, 1965; Geisler, Jousse, and Wynne-Jones, 1966; Goldberg and Freed, 1976; Seybold 1976; and Wilson, 1972). Yet the employment rates vary from 14 to 44 percent in the various studies, and the definition of what constitutes employment is not always clear. Thus, it is very difficult to compare one study with another. Obstacles to employment include financial disincentives to productivity, negative attitudes of employers, and lack of complete services by the state-federal Vocational Rehabilitation program. As with psychological factors, the research has focused exclusively on the characteristics of the person that lead to success. The emphasis is on the identification of winners and the attempt to screen out the losers rather than on the development of strategies that will identify marketable skills, train them, and place the person in a job which utlizes them. However, unless the financial disincentives to productivity are reduced, many persons with disabilities will not be able to afford to take a job even though they would like to work.

As with other attitudes, programs to educate the public or employers as a means of reducing prejudice toward the disabled are not recommended. Research in other areas (Bandura, 1969) demonstrates that we should emphasize behavior change as a means of producing attitude change rather than the reverse. Therefore, it is recommended that efforts be devoted to teaching disabled people to function successfully in the able-bodied world. This will create opportunities for able-bodied people to interact with the disabled and to behave in a normal, nonprejudicial fashion. As people change their behavior toward the disabled, their cognitions and emotions will gradually change.

SEXUALITY

Sexual function is an important part of life and continues following a spinal injury. There is some evidence to suggest that the sex drive may be slightly reduced following spinal injury (Hohmann, 1966), but age variables may play a powerful role. There is evidence that persons who abstain from sexual activities are no less well adjusted than those who do participate (Berkman, Weissman, and Frielich, 1978). However, whether one participates in sexual activities seems to be highly dependent on having a partner with whom a good relationship exists. In fact, in successful marriages where one partner is spinal cord injured, a significant proportion of the couples do not rely on sexual intercourse as their primary mode of sexual satisfaction (Berkman, Weissman, and Frielich, 1978). Thus, sexual function has many parameters which need to be evaluated, and methods of fostering sexual relationships need to be taught. People with spinal injuries should have the opportunity to participate in sexual relationships if they choose; and thus, training should be offered.

Treatment for sexual dysfunctions in spinal cord injury, judging from the literature, seems to consist of counseling-didactic sessions and sexual attitude reassessment workshops (Cole, Chilgren, and Rosenberg, 1973; Eisenberg and Rustad, 1976; Halstead, Halstead, Salhoot, Stock, and Sparks, 1977; Held, Cole, Held, Anderson, and Chilgren, 1975; and Romano and Lassiter, 1972). We have no evidence that these techniques lead to behavior change on the part of the participants, although most participants report that they thought the sessions were helpful. Therefore, we need to develop strategies for teaching people a variety of sexual behaviors, as well as research into the outcomes of these efforts. We have no data on the effect of disability on the partner or on the strategies to assist partners to cope with the disability. Much research is needed in this area.

THE IMPACT OF THE TREATMENT ENVIRONMENT

The treatment environment—the hospital or rehabilitation center—seems to have a profound effect on the behavior of the person with a disability. There is evidence that the hospital environment provides minimal opportunity for patient decision making, independence, or zest in any of the treatment activities which comprise a large part of rehabilitation (French, McDowell, and Keith, 1972; Miller and Keith, 1973; Vineberg and Willems, 1971; Willems, 1972; Willems, 1976; Willems and Vineberg, 1969). In fact, the treatment environment appears to account for more variability in patient behavior than individual patient characteristics do. A large part of a patient's day typically is spent in nontherapeutic activities or alone. Furthermore, of all rehabilitation personnel, aides and orderlies have the most patient contact time, but they are the ones who receive the least training in behavior change skills. Thus, we find that patients are often rewarded for dependent, nonassertive behaviors and ignored or punished when they try to be independent (Mikulic, 1971).

In the context of research activities or clinical evaluations, rehabilitation personnel are often asked to rate the behavior of the person with a disability. However, there is considerable evidence that they overestimate the degree of psychological distress. In addition, it appears that many personnel may have an unrealistic and negative stereotype of the disabled person which is not very different from that of the general population (Taylor, 1967). Since these personnel form part of the patient's environment, these unfavorable expectations as to how disabled persons should behave may be counterproductive influences during the rehabilitation process.

As a result of these studies regarding the treatment environment, we must examine the rehabilitation process to determine both its effect on patient behavior and whether that is the effect we desire. If not, then we must either change the procedures of rehabilitation centers or develop a multi-stage rehabilitation system: physical rehabilitation followed by training in functional skills for living.

INTERVENTION STRATEGIES

There has been considerable discussion in the literature about the importance of counseling, group counseling, and psychotherapy as treatment techniques following onset of a disability. However, there is no evidence to demonstrate that these techniques lead to improved functioning and behavior change. It is apparent that many of the goals are too globally defined, impossible to measure, and perhaps inappropriate for the technique in question. Thus, it is time to perform some carefully controlled studies to assess the effectiveness of counseling techniques as behavior change strategies.

Behavior therapy has been demonstrated to lead to behavior change in fluid intake, pushups, body positioning in bed, improved personal hygiene, and upper extremity strengthening (Malament, Dunn, and Davis, 1975; Roberts, Dinsdale, Matthews, and Cole, 1969; Rottkamp, 1976; Sand, Fordyce, and Fowler, 1973; Trotter and Inman, 1968). By using such techniques, "unmotivated" persons can achieve comparable levels of function to the "motivated" person. Since all of rehabilitation is a learning process, a behavior change process, intervention strategies must be evaluated for their ability to produce behavior change. In this regard, behavior therapy techniques have demonstrated this effect. If most behavior is learned through the principles of operant conditioning, then behavior therapy techniques could reasonably become the standard operating procedure of rehabilitation, and all personnel should become skilled in such strategies.

Social skills training shows promise as an intervention strategy, but there is only one research project which has studied its effect on behavior change in persons with spinal injury (Dunn, Van Horn, and Herman, 1977). Development of social skills training strategies should be a primary focus of research, along with the study of which types of settings are most appropriate for use of such techniques.

Because of the evidence of counterproductive effects of many hospital environments on patient behavior, we must study alternative methods of service delivery. The transitional living center concept shows promise and should be studied further (Manley and Armstrong, 1976; Stock and Cole, 1977). We must consider the possibility of a multi-stage rehabilitation process and study the cost-effectiveness of such an approach. This would entail learning the traditional physical rehabilitation skills in the medical rehabilitation center and learning social skills and survival skills in another setting, perhaps a transitional living center. The newly emerging independent living centers deserve to be studied with respect to their role in such a multi-stage rehabilitation process. They may prove to be a powerful community resource previously untapped.

CONCLUSIONS

The literature on the adjustment to spinal injury reveals that there has been more speculation and armchair reasoning then empirical research into the multitude of variables associated with outcome. The emphasis, in studies of psychological factors and vocational success, has been on the intrinsic characteristics of the injured person which lead to success, without a careful consideration of the variety of environmental variables which influence outcome. For example, the research into the social implications of the disability is meager; it often consists of statistics on divorce rather than an investigation of the complexity of interpersonal relationships following a severe physical disability. Furthermore, recent research reveals that the treatment environment itself has a tremendous impact on the behavior of the disabled person, an impact which is often counterproductive to the goals of independence and decision-making skill. Studies of vocational success usually do not mention financial disincentives to productivity or negative attitudes; instead, they focus on education and predisability employment as the key issues in obtaining full-time employment. And, of course, the focus of research is usually a direct reflection of professional attitudes and clinical approaches.

Therefore, a refocusing of our research efforts and clinical approaches is recommended. Rather than emphasizing the characteristics of the disabled person only, an integration of person and environment is proposed. That is, given the characteristics of a particular disabled person and the features of his or her environment, what strategies can be used to teach the behaviors needed to compete in an able-bodied world? Rather than searching for winners and attempting to screen out the losers, we should strive to teach all disabled persons the skills they need to achieve a psychosocial integration into their community. Within this approach, employment becomes one facet of such integration rather than the only goal of rehabilitation.

REFERENCES

Bandura, A. *Principles of behavior modification.* New York: Holt, Rinehart and Winston, 1969.

Berkman, A., Weissman, R., and Frielich, M. Sexual adjustment of spinal injured veterans living in the community. *Archives of Physical Medicine and Rehabilitation,* 1978, *59,* 29–33.

Berscheid, E., and Walster, E. Physical attractiveness. *Advances in Experimental Social Psychology,* 1974, *7,* 157–215.

Bors, E. Phantom limbs of patients with spinal cord injury. *Archives of Neurology and Psychiatry,* 1951, *66,* 610–631.

Bourestom, N., and Howard, M. Personality characteristics of three disability groups. *Archives of Physical Medicine and Rehabilitation,* 1965, *46,* 626–632.

Braakman, R., Orbaan, J., and Dishoeck, M. Information in the early stages after spinal cord injury. *International Journal of Paraplegia,* 1976, *14,* 95–100.

Brown, B., and Chanin, I. *Patterns of education and employment: Rehabilitants from severe spinal cord injury, FY 1972–73.* Rehabilitation Research Reports, No. 30, Department of Rehabilitation, Sacramento, CA., June 1, 1974.

Burke, D. Pain in paraplegia. *International Journal of Paraplegia,* 1973, *10,* 297–313.

Cogswell, B. Self socialization: Readjustment of paraplegics in the community. *Journal of Rehabilitation,* 1968, *34,* 11–13, 35.

Cole, T., Chilgren, R., and Rosenberg, P. A new programme of sex education and counseling for spinal cord injured adults and health care professionals. *International Journal of Paraplegia,* 1973, *11,* 111–124.

Conomy, J. Disorders of body image after spinal cord injury. *Neurology,* 1973, *23,* 841–850.

Diamond, M., Weiss, A., and Grynbaum, B. The unmotivated patient. *Archives of Physical Medicine and Rehabilitation,* 1968, *49,* 281–284.

Dinardo, Q. *Psychological adjustment to spinal cord injury.* Doctoral dissertation, University of Houston, 1971.

Dunn, M. Social discomfort in the patient with spinal cord injury. *Archives of Physical Medicine and Rehabilitation,* 1977, *58,* 257–260.

Dunn, M., Van Horn, E., and Herman, S. A comparison of three training procedures for spinal cord injury social skills. Paper presented at American Congress of Rehabilitation Medicine, Miami Beach, November 1977.

Dvonch, P., Kaplan, L., Grynbaum, B., and Rusk, H. Vocational findings in post disability employment of patients with spinal cord dysfunction. *Archives of Physical Medicine and Rehabilitation,* 1965, *46,* 761–766.

Eisenberg, M., and Rustad, L. Sex education and counseling program on a spinal cord injury service. *Archives of Physical Medicine and Rehabilitation,* 1976, *57,* 135–140.

El Ghatit, A., and Hanson, R. Outcome of marriages existing at the time of a male's spinal cord injury. *Journal of Chronic Disease,* 1975, *28,* 383–388.

El Ghatit, A., and Hanson, R. Marriage and divorce after spinal cord injury. *Archives of Physical Medicine and Rehabilitation,* 1976, *57,* 470–472.

Felton, J., and Litman, M. Study of employment of 222 men with spinal cord injury. *Archives of Physical Medicine and Rehabilitation,* 1965, *46,* 809–814.

Fordyce, W. Personality characteristics of men with spinal cord injury as related to manner of onset disability. *Archives of Physical Medicine and Rehabilitation,* 1964, *45,* 321–325.

Fordyce, W. Research on influencing level of patient participation in the rehabilitation process. *Selected research topics in spinal cord injury rehabilitation.* (Grant 16-P-56813/6-13.) Houston, Texas: Texas Institute for Rehabilitation and Research, July 1975.

French, D., McDowell, R., and Keith, R. A. Participant observation as a patient in a rehabilitation hospital. *Rehabilitation Psychology,* 1972, *19,* 89–95.

Geisler, W., Jousse, A., and Wynne-Jones, M. Vocational reestablishment of patients with spinal cord injury. *Medical Services Journal of Canada,* 1966, *22,* 698–710.

Goldberg, R., and Freed, M. The vocational development, interests, values, adjustment, and rehabilitation outlook of spinal cord patients: A four year follow-up. Paper presented at American Congress of Rehabilitation Medicine, San Diego, November 1976.

Goldiamond, I. A diary of self-modification. *Psychology Today,* November 1973, *7,* 95–102.

Halstead, L., Halstead, M., Salhoot, J., Stock, D., and Sparks, R. A hospital based program in human sexuality. *Archives of Physical Medicine and Rehabilitation,* 1977, *58,* 409–412.

Held, J., Cole, T., Held, C., Anderson, C., and Chilgren, R. Sexual attitude reassessment workshops: Effect on spinal cord injured adults, their partners, and rehabilitation professionals. *Archives of Physical Medicine and Rehabilitation,* 1975, *56,* 14–18.

Hohmann, G. Some effects of spinal cord lesions on experienced emotional feelings. *Psychophysiology,* 1966, *3,* 143–156.

Hohmann, G. Psychological aspects of treatment and rehabilitation of the spinal injured person. *Clinical Orthopedics,* 1975, *112,* 81–88.

Kalb, M. *An examination of the relationship between hospital ward behaviors and post-discharge behaviors in the spinal cord injury patients.* Doctoral dissertation, University of Houston, 1971.

Kemp, B., and Vash, C. Productivity after injury in a sample of spinal cord injured persons: A pilot study. *Journal of Chronic Disease,* 1971, *24,* 259–275.

Kerr, W., and Thompson, M. Acceptance of disability of sudden onset in paraplegia. *International Journal of Paraplegia,* 1972, *10,* 94–102.

Klas, L. *A study of the relationship between depression and factors in the rehabilitation process of the hospitalized spinal cord injured patient.* Doctoral dissertation, University of Utah, 1970.

Lawson, N. *Depression after spinal cord injury: A multi-measure longitudinal study.* Doctoral dissertation, University of Houston, 1976.

Malament, I., Dunn, M., and Davis, R. Pressure sores: An operant conditioning approach to prevention. *Archives of Physical Medicine and Rehabilitation,* 1975, *56,* 161–165.

Manley, S., and Armstrong, M. A transitional living experience for the severely disabled. *Rehabilitation Counseling Bulletin,* 1976, *19,* 551–555.

Mikulic, M. Reinforcement of independent and dependent patient behaviors by nursing personnel: An exploratory study. *Nursing Research,* 1971, *20,* 162–164.

Miller, R., and Keith, R. A. Behavioral mapping in a rehabilitation hospital. *Rehabilitation Psychology,* 1973, *20,* 148–155.

Roberts, A., Dinsdale, S., Matthews, R., and Cole, T. Modifying persistent undesirable behavior in a medical setting. *Archives of Physical Medicine and Rehabilitation,* 1969, *50,* 147–153.

Romano, M. Social skills training with the newly handicapped. *Archives of Physical Medicine and Rehabilitation,* 1976, *57,* 302–303.

Romano, M., and Lassiter, R. Sexual counseling with the spinal cord injured. *Archives of Physical Medicine and Rehabilitation,* 1972, *53,* 568–572.

Rottkamp, B. A behavior modification approach to nursing therapeutics in body positioning of spinal cord injured patients. *Nursing Research,* 1976, *25,* 181–186.

Sand, P., Fordyce, W., and Fowler, R. Fluid intake behavior in patients with spinal cord injury: Prediction and modification. *Archives of Physical Medicine and Rehabilitation,* 1973, *54,* 254–262.

Seligman, M. *Helplessness: On depression, development, and death.* San Francisco: W. H. Freeman, 1975.

Seybold, J. Rehabilitation and employment status report. *Paraplegia News,* 1976, *29*(330), 34–36.

Stock, D., and Cole, J. *Cooperative living: A cooperative self-support system for severely physically disabled young adults.* Final report of RSA grant 13-P-55487/6-01. Houston, Texas: Texas Institute for Rehabilitation and Research, 1977.

Swenson, E. *The relationship between locus of control expectancy and successful rehabilitation of the spinal cord injured.* Doctoral dissertation, Arizona State University, 1976.

Taylor, G. *Predicted versus actual response to spinal cord injury: A psychological study.* Doctoral dissertation, University of Minnesota, 1967.

Taylor, G. Moderator-variable effect on personality test item endorsements of physically disabled patients. *Journal of Consulting and Clinical Psychology,* 1970, *35,* 183–188.

Trieschmann, R. *The psychological, social, and vocational adjustment to spinal cord injury: A strategy for future research.* Final report of RSA grant 13-P-59011/9-01. Los Angeles: Easter Seal Society of Los Angeles County, April 30, 1978.

Trotter, A., and Inman, D. The use of positive reinforcement in physical therapy. *Physical Therapy,* 1968, *48,* 347–352.

Vineberg, S., and Willems, E. Observation and analysis of patient behavior in the rehabilitation hospital. *Archives of Physical Medicine and Rehabilitation,* 1971, *52,* 8–14.

Wilcox, N., and Stauffer, E. Follow-up of 423 consecutive patients admitted to the spinal cord centre, Rancho Los Amigos Hospital, January 1 to December 31, 1967. *International Journal of Paraplegia,* 1972, *10,* 115–122.

Willems, E. Interface of the hospital environment and patient behavior. *Archives of Physical Medicine and Rehabilitation,* 1972, *53,* 115–122.

Willems, E. Behavioral ecology, health status, and health care: Applications to the rehabilitation setting. In I. Altman and J. Wohlwill (eds.), *Human behavior and Environment.* New York: Plenum, 1976.

Willems, E., and Vineberg, S. Direct observation of patients: The interface of environment and behavior. *Psychological Aspects of Disability,* 1969, *16,* 74–88.

Wilson, W. *A study of quadriplegics in employment.* Woodrow Wilson Rehabilitation Center, Fisherville, Va., 1972.

12
Rehabilitation Following Severe Burns*

GARRY S. BRODY, M.D.
MARK A. JOHNSON, PH.D.

The severely burned patient represents a multidisciplinary challenge to obtain maximum rehabilitation potential. Dealing with both the physical and emotional scarring that results from severe burn injury requires support from a highly competent professional team, including a surgeon, psychologist, occupational therapist, physical therapist, and nursing staff. Ancillary services may include orthotics, liaison nursing, dermatology, and others. This chapter deals with what is now known about the physical and psychological factors associated with severe burn injury and rehabilitation of burn patients, emphasizing the actual and subjective experience of undergoing burn rehabilitation for the individual patient. The interaction of the burn injury with premorbid psychological or physical problems is also discussed.

There are more than 100,000 burn injuries requiring medical treatment in the United States each year. The Los Angeles County-University of Southern California Acute Burn Unit (the largest such facility in the world) treats up to 500 burn cases of all types per year. Of this population, about one in twenty requires significant long-term rehabilitative or reconstructive assistance. Epileptics, drug and alcohol abusers, battered children, suicide attempters, the infirm, and the careless are all at high risk of sustaining extensive burns. Therefore, of those patients requiring rehabilitation, 65 percent have severe, significant, preexisting psychological, social, or neurological disorders that can be directly related to the burn injury and are of clear concern to the rehabilitation process. This discussion will review both the *physical* and *psychological* aspects of rehabilitation for more severe burn victims.

Most of the current burn literature deals with the metabolic, physi-

*From the Burn Rehabilitation Service, Rancho Los Amigos/University of Southern California Medical Center.

cal, and bacterial aspects of the acute burn; literature on the rehabilitative phase of care is scanty. One purportedly complete bibliographic source (Feller, 1978) lists 2,298 citations published in 5,000 journals in 1977 in 27 languages that would be of interest to burn care specialists. Only two of these references (Jones and Feller, 1977; Hales, 1977) specifically deal with rehabilitation, and only a handful are concerned with burn reconstruction. There is, of course, extensive worldwide experience in the subject and much oral interchange among those dealing with the problem upon which this state of the art review is based.

The severe burn threatens both the physical and the emotional well-being of its victim. The patient must first survive the initial metabolic shock, bacterial invasion, debridement of dead tissue, and ultimate skin grafting. He or she is assaulted by innumerable needles, tubes in every orifice (including endotracheal intubation while awake if there are pulmonary complications), forced feeding, and exhortations to participate in active therapy when the inclination is to curl up in a corner and not move. The dead skin is picked at daily; the patient is doused in antibiotics, solutions, and ointments and isolated from normal human contact by dressings, gloves, masks, and gowns to minimize the risk of ever-threatening infection. The entire process is painful and terrifying.

The acute period ends with the burn areas almost entirely epithelialized and grafted. While the physical isolation and much of the pain is over, the patient is left with the realization of being debilitated and may be permanently scarred. There may be tight, contractured joints, amputated parts, or severely distorted features. The scars, like the injury, are both physical and emotional.

Rehabilitation begins with rebuilding of the depleted body reserves, followed by surgical reconstruction of the deformed parts and restoration of the patient's emotional well-being, with the ultimate goal of social and vocational self-sufficiency. Injured human skin scars in a fashion different than that of any known animal. When the body's epithelial cover is restored, its metabolic integrity is secure, but the scar undergoes a prolonged maturation characterized by an initial thickening and rigidity, called *hypertrophy,* and shrinkage called, *scar contracture.* (The term *keloid* is often incorrectly applied to all scars which are raised above the surface. This term should be reserved for a very special aberration of scar maturation. While burn scars may incidentally form keloid, the vast majority are merely hypertrophic, with or without contracture.)

The severity, rate of development, degree of contracture, and ultimate softening time of scars are highly variable, depending upon individual patient characteristics, extent of site of injury, mechanical forces, and subsequent treatment. As a general rule, the more racially inherited skin pigment a patient has, the greater the tendency to hypertrophy. Deep second-degree burns and seams between skin grafts seem to thicken the most. Scar contracture is most common and disabling over the flexor surfaces of joints and adjacent to body orifices where skin edges may have no counterfixation (e.g., eyelids, nostrils, mouth). Fingers, toes, and ears are the most likely parts to require amputation. Blindness, pulmonary damage, heterotopic ossification, unrelenting pruritus, peripheral nerve entrapment phenomena (carpel tunnel, etc.), septic arthritis, and even—rarely—late (twenty to thirty years later) squamous malignancies in unstable skin can complicate the problem.

Restoration of maximum physical, social, and emotional well-being requires a coordinated, multidisciplinary team of professionals. The process of rehabilitation can be divided into two major facets, but each team member must be intimately concerned with all aspects of care.

PHYSICAL REHABILITATION

Physical rehabilitation begins with a total patient evaluation and separation of the true physical limitations from their emotional overlay. The patient should be encouraged to restore proper nutrition with a high-calorie, well-balanced diet. Vitamin supplements should not be required. Skin care is essential, as the patient may still have a few small open areas or folliculitis in entrapped hair follicles. The skin lacks sebaceous glands and will require daily lubrication. Severe overheating must be avoided in patients with extensive scars (60 percent or more), as they may have insufficient residual sweat glands to cool the body. Pruritus can be very troublesome and may be resistant to all medication, though this condition usually subsides to a tolerable level with time. Judicious management of analgesic medication may require both Solomonic wisdom and Jobian patience by the rehabilitation team, as burn victims frequently become drug dependent and can be quite manipulative in their efforts to have pain-killing medication continued.

Active occupational and physical therapy can frequently correct or improve certain degrees of scar contracture, especially in the major joints. Dynamic and passive splinting will aid in increasing range, reeducation in functional activities, and compensation for amputated parts. Resolution and softening of the hypertrophic scars can be increased and accelerated by total contact splints and customized elastic pressure garments (custom-made by Jobst®). In a major burn, however, so much equipment may be required that patient tolerance may be overtaxed. The type of patient who gets burned not uncommonly has poor self-discipline, so that a commonsense appraisal must be made in each case to avoid drawers full of unused, expensive appliances.

While the patient must realize that residual scarring is inevitable, much improvement can be gained in both appearance and function with surgical intervention. Current popular imagery expects plastic surgeons to magically wipe away scars, and it is almost impossible to create for patients a precise word image about what results may realistically be anticipated. Conversations with other burn patients may help, but the enthusiast may oversell or the disaffected unduly discourage the uncertain surgical candidate. The best preparation the surgeon can provide is a frank, compassionate, and unhurried conversation with the patient close to the time of surgery.

Skin grafting is the *sine qua non* of surgical reconstruction. Transection of tight, thickened bands across joints permits restoration of limb range, thus creating a defect to be filled with a graft. The release of tension on the tight scar permits it to soften and thin, though surface irregularities and pigmentary variations may still persist. Irregularly pitted and corrugated skin surfaces can be smoothed by careful regrafting in areas of cosmetic concern, and this smooth skin will later accept cosmetic coverage of residual discoloration. Deformed noses and eyelids and partial ear losses require specialized techniques individualized to the peculiarities of each patient's deformity.

Burned hands are especially challenging. The proximal interphalangeal joints fare poorly with burns, and frequently one can only arthrodese them in an optimal position. Restoration of opposition may require deepening of webs or even digital transposition. Skin grafts never fully recover normal fine discriminatory sensation, especially in adults, so that highly tactile areas, especially on the hands and fingers, can be significantly handicapped.

After each operative procedure, the resultant scars and donor sites must mature over a prolonged period of time, ranging from months to years. The use of splints and elastic compression garments during the early active phases of maturation will help to preserve the surgical gains.

Once a scar has matured, and if it is free of repetitive stresses, such as in contractures about joints, it can be assumed to be serviceable and unchanging for life. In the young burn victim, the scar grows as the child grows, and only presents late problems with female breast development. At puberty, chest scars may produce a carapace of restricted skin, severely deforming the developing breast. Surgical release, reshaping and grafting must be done at this age and cannot be predictively treated before the breasts are formed.

Entrapped nerves must be released promptly and heterotopic bone excised when mature. Mature skin grafts tolerate prostheses well with a modicum of care, so that prosthetic replacement of major amputated parts represents little problem in this regard.

PSYCHOLOGICAL REHABILITATION

The prolonged period of reconstructive surgery becomes an agonizing testament to the postburn patient's ability to cope with the sequels of surgical intervention, including continuing changes in cosmesis, recurrent physical pain, mental anguish, and social displacement. (Andreasen et al., 1971; Andreasen et al., 1972; Bernstein, 1976; Brodland and Andreasen, 1974; Goodstein and Hurwitz, 1975; Steiner and Clark, 1977). In addition, burn patients must at some point begin to deal with the fact that their life has been unalterably changed and come to grips with the feeling of stigma created by the injury. Recent research completed by one of the authors (Johnson) confirmed that burn trauma, especially to the face or hands, can result in poorer body images and self-concepts. Thus, it would seem that a disabling burn is highly stigmatizing because its "known aboutness," "obtrusiveness," and "perceived focus" (Goffman, 1963) would necessarily be intensified as the result of residual physical scarring, especially if visible body parts were involved. Severe burn patients can then become the modern equivalent of the biblical leper.

Coping styles, as they evolve, appear to reflect varying aspects of the patient's injury, as well as the premorbid personality and certain exogenous variables such as age, sex, and ethnic group (Levine, 1971). Bearing each of these concomitants in mind, one still finds, however, that the patient struggles through a fairly recognizable set of psychological events (or stages) toward personal adjustment. Selye's *general adaptation syndrome* (Selye, 1956) provides a conceptual framework for achieving some understanding of the patient's adaptive capacity and relative progress toward adjustment to the injury. In brief, this syndrome, as Selye described it, comprises three psychobiological stages: (1) alarm, (2) resistance, and (3) exhaustion. We would add a fourth: reconstitution. These stages are roughly analogous to those postulated by Kübler-Ross for the dying patient (Kübler-Ross, 1974). Selye's construct was chosen, however, because it helps us to appreciate more fully the patient's dilemma within the context of both psychological and biological changes brought to bear on emotional resources. Selye suggested that the adaptive capacity of any biological system is limited: those resources utilized to meet the adjustive demands of a stressful situation are not available to meet other types of demands.

Having passed through the acute state of recovery, the patient is introduced into a milieu in which numerous adjustive demands are made almost immediately by the treatment team. With each subsequent surgery, the patient is required to accept an arduous routine having both physical and emotional analogs, at least with regard to the ability to cope. While the body is physically violated by the scalpel and forced to adapt to further biological changes, so too is the psyche required to adapt to the additional emotional stresses accompanying the recovery process. This situation ultimately culminates in an environmentally induced crisis which forces the patient to: (1) relinquish many already tenuous ego defenses and (2) hopefully begin to acknowledge the ramifications of the catastrophic injury.

Stage I: Alarm

Having recently survived acute treatment (perhaps with a brief interlude at home), the patient comes to realize that much of what happened seems to make no sense. This confusion is the result of having recently passed through a traumatic set of events in a somewhat dissociated mental state, leaving the patient disoriented and extremely apprehensive. Cognitive dissociation follows from the conscious mind's unwillingness or inability to fully comprehend the magnitude of what has happened (initially the patient may enter a state of shock) and also from the altered state of consciousness induced by the utilization of high levels of pain medication.

Cogent issues at this stage of rehabilitation seem to focus on reeducation, with subsequent reduction of inappropriate fears. One patient presented a rather false sense of bravado upon admission and said that his burn scars, contractures, and obviously painful open areas were of no real concern to him. Yet he found that he couldn't tolerate looking at a painted picture of clowns, which hung in the lobby of the treatment area, without feeling extremely anxious. It was discovered during the course of psychotherapy that he had perceived the attending physicians in the earliest days of his recovery as circus clowns dressed in appropriate attire. Obviously the perceptual image drawn from memory held a strongly negative association and continued to elicit fear.

Another patient continued to complain about having nightmares in which she viewed herself as a "ham in an oven" which was incessantly poked and prodded with knives and forks by "someone outside." Such imagery constituted the patient's attempt at reassimilating those painful experiences which were held in the unconscious and which could be alluded to by the conscious mind only in terms of vague reflections and nightmarish accounts of what had really happened.

With pending surgery the treatment team may find the patient becoming increasingly anxious as he or she borrows from old experiences, old images, and a residue of feelings which may no longer be appropriate. The goal of successful treatment during this stage then becomes an attempt to get the patient to look at things as they really are and to facilitate the efforts to acknowledge fear. The patient is asked to begin attaching feelings to certain events in the environment in a more congruent and realistic manner, and hopefully to reorient the self to the world. In some cases, the patient has internalized faulty beliefs and mistaken ideas which are maintained through a kind of "self talk"—an internal dialogue in which the patient continually reaffirms these faulty assumptions. It is hoped that the patient will become less fearful and increasingly desensitized to the world through rational explanation of personal feelings. In essence, the treatment team becomes responsible for making some sense out of these experiences, which until now may have seemed totally senseless to the patient.

Stage II: Resistance

The patient faces continued stress brought on by the physical distress accompanying surgery or ongoing therapy. Adaptation at this stage of adjustment is aimed primarily at reducing discomfort (at least psychologically) rather than resolving it. A kind of defensive retreat may be instituted, although the patient may not be consciously aware of it. The aim becomes avoidance of both physical and emotional pain, many times through psychological mechanisms such as denial. A characteristic behavior is the avoidance of mirrors to deny the existence of the gross dissimilarities between the patient's past and present appearance. With regard to behavioral concomitants, there may be no need to remove mirrors from the patient's room, since in most cases the patient simply doesn't see them, but rather psychologically removes them from his or her perceptual field. When the patient finally begins to take notice of the mirrors, the treatment team may have some clinical indications that the patient is moving beyond denial to some degree of acknowledgment.

Another aspect of self-perception which occurs somewhat later (when the patient finally begins to acknowledge the existence of personal deformities) appears to be a kind of tunnel vision. The patient may become fixated on some aspect of his or her cosmesis and will openly refuse to accept the self within the context of "limited improvement." Noting that things aren't as they used to be, the patient begins to ruminate about even the most minuscule defects (especially of the face) and rejects the idea that he or she is getting better. The patient's own negativity begins to adversely affect the self-concept; while the staff may report that there has been vast improvement cosmetically, this idea cannot be accepted. This is a perceptual phenomenon involving some distortion of objective reality; that distortion experientially becomes part of the patient's subjective reality and has to be dealt with as such.

Other aspects of the patient's resistance typically involve the family, loved ones, or other significant friends. He or she may take on a "sick" role for the purposes of secondary gain and establish an implicit contract with others (in a kind of "survival pact") suggesting that recent events and their obvious implications are not to be discussed. These dynamics reflect the patient's desire to be viewed as a helpless, perhaps childlike individual who is to be taken care of rather than viewed as he or she really is: a disfigured human being who must ultimately take responsibility for the disability and feelings of self-devaluation.

Each of these aspects of resistance must be dealt with by the treatment team and can perhaps be most quickly ameliorated through setting up an "extended family"; the treatment team then becomes a support system for the patient. Within this therapeutic context, the team can begin to foster emotional growth through a kind of pseudo-parenting, creating an emotional atmosphere suggesting that physical loss does not necessarily mean loss of social significance. Acceptance of the patient by the staff becomes crucial. In addition, the tenet that self-expression promotes self-acceptance becomes equally important. While self-denigrating comments need not necessarily be reinforced, patients need to feel heard; trying to dissuade them from thinking that they are in a miserable condition may be counterproductive. Instead, active listening and a full—and expressed—appreciation of the patient's predicament from his or her point of view may facilitate greater acknowledgement of these feelings of minimal self-worth, and beyond that promote a healthier coping style.

If acting-out behavior becomes an issue for staff and ultimately leads to their feeling a need to distance themselves from the patient, the behavioral scientist on the rehabilitation team may want to intervene and provide staff in-service training concurrent with individual and family counseling for the patient. This team member, hopefully, can function as a liaison, and more importantly as a model of communication, thereby suggesting to all concerned that the patient is "dealing with it" as well as possible. Reeducating the patient and staff as to how to communicate effectively becomes essential. The establishment of an understanding that the patient's intentions may be good—the feelings may be appropriate but the way they are expressed is ineffective (i.e., message sent may not be message received)—becomes the immediate behavioral goal, followed by learning of new and more effective communication methods.

Stage III: Exhaustion

At this point, the patient suddenly faces a psychological crisis resulting from reality's painful and unyielding encroachment. Repetitive surgical procedures and continuing demands by staff on the patient's time and energy reserves ultimately force the patient to make an existential choice: "Do I face up to what has happened or try to escape from reality by dissociating myself from what's going on around me?" For the patient who chooses to "face up," the affective response may be one of anger, remorse, or extreme despair, concurrent with feelings of shame. For the patient who cannot accept the harsher side of reality, a chronic state of denial may begin and schizoid mentality can be increasingly observed.

The latter state is typified by a female patient who always appeared euphoric and whose more manic qualities and laughter were usually well received by staff. When confronted with this rather incongrous state of affairs, the patient simply replied that it was "better to laugh than to cry." Such may not be the case—and in fact, for this particular patient, was far from the truth. Her mental anguish became so great and her unwillingness to deal with her reality so profound that she quietly slipped into a psychosis which required immediate psychiatric placement. If the patient chooses to acknowledge the full significance of the injury, however, he or she will most likely go through a period of mourning or grieving which constitutes a "giving up" (Wright, 1960). This giving up involves saying goodbye to an old part or image of the self which no longer "fits." This grieving may be manifested, for example, in the patient's obsessively looking at old photographs of himself which he will suddenly begin to point out to everyone. The staff often voices concern over the patient's ruminations, but they must understand that the patient is doing exactly what is necessary in mourning this loss. It is comparable to saying goodbye to a loved one who has suddenly departed and in so doing having to "cry it through."

When depressive overlay becomes too great, the patient may become involutional and begin to withdraw more and more. Outside the immediate support system of the hospital (i.e., upon discharge) the patient may retreat into a kind of "social death" (Bernstein, 1976), announcing to the world the inability to cope. Feelings of shame may also become paramount; physical defacement can be translated into an attitude of general self-loathing. Moreover, patients may become fearful that they will be loathed by others, and for more than their physical deformities. One patient put it rather poignantly when he said he was afraid that the "mud on his face would be mistaken for mud on his heart." In essence, he was saying that his facial scars had left him feeling fearful that others would see some ugliness inside that wasn't really there.

Behavioral goals for the treatment team at this point seem to involve facilitating the healthy resolution of the patient's grief. Borrowing from Kübler-Ross (1974): "With very depressed patients who have given up hope, it helps to let them talk about their sense of futility and hopelessness." Empathic understanding may provide a therapeutic milieu in which the patient can afford to express anguish. Team members, hopefully, will have worked through their own feelings of helplessness in dealing with the severe burn patient (perhaps via team encounter or sensitivity groups). It becomes essential to avoid trying to implement "hidden agendas," such as: (1) providing the patient with false hope; (2) denying the significance of the injuries; or (3) reinforcing the patient's attempts at bargaining (i.e., "Let me convince you and thus myself that the next surgery will finally restore my self-confidence and allow me to feel good about myself"). Each of these misconceived maneuvers will do nothing more than prolong the process of letting go.

Stage IV: Reconstitution

Having moved through these various stages toward adjustment, the patient may now establish adaptive capacities to alleviate stress, so that the process of decompensation is reversed and recompensatory trends are set in motion. With psychological surrender to one's grief comes some degree of resolution and, in many cases, the generation of real hope. The question "Why me?" may be raised, at which point the team member must help the patient, again through active listening. This team member may want to express appreciation of the patient's anger and envy, and that if positions were reversed, the team member would be angry too. In other words, the health professional can try to "fuel the fire" (Kübler-Ross, 1974), to let the traumatized individual ventilate anguish without feeling guilty.

Most patients are angry that their future has been seemingly taken away. Gradually, however, they realize that they are still living today and still have a tomorrow. "Tincture of time" becomes part of the treatment. Successive surgeries seem to become less threatening once the patient can begin to acknowledge that he or she can survive psychologically without them. Part of the healing process seems to involve the patient's reducing the level of expectations and learning to accept compromise with perfection. The "body ideal" becomes altered just as the body image has been altered. As actual body proportions approach the appearance of the recently diminished body ideal, the patient begins to think better of his or her physical and/or nonphysical self (Hamachek, 1971).

Members of the health team must remember that for a long time the patient may need to touch base with the great "stone mother" which the hospital comes to represent. Outreach groups become important to patients because they provide an environment of total acceptance and mutual support. The burn victim's struggle will always be that of a stigmatized individual who, like any social creature, needs to be with others while fighting off an opposing need to hide. Of special concern to the treatment team is determining the patient's need to enter a vocational rehabilitation program upon discharge (initial referral and contact with a vocational counselor typically occurs shortly after the patient's admission). As Bernstein and others have pointed out, the results of intensive care and an outstanding medical treatment may be negated by the lack of appropriate rehabilitation counseling, guidance, and support during transition back to the community (Bernstein, 1976; Granite and Goldman, 1975; Miller and Gardner, 1976).

OVERVIEW

In essence, patients who are forced to return to the world at large, already bearing the plight of a stigmatizing injury, will be rendered a tremendous disservice if they have not been adequately prepared to take up an active and productive role in society—a role that may be very different than the preinjury one. Their relatively poor self-image will be magnified if they can't find something useful to do, and learn how to contend with all of the consequences of their burn injury, including the vocational ones (Spencer, 1963).

Of further importance is the realization that some patients appear to be functioning at a higher psychological level after discharge than they may have been premorbidly (at least, on the basis of "case work analysis"). While such results obviously need to be more fully documented and empirically investigated, it may be of some heuristic value for the reader to keep in mind that upon admission the patient is introduced into a treatment milieu which provides certain emotional supports that may not have existed in the outside world.

Tragic as it may sound, the patient may have to get sick before getting better, face death before being reborn. Then the social, emotional, medical, and financial resources offered by a community agency may be mobilized to assist the patient achieve some degree of self-actualization, as well as to adjust to the after effects of the injury. This viewpoint stresses the need for emphasis on the psychological (and vocational) aspects of rehabilitation.

In summary, in most cases of simple minor burns, reasonably stable and secure people do well, and there is little need for multidisciplinary professional rehabilitative services. The severe burn, frequently complicated by premorbid, psychosocial, or neurological pathology, represents a supreme rehabilitative challenge. Only a well coordinated multidisciplinary team of nurses, therapists, social workers, vocational counselors, psychologists, and surgeons familiar with the particular problems of such patients have a chance to restore the burn victim to physical, social, and emotional well-being.

REFERENCES

Andreasen, N. J. C., Norris, A. S., and Hartford, C. E. Incidence of long-term psychiatric complications in severely burned adults. *Annals of Surgery,* 174:785–793, November 1971.

Andreasen, N. J. C., Noyes, R., Hartford, C. E., Broadland, G., and Proctor, S. Emotional reactions in burned adults. *New England Journal of Medicine,* 286:65–69, January 1972.

Annual Research Progress Report. Fort Sam Houston, U.S. Government Printing Office, Brooke Army Medical Center, U.S. Army Institute of Surgical Research, 1977.

Baur, P. S., et al. Ultrastructural analysis of pressure-treated human hypertrophic scars. *Journal of Trauma,* 16:(12), 958–67, December 1976.

Bernstein, N. R. (Ed.). *Emotional Care of The Facially Burned and Disfigured.* Boston: Little, Brown, 1976.

Black, E. A.. Burn research in the USA—The Center Concept. *Burns,* 1:(3), 233–36, April 1975.

Boswick, J. A., Jr. Home care nursing program for burn patients. *Kango,* 24:151–5, December 1972 (Japan).

Brodland, G. A., and Andreasen, N. J. C. Adjustment problems of the family of the burn patient. *Social Case Work,* 55:13–18, 1974.

Chavigny, K. H. Nurse epidemiologist in the hospital. *American Journal of Nursing,* 75:(4), 638–42, April 1975.

Feller, I. Facing the burn care issue—Burn units. *Emerg Prod News,* 9:(4), 12, June 1977.

Feller, I. *International bibliography on burns.* National Institute for Burn Medicine, Ann Arbor, MI, 1969, with yearly supplements for 1970, 1971, 1972, 1973, 1974, 1975, 1976, 1977, and 1978.

Feller, I., Flora, J. D., and Bawol, R. Baseline results in therapy for burned patients. *Journal of the American Medical Association,* 236 (17), 1943–7, October 1976.

Feller, I., et al. A Michigan burn information and tri-age system. *Michigan Hospitals,* 13:(12), 10–15, December 1977.

Goffman, E. *Stigma.* Englewood Cliffs, N.J.: Prentice-Hall, 1963.

Goldberg, R. T. Rehabilitation of the burn patient. *Rehabilitation Literature,* 35:73–8, March 1974.

Goodstein, R. K., and Hurwitz, T. D. The role of the psychiatric consultant in the treatment of burn patients. *International Journal of Psychiatry in Medicine,* 6:413–421, July–September 1975.

Granite, V., and Goldman, S. B. Rehabilitation therapy for burn patients and spouses. *Social Case Work,* 56:593–598, 1975.

Hales, M. Physical treatment and rehabilitation for burns. *Physiotherapy,* 63(5):157–8, May 1977.

Hamachek, D. E. *Encounters With the Self.* New York: Holt, Rinehart & Winston, 1971.

Hunter, J. A., and Finlay, J. B. Scanning electron microscopy of normal human scar tissue and keloids. *British Journal of Surgery,* 63:(10), 826–30, October 1976.

Imbus, S. H., and Zawacki, B. E. Autonomy for burned patients when survival is unprecedented. *New England Journal of Medicine,* 297:(6), 308–11, August 1977.

International Congress on Research in Burns. *Abstracts.* First National Naval Medical Center, Washington, D.C., September 19–20, 1960.

Jones C. A., and Feller, I. Burns—The home stretch. *Rehabilitation Nursing,* 77:(12), 54–7, December 1977.

Jorgensen, J. A., and Brophy, J. J. Psychiatric treatment of severely burned adults. *Psychosomatics,* 14:331–335, November–December 1973.

Kenner, C., and Marvin, J. Advanced preparation for clinical specialists in burns. *Jen,* 1:(3), 22–3, May–June 1975.

Konn, G., and Brandt, J. Causes of death in burns. *Monatsschr Unfalldeilkd,* 77:(11), 530–7, November 1974 (Ger).

Kübler-Ross, E. *Questions and Answers on Death and Dying.* New York: Macmillan, 1974.

Larson, D. L., et al. Mechanisms of hypertrophic scar and contracture formation in burns. *Burns,* 1:(2), 119–27, January 1975.

Levine, L. S. Psychological and social aspects of disability. *In* Harold A. Moses and C. H. Patterson (Eds.), *Readings in Rehabilitation Counseling.* Champaign, Ill. Stipes, 1971.

Lynch, J. B. Current status of treatment of burns. *Southern Medical Journal,* 69:(8), 1085–9, August 1976.

Lynch, J. B., and Lewis, S. R., (Eds.). *Symposium on The Treatment of Burns.* Vol. 5. St. Louis: C.V. Mosby, 1973.

Miller, W. C., Gardner, B. A., and Mlott, S. R. Psychosocial support in the treatment of severely burned patients. *Journal of Trauma,* 16:722–725, September 1976.

Mlott, S. R., Lira, F. T., and Miller, W. C. Psychological assessment of the burn patient. *Journal of Clinical Psychology,* 33:(2), 425–30, April 1977.

Montandon, D., D'Andiran, G., and Gabbiani, G. The mechanism of wound contraction and epithelialization. *Clinical Plastic Surgery,* 4:(3), 325–46, July 1977.

Murazian, R. I. Mortality in burns. *Khirurgiia (Mosk)*, (9), 30–6, September 1974 (Rus).

Petersen, P. A conformer for the reduction of facial burn contractures. *American Journal of Occupational Therapy,* 31:(2), 101–4, February 1977.

Polk, H. C., Jr., Trunkey, D., and Curreri, P. W. Better definition of the usefulness of burn units. *Journal of Surgical Research,* 23:(1), 6–7, July 1977.

Pruitt, B. A., Jr. *The burn patient.* New York, Monographs for Medicine, Inc., 1977.

Roding, H. Results in the treatment of burns and their comparability. *Z Aerztl Fortbild (Jene)*, 68:(17), 924–9, September 1975 (Ger).

Rudolph, R. The effect of skin graft preparation on wound contraction. *Surgery, Gynecology and Obstetrics.* 142:(1), 49–56, January 1976.

Schmid, E. Treatment of burn scar contractures. *Annal Chirurgica Plastica,* 22:(2), 147–52, 1977 (Fre).

Selye, H. *The Stress of Life.* New York: McGraw-Hill, 1956.

Shriners Burns Institute, Boston Unit. *An Annotated Bibliography for the Non-Burn Specialist—Selected Literature Related to Childhood Burn Injuries,* February 1974.

Solheim, K. Editorial—Centralized treatment of burns. *Tidsskr Nor Laegeforen,* 96:(15), 861–2, May 1976 (Nor).

Spencer, W. A. Rehabilitation—the road to independence. *Rehabilitation Record,* 4:(3), 22–25, July–September 1963.

Steiner, H., and Clark, W. K. Psychiatric comparison of burned adults: A classification. *Journal of Trauma,* 17:134–143, February 1977.

Stiffman, L. (s): The impact of injuries on the medical system. *In* C. F. Frey (Ed.), *Initial Management of the Trauma Patient.* Philadelphia: Lea & Febiger, 1976.

Total care for burn patients—a guide to hospital resources. *American Burn Association, Bulletin,* 62:(10), 6–14, October 1977.

Vladovic-Relja, T., Montani, D., and Zevic, D. Mortality in burn injury over a period of ten years. *Acta Chir Plast (Praha),* 15:(4), 231–7, 1973.

Waisbren, B. A. Burn information exchange. *Journal of the American Medical Association,* 236:(17), 1981–2, October 25, 1976.

Waisbren, B. A., Stern, M., and Collentine, G. E. Methods of burn treatment—comparison by probit analysis. *Journal of the American Medical Association,* 231:(3), 255–8, January 1975.

Wallace, A. B. Training in the care of burn injuries. *Burns,* 1:(4), 281–84, July 1975.

Wright, B. A. *Physical disability—a psychological approach.* New York: Harper & Row, 1960.

Wright, L., and Fulwiler, R. Long range emotional sequelae of burns: Effects in children and their mothers. *Pediatrics,* 8:931–934, December 1974.

13
Chronic Pulmonary Diseases

WILLIAM F. MILLER, M.D.

Prior to 1958, most interest in pulmonary diseases centered on the predominantly restrictive disorder of pulmonary fibrosis due to chronic infections, especially tuberculosis. From 1958 to 1968, interest was focused on the obstructive disorders resulting from a variety of factors causing loss of integrity of the airways. In the past ten years, the principal period covered by this chapter, there has been mainly an expansion of medical awareness of the need for and the role of rehabilitation.

Dr. Miller focuses on this awareness and documents the important advances in the pharmacological therapy for pulmonary diseases. Psychosocial responses and the physiological nature of exercise rehabilitation with respect to the respiratory system are also discussed.

Chronic pulmonary diseases causing impairment of function and disability are classified functionally as either *volume restrictive* disorders, which limit the expansion of lung units, or *flow obstructive* disorders, which limit the rate of movement of air into or out of lung units. In most cases, both types of conditions are present to some degree. By far the more common are the chronic obstructive pulmonary diseases such as asthma, bronchitis, and emphysema. Impairments resulting from these diseases may be of a physical, mental, emotional or vocational nature, and rehabilitation is thus concerned with all of these impairments. Medical and physical aspects of rehabilitation have certain special elements relating to the nature of the disease state, and these will be the principal focus of this chapter.

Before 1958 most interest centered on the restrictive disorders of pulmonary fibrosis due to chronic lung infections, especially tuberculosis. From 1958 to 1968, interest was focused for the first time on the obstructive disorders resulting predominantly from a variety of environmental factors causing the loss of integrity of the airways. In the past ten years, the principal period covered by this chapter, there has been an increased medical awareness of the need for rehabilitation and an improved definition of the role of rehabilitation in comprehensive care. Some specific developments include:

- Important advances in pharmacologic therapy.
- Documentation of the nature of the psychosocial responses to these diseases.
- Further definition of the physiological nature of these conditions, especially the responses of the chronic obstructive pulmonary disease (COPD) patient to physical exercise.
- Definition of the role of physical exercise in the rehabilitation of these patients.

Since this chapter covers more than 1,000 publications which have appeared in the past twenty years, it was necessary to be selective to provide a fairly complete, yet concise, overview of the developments in this field. In so doing, some publications may inadvertently have been overlooked or given less emphasis than was appropriate.

A number of excellent reports on studies characterizing the course and prognosis of COPD have appeared (Boushy et al., 1964; Boushy et al., 1973; Burrows and Earle, 1969; Cotes, 1960; Emirgil et al., 1969; Fletcher et al., 1976; Kreukniet and Bangma, 1966; Mitchell et al., 1964; Renzetti et al., 1966). Unique among these is the monograph by Fletcher and his colleagues (1976) covering an eight-year study of the natural history of early chronic bronchitis and pulmonary emphysema in working men in London. This study reveals that there are two distinct but commonly associated components of these disorders: the *obstructive disorder* and the *hyper-secretory disorder.* Both of these are the consequences of inflammatory reactions in the airways due to a variety of irritants, principally cigarette smoking. Some people develop predominantly the obstructive disorder, while others develop predominantly the hyper-secretory disorder, often accompanied by less severe obstruction; some develop both manifestations. The factors responsible for these differences remain unclear. Most patients who come to a physician for diagnosis and treatment are between the ages of fifty-five and sixty; they have impairments of ventilatory flow functions that, on the average, are reduced to about one-third of normal. With the passage of time, there is a natural progressive decline of flow functions. The most frequently used is the forced expiratory volume at one second, $(FEV)_1$. In normal persons, decline occurs at the rate of 20 to 30 cc per year. In nonsmoking patients with COPD, the decline is slightly greater, 30 to 50 cc per year. In patients with COPD who continue to smoke, the progressive decline in the FEV_1 accelerates to 75 to 90 cc per year. The overall prognosis tends to worsen with the degree of functional impairment observed regardless of the functions examined. However, there is considerable variability in the prognosis and functional impairment.

The late Alvan Barach pioneered the concepts of symptom control and rehabilitation for patients with COPD (Barach, 1938, 1948; Barach, Bickerman, and Beck, 1952). Subsequently, Miller (1954, 1958), Cotes (1956, 1960), and Rusk (1971), as well as others in Australia and Europe (Becklake et al., 1954; Bolton et al., 1956; Campbell and Friend, 1955; McNeill and McKenzie, 1955; Sinclair, 1955) expanded on Barach's effort with specific details on techniques and studies to evaluate the physiological consequences of the application of therapies so astutely proposed by Barach. Haas and Cardon (1969), Rusk (1971), and Petty (1971), as well as others have extended and popularized these concepts that are now being applied throughout the world.

The magnitude of this problem is reflected in the recent estimates of the Social Security Administration, which for 1977 reported that 185,000 persons under age sixty-five were receiving disability benefits because of COPD. An additional 75,000 or more persons over age sixty-five are disabled by chronic pulmonary disease. The total cost of disability from COPD exceeds $1 billion per year.

A working definition of *pulmonary rehabilitation* was proposed by the Committee on Pulmonary Rehabilitation of the American College of Chest Physicians (1975). "Pulmonary rehabilitation may be defined as an art of medical practice wherein an individually tailored multidisciplinary program is formulated which, through accurate diagnosis, therapy, emotional support, and education, stabilizes or reverses both the physiology and psychopathology of pulmonary diseases and attempts to return the patient to the highest possible functional capacity allowed by his pulmonary handicap and overall life situation" (p. 35).

The various approaches to comprehensive care have been presented in a number of review articles and monographs (Barach, 1948; Barach and Bickerman, 1956; Bergofsky, 1973; Haas and Cardon, 1969; Hodgkin et al., 1975; Lertzman and Cherniack, 1976; Miller, 1967; Petty, 1971; Petty, 1978; Shephard, 1977; and White et al., 1963). The most complete and concise reviews available are the Hodgkin et al. article of 1975 and the Petty monograph of 1978. The same team that wrote the 1975 article has developed an expanded, updated, detailed monograph which will appear soon. The basic ingredients of the recommended therapies are virtually identical from one treatment center to another, with variations being largely a matter of style and, to some extent, intensity.

A philosophically oriented article of particular interest is "Rehabilitation: An Evolving Concept" by Dr. Charles Gilette Eustace (1966).

Eustace begins by pointing out that rehabilitation is concerned with the impulse of people of goodwill to make other people whole. He further states that rehabilitation problems must be worked out in terms of the culture in which they are bred. The many disciplines involved in medical rehabilitation, each with its vested interest in helping the patient, have tended to shift control from physicians to nonphysicians, a situation that is deplored both on ethical and practical grounds. Vocational rehabilitation, on the other hand, is almost entirely the responsibility of nonphysicians. All the handicapped do not have adequate potential and motivation for rehabilitation. Eustace states, "We cannot escape the fact that the quality of a finished product will depend upon the quality of the raw material that went into it" (p. 1131). He warns that those whose task is rehabilitation must emphasize to patients that the greatest resource for help is *self-help,* a concept that Eustace credits to Dr. Howard Sprague of Boston. The greatest danger the disabled patient faces is not necessarily the loss of earning power but boredom, apathy, and despair wherein an awareness of self-worth and dignity are lost. While Eustace emphasizes the virtues of humility, tolerance, and compassion, he urges that all should heed Sir William Osler's conclusion that some patients never have and never will be able to stand entirely on their own feet. Thus, in spite of the obvious importance—and frequent success—of rehabilitation efforts, according to Osler, if reasonable examination and evaluation indicate that a patient does not have appropriate rehabilitation potential, then to waste valuable time, talent, money, and facilities on such a patient shows a distinct lack of intelligence and courage.

PATIENT AND FAMILY EDUCATION

The success of any rehabilitation program depends on both patient and family fully understanding the nature of the problem, the cause of symptoms, and the role of the various modes of therapy. The goal for each therapeutic procedure must be made perfectly clear, and the means of self-assessment must be demonstrated to the patient.

In recent years an abundance of educational material in the form of booklets, pamphlets, movies, tapes, and charts has become available. A list of educational materials has been compiled by the American Lung Association (1978). Among the several published booklets are *For Those Who Live and Breathe, A Manual for Patients with Emphysema and Chronic Bronchitis* by Thomas Petty, M.D., and Louise Neff, R. N., (1972), and *Better Living and Breathing: A Manual for Patients* by M. Modrak (1975).

MEDICAL THERAPY

The details of current medical therapy have been outlined exhaustively in a number of monographs (Hodgkin et al., 1975; Petty, 1978; Stein, 1975; Weiss and Segal, 1976).

Bronchodilators

Basic medical therapy begins with the use of bronchodilator drugs. The status of bronchodilator and other pharmacologic therapy has recently been reviewed by Miller and Geumei (1978). There are two types of bronchodilator agents: the $beta_2$ adrenergic agonists and the methyl xanthines. The B_2 sympathetic receptor stimulants, such as isoetharine, metaproterenol, terbutaline, carbuterol, fenoterol, and salbutamol, produce more specific bronchial dilation without cardiogenic or central nervous system side effects of any consequence; this is especially true when administered by the aerosol route. The dosing and the frequency of administration must be individualized. The specific goal of aerosol bronchodilator therapy is to administer a minute amount of a highly potent substance as an ultra-fine particle aerosol. Ideally, the inhaled particles should be less than 3 microns in size, although current evidence suggests that particles less than 1 micron in size are more appropriate (Ariens, 1964; Dautrebande, 1962). The breathing pattern must be slow and deep, with a prolonged inspiratory pause to allow adequate time for deposition of the very fine particles which would otherwise be exhaled. A number of studies clearly indicate that bronchodilator therapy should be continuous as long as there is evidence of bronchial reactivity (Ayres et al., 1974; Curtis et al., 1966; Gandevia and Rogers, 1963; McFadden et al., 1973). These studies further report that tolerance or resistance to inhaled bronchodilator agents does not develop. The new B_2 agents—metaproterenol, terbutaline, carbuterol, fenoterol, and salbutamol—can be administered orally. Although very effective, they have as their principal side effects hand tremor and after a prolonged period of use, development of tolerance (Miller and Geumei, 1978; Vale, 1970).

Theophylline Derivatives

The large numbers of theophylline-containing preparations available have created great confusion for the practitioner. These have been listed by Miller and Geumei (1978), showing their anhydrous theophylline equivalence. Fortunately, it is clear that the efficacy of these agents depends on the bioavailability of the anhydrous theophylline equivalent of each preparation and the theophylline blood level that is achieved. Clinically satisfactory therapeutic effects are seldom seen with blood levels below 5 μg/ml, and toxicity is seldom seen at levels below 20 μg/ml. The recommended therapeutic level is between 10 and 20 μg/ml. Current studies clearly indicate the need to monitor blood levels rather than use empirical dosages because of the multiple factors which influence the rate of metabolism (Jacobs et al., 1976; Jenne et al, 1972; Powell et al, 1977). Age, chronic liver disease (Piafsky et al., 1977a), heart failure (Piafsky et al., 1977b), and acute viral infections are among the conditions known to impede metabolism and increase blood levels for any given administered dose. Concomitant administration of erythromycin (Cummins et al., 1977) or troleandomycin (Weinberger et al., 1977) prolongs the half-life and increases the likelihood of toxicity with theophylline preparations. The earliest signs of toxicity include irritability, insomnia, itching, headache, anorexia, diarrhea, persistent tachycardia, nausea, and vomiting. Again, it must be emphasized that until more is known of the pharmacodynamics of theophylline preparations, careful monitoring of the blood level is essential. Many sustained-release theophylline preparations are available. These allow less frequent dosing of the patient, in most instances requiring doses at twelve-hour intervals, and have greatly improved clinical effectiveness as well as patient compliance. Now theophylline levels can be maintained essentially constant throughout each twenty-four-hour period (Jenne et al., 1972; Mitenko and Agilvie, 1974; Spangler et al., 1978).

Both sympathomimetics and methyl xanthines act either directly on the smooth muscle receptors or by producing an increased intracellular phosphorylase activity (Ariens, 1964). Beta adrenergic agonists stimulate the conversion of adenosine triphosphate (ATP) to 3',5' cyclic adenosine monophosphate (cAMP) through the enzyme adenylate cyclase. Methyl xanthines, on the other hand, inhibit the hydrolytic degradation of cAMP by the enzyme phosphodiesterase (PDE). Increases in cAMP increase cell membrane stability, which has been shown to block mediator release from mast cells and relax smooth muscles. This two-pronged pharmacologic approach to increasing cAMP suggests that there is a logical basis for combined use of submaximal doses of adrenergic agonists and methyl xanthine agents for bronchodilator therapy to achieve the best results with the fewest side effects.

Atropine Derivatives

Crompton (1968) and Klock et al. (1975), as well as others (Cavanaugh and Cooper, 1976; Gross, 1975; Vlagopoulos et al., 1976) have shown that inhalation of atropine is an effective bronchodilator agent in doses of 0.05 to 0.1 ml/kg. However, the side effects of irritation and drying of the respiratory mucous membrane, as well as systemic anticholinergic effects of dry mouth and tachycardia, cannot be entirely avoided. There is hope that similar anticholinergic substances may offer more clinical promise (Gross, 1975; Storms et al., 1975; Vlagopoulos et al., 1976). Recommendations for clinical use cannot be clearly delineated at this time.

Antiinflammatory Agents

Adrenal corticosteroids were introduced for the treatment of bronchial asthma more than twenty-five years ago. Since that time, a number of corticosteroid derivatives have been developed and are widely used to treat reversible airways obstruction. They are generally effective in allergic asthma and occasionally effective in nonallergic inflammatory airways disease, but are definitely not effective in emphysema (Beerel et al., 1963; Blumberg and Buckley, 1975; Clifton and Stuart-Harris, 1972; Cullen and Reidt, 1960; Evans et al., 1974; Franklin et al., 1958; Freedman, 1963; Fuleihan et al., 1967; Horn et al., 1975; Klaustermeyer and Hale, 1976; Klein et al., 1969; Lowell, 1975; Mages and Kershaw, 1957; Morgan and Rusche, 1964; Oppenheimer et al., 1968; Petty et al., 1970; Watanabe et al., 1972). It is important to monitor spirometric flow function and total eosinophile count before and during the course of a trial on steroid therapy to determine the need for therapy as well as efficacy.

The most important recent advance in corticosteroid therapy is the availability of poorly soluble aerosol preparations which are safer than systemic therapy and have been demonstrated to be effective in steroid-responsive patients (Brown et al., 1972; Clark, 1972; Godfrey and Konig, 1973; Lourenco et al., 1967; Mintz et al., 1975; Ruff et al., 1975; Williams et al., 1974). In 1977–1978, more than fifty papers reported experience with aerosol corticosteroids, principally beclamethasone diproprionate and triamcinolone acetonide. Reports have all been generally favorable.

Because of the well-known side effects of corticosteroids (Dale and Petersdorf, 1973; David et al., 1970; Dujovne and Azarnoff, 1973; Shatz et al., 1976; Streeten, 1975), it is imperative that all other measures of therapy be exploited to the fullest extent before steroid therapy is started and that it be withdrawn as quickly as is clinically feasible to minimize the adrenal suppression and other undesirable steroid effects. It is imperative, whenever possible, that only short-acting agents be used and that either a single daily dose be given in the morning or alternate day therapy be used (Ackerman and Nolan, 1968; Harter et al., 1963; Morris and Jorgensen, 1971; Reimer et al., 1975; Siegel et al., 1972; Soyka, 1972). Fauci (1978) has recently summarized the current state of the art of alternate-day corticosteroid therapy, emphasizing that it is inappropriate to empirically continue daily therapy on a patient in whom a remission has been successfully induced. It is similarly naive to attempt to induce a remission with alternate-day therapy on a patient with aggressively active disease. Conversion from daily steroid therapy to alternate-day therapy in difficult cases requires patience and flexibility.

Cromolyn Sodium

This unique substance has no therapeutic effect on the inflammatory response or the symptoms resulting from the inflammatory reaction (Bernstein, 1972; Howell and Altounyan, 1967; Lopez et al., 1969; Methison et al., 1971; Pepys, 1973). It is presumed that the principal effect is to inhibit degranulation of sensitized mass cells when they are exposed to a specific antigen or other substances likely to induce chemical mediator release. It has no other known pharmacologic effects. Because of its unique nature, it is effective only when administered prior to exposure to the offending agent. It effectively reduces the frequency and severity of asthmatic episodes but has exhibited no demonstrable effect in bronchitis or emphysema patients (Bruderman, 1975; Toogood et al., 1978).

The use of adjunct medical therapy, including other drugs, has been reviewed elsewhere (Miller and Geumei, 1978).

Respiratory and Physical Therapy

Bronchopulmonary Clearance

Bronchodilator agents enhance bronchopulmonary clearance, not only by stimulating the mucociliary apparatus but also by improving ventilation, thus enhancing cough effectiveness.

Bronchopulmonary clearance may be improved by the inhalation of high-density aerosols of bland solutions such as saline, sodium bicarbonate, and propylene glycol (Miller, 1973; Miller et al., 1968). They are used principally to provide a less viscid, less stickly liquid vehicle in the airways, which creates an expectorant effect as an aid to bronchopulmonary clearance.

In some instances where vigorous therapy with bland aerosols (Miller 1958, 1973) fails to achieve desired clearance of secretions, aerosols of 10 to 20 percent N-acetylcysteine (NAC) does so by attacking the sulfhydryl bonds responsible for much of the viscosity and tenaciousness of inflammatory secretions (Barton and Lourenco, 1973; Hirsch et al., 1969).

Strict cleanliness and care of high-density aerosol equipment are essential to prevent nosocomial contaminations and serious gram-negative bacterial infection in the patients who are using these devices (Pierce and Sanford, 1966).

Physical therapy measures, such as *chest percussion* and gravitational bronchial *postural drainage,* have been used clinically on an empirical basis for many years. Recent objective investigations confirm the value of these procedures as adjuncts to other measures for bronchopulmonary clearance (Barach et al., 1952; Chopra et al., 1977; Clarke et al., 1973; Conkie et al., 1972; Denton, 1962; Gaskell and Welsher, 1973; Grimby, 1974; Haas et al., 1976; Lorin and Denning, 1971; March, 1971; Mellins, 1974; Pham et al., 1973; Tecklin and Halsclaw, 1975, 1976). Anthonisen (1964) reported negative results, but these were probably a result of poor case selection, since it was a random selection of COPD patients irrespective of the magnitude of sputum production and functional impairment. Barach, Bickerman, and Beck (1952) reviewed the then used techniques for chest physical therapy, which were described in detail and popularized by the British (Gaskell and Welsher, 1973).

The value of *controlled coughing* as an adjunct to these measures was described by Miller (1958), who emphasized that the typical techniques of coughing are exhausting and ineffective for the patient with severe small airways obstruction and limited ventilatory reserve. Vigorous, forced coughing from a large lung volume causes abrupt airway collapse and prevents secretions from moving while expending a great deal of the patient's energy. By contrast, slow, deep inhalations followed by controlled, sustained exhalations through pursed lips to empty the lung of excess residual volume has a gentle, dynamic, compressive effect on the airways which helps to move secretions into the proximal airways. Continued exhalation with short, gentle bursts at lower lung volume requires less energy and is more effective in mobilizing secretions.

In addition to other physical measures, exercise maneuvers such as treadmill walking, stationary bicycling, or stepping up in place, combined with inhaled high-density aerosols, are valuable adjuncts to enhancing bronchial evacuation.

The ultimate goals of therapy are complete eradication of cough and sputum production and the achievement of a stable, optimal level of ventilatory and gas exchange functions. The requirements of individual patients in terms of frequency and duration of treatment depend on the magnitude of the secretion problem, the degree of pulmonary function impairment, and the severity of the environmental challenge in the form of irritation or dehydration. Patients with cystic fibrosis are a special example of persons who usually require vigorous bronchopulmonary clearance measures.

Role of Ventilatory Assistance

Recently, the value of inspiratory positive pressure breathing (IPPB), used intermittently in patients with COPD as an adjunct to aerosol administration and bronchial evacuation procedures, has been vigorously challenged. It is not the purpose of this brief review to detail this controversy, the status of which has been succinctly summarized in recent comments by Demers (1978) and Miller and Geumei (1978). Studies done in our laboratory (Wu et al., 1955) caused us to conclude that those patients who have chronic cough and sputum production associated with severe chronic respiratory failure, characterized by hypoxemia, carbon dioxide retention, and very limited ventilatory capacity, usually control their problem and have fewer hospitalizations if mechanical ventilatory assistance is used as an adjunct to other respiratory measures. When properly used, this aid will facilitate bronchial clearance and help maintain functional integrity, thus improving the quality of life by enhancing the patient's ability to cope with the disease. It will not alter the overall course or mortality of COPD, as reflected by studies to date (Cherniack and Svanhill, 1976; Murray, 1974). Carefully controlled clinical trials are currently underway in an effort to determine more precisely the proper role of ventilatory assistance in the care of these patients.

Relaxation and Breathing Retraining

The principal goal of relaxation and breathing retraining is to control dyspnea by helping the patient develop a more efficient pattern of breathing and cope better with the disease. If physical training measures are to be effective, the patient must be relaxed. The classic relaxation techniques of Jacobson (1938) and the more recent works of Benson (1975) and Benson and colleagues (1977) have been used effectively for many years. An outstanding review of the psychosocial concomitants of COPD was prepared by Dudley, et al. (1978). These authors found that the number and severity of psychosocial problems correlate directly with the severity and duration of COPD. The response of both physical and psychological disturbances to therapy tends to be inversely related to the severity and duration of the lung disease and directly related to the patient's psychosocial assets. The principal psychological reactions to disability are anxiety, dependency, loss of self-esteem, and depression. Improvement of the physical aspects of the disease is usually reported to have a greater effect on psychological improvement than does psychotherapy. The COPD patient tends to blunt the emotional responses of anger, anxiety, and euphoria, or tries through isolation to avoid circumstances causing these emotional reactions because they tend to increase metabolic demands and stimulate breathing, thus aggravating respiratory symptoms. The ability to express anger or resentment may be further blunted because of fear of alienation from those who provide care. This intensifies the anxiety problem. When anxiety and depression co-exist, the latter may go unrecognized and untreated.

Behavior modification may offer the best hope for helping COPD patients. This is accomplished by reassuring the patient and family and explaining symptoms and expectations of therapy, along with teaching the patient proper breathing and relaxation techniques. In some instances, deep meditation, hypnosis, and biofeedback have also been used.

Highly individualized use of psychoactive drugs is often the only feasible approach to management of symptoms in patients with advanced disease and firmly entrenched psychological problems. Doses of medications need to be smaller than usual to avoid aggravating or causing respiratory depression. Doxepin given at night is the agent of choice for agitated, depressed patients, and protriptyline given in the morning is the drug of choice for retarded, depressed patients.

The techniques of biofeedback have been introduced as valuable adjuncts to relaxation and breathing training (Agle et al., 1973; Chong, 1977; Davis et al., 1973; Feldman, 1976; Green and Green, 1977; Johnston and Lee, 1976; Kass et al., 1975; Vachon and Rich, 1976). The most authoritative current review is that by Green and Green (1977). Whereas the conventional approach to biofeedback involves the use of sensitive devices to demonstrate significant changes in the physical state of the target system, in patients with COPD the awareness of tightness in the chest or difficulty in breathing is so sensitive and so obvious to the patient that there is seldom need for reinforcement. The patient needs only to be aware of the breathing rate; therefore, some simple device to indicate rate or to sensitize the patient to an increased breathing rate suffices. In this regard, an expiratory resistor placed in a mouthpiece can serve to provide effective feedback through the back pressure which develops in the upper airway when breathing becomes forced.

Barach (1938) was the pioneer in teaching patients the techniques to help control dyspnea, based on work done by Hofbauer (1925), Livingstone and Gillespie (1935), and Schutz (1935). Cournand and colleagues (1936) presented a physiological basis for breathing retraining and demonstrated the inefficiency and lack of coordination in breathing in COPD patients. Barach summarized his methods in a classic book on physiological therapy in pulmonary disease (Barach, 1948), and Miller reviewed the state of the art ten years later (Miller, 1958). Following the report of a physiological evaluation of breathing retraining (Miller, 1954), there appeared a series of short-term evaluations (Becklake et al., 1954; Campbell and Friend, 1955; McNeill and McKenzie, 1955; Sinclair, 1955), all of which questioned the effectiveness of these techniques. These authors were looking for lasting physiological changes in patients who also, for the most part, were not properly trained, as shown by the failure of the patients to demonstrate evidence during the post-training evaluations of having learned breathing control. There is no reason to expect a change in the underlying disease from such training, but breathing control, when used properly, will help the patient control dyspnea and thereby improve activity tolerance and need for medication. Subsequent studies (Barach, 1955; Levison and Cherniack, 1968; Motley, 1963; Mueller et al., 1970; Pfeiffer et al., 1964; Thoman et al., 1966; Williams and Kane, 1964) did show evidence of slower respiratory frequency, improved distribution of ventilation, improved gas exchange, relief of dyspnea, and improved exercise tolerance. Barach and Bickerman (1956) proposed, as an adjunct to the training techniques, the use of the head-down position and abdominal weights. Tucker and Sieker (1960) were not enthusiastic about the results of this technique, but in better studies by Gayrard, Becker, and Bergofsky (1968) the favorable effects previously reported by Barach were confirmed.

At almost the same time, three separate pieces of work suggested a physiological advantage to forward bending in the upright or prone position in improving breathing efficiency and diaphragmatic function in the COPD patient (Barach, 1974; Brach et al., 1977; Bryan, 1974; Cole et al., 1962; Grant and Capel, 1972; McKinley et al., 1961; Petersen et al., 1967; Sharp et al., 1974).

Recent investigators, persisting in efforts to find long-term effects of breathing training on pulmonary function, predictably still find no changes (Cole et al., 1962; McKinley et al., 1961; Petersen et al., 1967; Sackner et al., 1974).

In conclusion, little has been added to knowledge of these procedures since the report of 1958 (Miller, 1958), with the exception of the forward-bending technique described by Grant and Capel (1972) and Barach (1974). Sharp and colleagues (1974) have authoritatively reviewed the physiological relationships involved, and Brach and colleagues (1977) reported the most recent physiological assessment using radioactive zenon.

Exercise Conditioning

In recent years a great deal of interest has developed in both exercise testing and therapeutic exercise. Notable among the monographs that have a great deal to offer are Jones et al, *Clinical Exercise Testing,*

(1975), and Naughton and Hellerstein's *Exercise Testing and Exercise Training in Coronary Heart Disease,* (1973). Publications of both lay and professional interest include Cooper's *The New Aerobics* (1970) and Morehouse and Gross' *Total Fitness in 30 Minutes a Week* (1975). The concept of therapeutic exercise is not new; of historical interest is the monograph by Cristabol Mendez entitled *Book of Bodily Exercise*, orginally published in 1553, translated and republished in 1960. The modern era of therapeutic exercise for pulmonary disease was first promoted by Barach (1948). In 1952, Barach extended his observations and included more emphasis on oxygen supported exercise.

Published data on exercise conditioning in COPD patients first appeard from Miller (Miller et al., 1962, 1963), Pierce et al., (1964), and Paez et al. (1967). It was clearly demonstrated that a training effect similar to that observed in normal individuals could be induced in patients with chronic obstructive airways disease, with emphasis on breathing control as an important factor in exercise tolerance. Paez and associates (1967) demonstrated that the training results produced on the treadmill were not transferrable to the bicycle ergometer, suggesting that there was a specific learning effect involved in treadmill training in his patients. Christie (1968) found a definite decrease in the work of breathing associated with decrease in repiratory frequency accompanied by improved abdominal breathing and an increase in tidal volume. This was subsequently confirmed by Haas and Cardon (1969) and Woolf and Suero (1969). Other studies demonstrating positive training effects in patients with COPD include exercise rehabilitation on the bicycle as well as the treadmill for both continuous or sustained and interval work. The latter is characterized by brief periods of submaximal work followed by periods of rest done repetitively for a total exercise and rest time of approximately thirty minutes. It is not clear whether this type of exercise produces the same order of physiological improvement as sustained exercise (Laros and Swierenga, 1972; Vyas et al., 1971). Mertens, Shephard, and Kavanaugh (1978) reported additional effects of an exercise conditioning program, including fewer respiratory infections; decreased cough and sputum; increased libido; improved sleeping; and improved oxygen exchange, which has also been reported by others (Miller et al., 1962, 1963; Paez et al., 1967; Pierce et al., 1964; Woolf and Suero, 1969).

The optimal benefits of exercise conditioning in patients with COPD definitely depend on the development of control of a slow, deep breathing pattern which not only permits the patient to carry out the exercise that produces the characteristic physiological conditioning effects but also decreases the work of breathing, increases tidal volume, and improves gas exchange.

Further studies have clearly demonstrated that patients with limited gas exchange capacity owing to advanced destructive disease with hypoxemia, either during rest or exercise, have the same effects during oxygen-supported exercise as patients breathing room air. Oxygen-supported exercise was first recommended for these patients by Barach (1938). The first evaluation data was obtained by Cotes (Cotes, 1960; Cotes and Gilson, 1956; Cotes et al., 1963). Cotes found that, compared with exercise performed without oxygen, exercise conditioning supported by oxygen resulted in a 26.5 percent reduction in exercise ventilation, 7.5 percent reduction in cardiac output, 9.6 percent reduction in the heart rate, 5.2 percent reduction in blood pressure, and 10.1 percent reduction in pulmonary artery pressure. Similar studies further illustrating the training effect of oxygen-supported exercise were conducted by Miller et al. (1963), Paez et al. (1967), and Christie (1968). These observations have been recently confirmed (Haas and Cardon, 1969; Vale, 1970; Woolf and Suero, 1969). Like others dating back to Barach, these workers found that the carbon dioxide retention that developed during exercise created no difficulties and subsided during periods of rest.

The long-term use of oxygen as a supplement, not only for conditioning exercises but for other forms of activity, has been studied extensively, confirming both the efficacy and safety of this procedure (Alpert et al., 1974; Bass et al., 1970; Bergofsky, 1973; Brundin I and II, 1974; Degre et al., 1974; Lustig et al., 1972; Nicholas et al., 1970; Zohman, 1968). Very significant is the fact that studies have shown a progressive decrease in pulmonary artery pressure in many patients with prolonged effective oxygenation (Alpert et al., 1974; Bass et al., 1970; Nicholas et al., 1970; Zohman, 1968). Oxygen concentrations administered have varied from 35 to 100 percent inspired oxygen. The need for higher concentrations is more apparent in the patients with markedly limited diffusing capacities or cardiac function. If a convenient, economical demand system were available, the use of higher concentrations of oxygen would be economically more feasible. With continuous-flow oxygen the prolonged expiratory phase of COPD patients results in a considerable waste of oxygen.

The overall effects of the exercise conditioning with breathing control in patients with COPD are a 15 to 30 percent reduction in all physiological stress parameters, including breathing frequency, ventilation, oxygen consumption, CO_2 production, heart rate, work of breathing; more efficient work performance, as indicated by a greater percentage of oxygen cost being effected during actual work; a lessened oxygen debt; and a lessened lactic acid accumulation. Even more important is the clear-cut evidence of improved work capacity indicated by both the increased mechanical work and metabolic work, including both maximal oxygen consumption, maximum heart rate, and maximal tolerated lactic acid.

Details concerning the most effective form of exercise and the amount of exercise necessary to produce optimal training effects in these patients remain to be determined.

Comprehensive rehabilitation programs for patients with severe, chronic airways obstruction have thus been shown to produce objective improvement in both exercise tolerance and capacity, as well as significant psychological and symptomatic benefits (Fishman and Petty, 1971; Kimbel et al., 1971), in spite of irreversible abnormalities in pulmonary function in many cases. In addition to an improved quality of life, a significant reduction in overall costs of medical care, including a reduction in the number of days of hospitalization, has been clearly demonstrated (Hudson et al., 1976).

REFERENCES

Ackerman, G. L., and Nolan, C. M. Adrenocortical responsiveness after alternate-day corticosteroid therapy. *N Engl J Med,* 1968, 278:405–409.

Agle, D. P., Baum, G. L., Chester, E. H., et al. Multidiscipline treatment of chronic pulmonary insufficiency. 1. Psychologic aspects of rehabilitation. *Psychosom Med,* 1973, 35:41–49.

Alpert, J. S., Bass, H., Szucs, M. M., et al. Effects of physical training on hemodynamics and pulmonary function at rest and during exercise in patients with chronic obstructive pulmonary disease. *Chest,* 1974, 66:647–651.

American Lung Association-Dallas Area. *Resource Directory for Respiratory Patient Education.* Dallas, Texas, 1978.

Anthonisen, P., Riis, P., and Sigaard-Andersen, T. The value of lung physiotherapy in the treatment of acute exacerbations of chronic bronchitis. *Acta Med Scand,* 1964, 175:715–719.

Ariens, E. J. Pharmacology of bronchodilating and bronchoconstricting drugs. In *Bronchitis II.* Edited by N. G. M. Orie and H. J. Sluiter. Netherlands: Royal Van Gorcum, Ltd., 1964, pp. 209–238.

Ayres, S. M., Griesbach, S. J., Reimold, F., et al. Bronchial component in chronic obstructive lung disease. *Am J Med,* 1974, 57:183–191.

Barach, A. L. Physiological methods in diagnosis and treatment of asthma and emphysema. *Ann Intern Med.* 1938, 12:454–481.

Barach, A. L. *Physiologic Therapy in Respiratory Diseases.* Philadelphia: J. B. Lippincott, 1948.

Barach, A. L. Breathing exercises in pulmonary emphysema and allied chronic respiratory disease. *Arch Phys Med & Rehab,* 1955, 36:379–390.

Barach, A. L. Chronic obstructive lung disease: Postural relief of dyspnea. *Arch Phys Med & Rehab,* 1974, 55:494–504.

Barach, A. L., and Beck, G. J. The ventilatory effects of the head-down position in pulmonary emphysema. *Am J Med,* 1954, 16:55–60.

Barach, A. L., and Bickerman, H. A. *Pulmonary Emphysema.* Baltimore: Williams & Wilkins, 1956.

Barach, A. L., Bickerman, H. A., and Beck, G. J. Advances in treatment of non-tuberculous pulmonary disease. *Bull N Y Acad Med,* 1952, 28:353–384.

Barton, A. D., and Lourenco, R. V. Bronchial secretions and mucociliary clearance: Biochemical characteristics. *Arch Intern Med,* 1973, 131:140–144.

Bass, H., Whitcomb, J. F., and Forman, R. Exercise training: Therapy for patients with chronic obstructive pulmonary disease. *Chest,* 1970, 57:116–121.

Becklake, M. R., McGregor, M., Goldman, H. I., et al. A study of the effects of physiotherapy in chronic hypertrophic emphysema using lung function tests. *Dis Chest.,* 1954, 26:180.

Beerel, F., Jick, H., and Tyler, J. M. A controlled study of the effect of prednisone on airflow obstruction in severe pulmonary emphysema. *N Engl J Med,* 1963, 268:226–230.

Benson, H. *The Relaxation Response.* New York: William Morrow, 1963.

Benson, H., Kotch, J. B., and Crassweller, K. D. The relaxation response: A bridge between psychiatry and medicine. *Med Clin N Am,* 1977, 61:929–938.

Bergofsky, E. H. Rehabilitation medicine and prospects for the prevention of disability from chronic obstructive lung disease. *Prev Med,* 1973, 2:43–56.

Bernstein, J. L. (Chairman of the Drug Committee of the American Academy of Allergy). A controlled study of cromolyn sodium. *J Allergy Clin Immunol,* 1972, 50:235–245.

Blumberg, M. Z., and Buckley, J. M. The total eosinophil count and adrenal function in asthmatic children. *Ann Allergy,* 1975, 35:377–381.

Bolton, J. H., Gandevia, B., and Ross, M. Rationale and results of breathing exercises in asthma. *J Australasia,* 1956, 2:675–679.

Boushy, S. F., Adhikari, P. K., Sakamoto, A., et al. Factors affecting prognosis in emphysema. *Dis Chest,* 1964, 45:402–411.

Boushy, S. F., Thompson, H. K., North, L. B., et al. Prognosis in chronic obstructive pulmonary disease. *Am Rev Respir Dis,* 1973, 108:1373–1383.

Brach, B. B., Chao, R. P., Sgroi, V. L., et al. ^{133}Xenon washout patterns during diaphragmatic breathing. Studies in normal subjects and patients with chronic obstructive pulmonary disease. *Chest,* 1977, 71:735–739.

Brown, H. M., Storey, G., and George, W. H. S. Beclomethasone dipropionate: A new steroid aerosol for the treatment of allergic asthma. *Br Med J,* 1972, I:585–590.

Bruderman, I. Cromolyn therapy. *New Directions in Asthma,* ed. M. Stein, chap. 27. Sweden: Rahms, 1975.

Brundin, A. Physical training in severe chronic obstructive lung disease. I. Clinical course, physical working capacity and ventilation. *Scand J Respir Dis,* 1974, 55:25–36.

Brundin, A. Physical training in severe chronic obstructive lung disease. II. Observations on gas exchange. *Scand J Respir Dis,* 1974, 55:37–46.

Bryan, A. C. Comments of a Devil's advocate. *Am Rev Respir Dis,* 1974, 110 (Suppl):143–144.

Burrows, B., and Earle, R. H. Course and prognosis of chronic obstructive lung disease. A prospective study of 200 patients. *N Engl J Med,* 1969, 280:397–404.

Campbell, E. J. M., and Friend, J. Action of breathing exercises in pulmonary emphysema. *Lancet,* 1955, I:325.

Cavanaugh, M. J., and Cooper, D. M. Inhaled atropine sulfate: Dose response characteristics. *Am Rev Respir Dis,* 1976, 114:517–524.

Cherniack, R. M., and Svanhill, E. Long-term use of intermittent positive-pressure breathing (IPPB) in chronic obstructive pulmonary disease. *Am Rev Respir Dis,* 1976, 113:721–728.

Chong, T. M. The management of bronchial asthma. *J Asthma Res*, 1977, 14:73–89.
Chopra, S. K., Taplin, G. V., Simmons, D. H., et al. Effects of hydration and physical therapy on tracheal transport velocity. *Am Rev Respir Dis,* 1977, 115:1009–1014.
Christie, D. Physical training in chronic obstructive lung disease. *Br Med J,* 1968, 2:150–151.
Clark, T. J. H. Effect of beclomethasone dipropionate delivered by aerosol in patients with asthma. *Lancet,* 1972, I:1361–1364.
Clarke, S. W., Cochrane, G. M., and Webber, B. The effects of sputum on pulmonary function. *Thorax,* 1973, 28:262.
Clifton, M., and Stuart-Harris, C. H. Steroid therapy in chronic bronchitis. *Lancet,* 1962, I:1311–1313.
Cole, M. B., Stansky, C., Roberts, F. E., et al. Studies in emphysema: Long-term results of training in diaphragmatic breathing on the course of obstructive emphysema. *Arch Phys Med & Rehab,* 1962, 43:561–564.
Committee Reports. Bulletin of the American College of Chest Physicians, 1975, 14:35.
Conkie, B., et al. Moyens de controle en reeducation respiratoire. *Bull Physiopathol Respir,* 1972, 8:884.
Cooper, K. H. *The New Aerobics.* New York: Bantam Books, 1970.
Cotes, J. E. Respiratory function and portable oxygen therapy in chronic non-specific lung disease in relation to prognosis. *Thorax,* 1960, 15:244–251.
Cotes, J. E., and Gilson, J. C. Effect of oxygen on exercise ability in chronic respiratory insufficiency. Use of portable apparatus. *Lancet,* 1956, I:872.
Cotes, J. E., Pisa, Z., Thomas, A. J. Effect of breathing oxygen upon cardiac output, heart rate, ventilation, systemic and pulmonary blood pressure in patients with chronic lung disease. *Clin Sci,* 1963, 25:305–321.
Cournand, A., Brock, H. J., Rappaport, I., et al. Disturbances of the respiratory muscles as a contributing cause of dyspnea. *Arch Intern Med,* 1936, 57:1008.
Crompton, G. K. A comparison of responses to bronchodilator drugs in chronic bronchitis and chronic asthma. *Thorax,* 1968, 23:47.
Cullen, J. H., and Reidt, W. U. A study of the respiratory effects of prednisone in diffuse airway obstruction. *Am Rev Respir Dis,* 1960, 82:508–515.
Cummins, L. H., Kozak, P. P., and Gilman, S. A. Erythromycin's effect on theophylline blood level. *Pediatrics,* 1977, 59:144–145.
Curtis, J. K., Liska, A. P., Rasmussen, H. K., et al. The bronchospastic component in patients with chronic bronchitis and emphysema. *JAMA,* 1966, 197:693–696.
Dale, D. C., and Petersdorf, R. G. Corticosteroids and infectious diseases. *Med Clin N Am*, 1973, 57:1277–1287.
Dautrebande, L. *Microaerosols.* New York: Academic Press, 1962.
David, D. S., Grieco, M. H., and Cushman, P., Jr. Adrenal corticosteroids after twenty years: A review of their clinically relevant consequences. *J Chronic Dis,* 1970, 22:637–711.
Davis, M. H., Saunders, D. R., Creer, T. L., et al. Relaxation training facilitated by biofeedback apparatus as a supplemental treatment in bronchial asthma. *J Psychosom Res,* 1973, 17:121–128.
Degre, S., Sergysels, R., Messin, R., et al. Hemodynamic responses to physical training in patients with chronic lung disease. *Am Rev Respir Dis,* 1974, 110:395–402.
Demers, R. R. IPPB treatments: Indications and alternatives. *Respir Care,* 1978, 23:758–759.
Denton, R. Bronchial secretions in cystic fibrosis. *Am Rev Respir Dis,* 1962, 86:41–46.
Dudley, D. L., Hudson, L. D., and Smith, C. K. *Psychological Aspects of Chronic Obstructive Lung Diseases.* North Chicago, Ill.: Abbott Laboratories, 1973.

Dudley, D. L., Glaser, E. M., Jorgensen, B. N., and Logan, D. L. Psychosocial concomitants to rehabilitation in chronic obstructive pulmonary disease. *Chest,* in press.

Dujovne, C. A., and Azarnoff, D. L. Clinical complications of corticosteroid therapy. A selected review. *Med Clin N Am,* 1973, 57:1331–1342.

Emirgil, C., Sobol, B. J., Norman, J., et al. A study of the long-term effect of therapy in chronic obstructive pulmonary disease. *Am J Med,* 1969, 47:367–377.

Eustace, C. G. Rehabilitation: An evolving concept. *JAMA,* 1966, 195:1129–1132.

Evans, J. A., Morrison, I. M., Saunders, K. B. A controlled trial of prednisone, in low dosage, in patients with chronic airways obstruction. *Thorax,* 1974, 29:401–406.

Fauci, A. S. Alternate-day corticosteroid therapy. *Am J Med,* 1978, 64:729–731.

Feldman, G. M. The effect of biofeedback training on respiratory resistance of asthmatic children. *Psychosom Med*, 1976, 38:27–34.

Fishman, D. B., and Petty, T. L. Physical, symptomatic, and psychological improvement in patients receiving comprehensive care for chronic airway obstruction. *J Chronic Dis,* 1971, 24:775–785.

Fletcher, C., Peto, R., Tinker, C., et al. *Natural History of Chronic Bronchitis and Emphysema.* New York: Oxford University Press, 1976.

Franklin, W., Michaelson, A. L., Lowell, F. L., et al. Bronchodilators and corticosteroids in treatment of obstructive pulmonary emphysema. *N Engl J Med,* 1958, 258:774.

Freedman, B. J. Bronchodilators and corticosteroids in chronic bronchitis and emphysema. *Br Med J,* 1963, 2:1509–1512.

Fuleihan, F. J. D., Feisal, K. A., Malouf, N. N. Effect of corticosteroids on pulmonary function in chronic bronchitis with airway obstruction. *Am Rev Respir Dis,* 1967, 96:678–684.

Gandevia, B., and Rogers, N. Effect of bronchodilator aerosol on ventilatory capacity in chronic lung and heart disease. *Br Med J,* 1963, 2:1097–1199.

Gaskell, D. V., Welsher, B. A. *The Brompton Hospital Guide to Chest Physiotherapy,* 2nd ed. Philadelphia: F. A. Davis, 1973.

Gayrard, P., Becker, M., Bergofsky, E. H. The effects of abdominal weights on diaphragmatic position and excursion in man. *Clin Sci,* 1968, 35:589–601.

Godfrey, S., and Konig, P. Beclomethasone aerosol in childhood asthma. *Arch Dis Child,* 1973, 48:665–670.

Grant, B. J. B, Capel, L. H. Walking aid for pulmonary emphysema. *Lancet,* 1972, II:1125–1127.

Green, E., and Green, A. *Beyond Biofeedback.* New York: Dell, 1977.

Grimby, G. Aspects of lung expansion in relation to pulmonary physiotherapy. *Am Rev Respir Dis,* 1974, 110(Suppl):145–153.

Gross, N. J. Sch 1000: A new anticholinergic bronchodilator. *Am Rev Respir Dis,* 1975, 112:823–828.

Haas, A., and Cardon, H. Rehabilitation in chronic obstructive pulmonary disease: A 5-year study of 252 male patients. *Med Clin N Am,* 1969, 53:593–606.

Haas, A., Castillo, R., and Lustig, F. The application of rehabilitation medicine to bronchial asthma. In *Bronchial Asthma,* E. B. Weiss and M. S. Segal (Eds.). Boston: Little, Brown, 1976.

Harter, J. C., Reddy, W. J., and Thorn, G. W. Studies on an intermittent corticosteroid dosage regimen. *N Engl J Med,* 1963, 269:591–596.

Hirsch, S. R., Zastrow, J. E., and Kory, R. C. Sputum liquefying agents: A comparative in vitro evaluation. *J Lab Clin Med,* 1969, 74:346–353.

Hodgkin, J. E., Balchum, O. J., Kass, I., et al. Chronic obstructive airway diseases. Current concepts in diagnosis and comprehensive care. *JAMA,* 1975, 232:1243–1260.

Hofbauer, L. Pathologische Physiologie der atmung. In *Handbuch der normalen und pathologischen Physiologie,* ed. by A. Bethe et al. Volume 2. Berlin: Julius Springer, 1925, p. 337.

Horn, B. R., Robin, E. D., and Theodore, J. Total eosinophil counts in the management of bronchial asthma. *N Engl J Med,* 1975, 292:1152–1155.

Howell, J. B., and Altounyan, R. E. A double-blind trial of disodium cromoglycate in the treatment of allergic bronchial asthma. *Lancet,* 1967, II:539–542.

Hudson, L. D., Tyler, M. L., and Petty, T. L. Hospitalization needs during an outpatient rehabilitation program for severe chronic airway obstruction. *Chest,* 1976, 70:606–610.

Jacobs, M. H., Senior, R. M., and Kessler, G. Clinical experience with theophylline: Relationships between dosage, serum concentration, and toxicity. *JAMA,* 1976, 235:1983–1986.

Jacobson, E. *Progressive Relaxation: A Physiological and Clinical Investigation of Muscular States and Their Significance in Psychology and Medical Practice,* 2nd ed. Chicago: Chicago University Press, 1938.

Jenne, J. W., Wyze, M. S., Rood, F. S., et al. Pharmacokinetics of theophylline. Application to adjustment of the clinical dose of aminophylline. *Clin Pharmacol Ther,* 1972, 13:349–360.

Johnston, R., and Lee, K. Byofeedback. A new method of teaching breathing exercises in emphysematous patients. *Phys Ther,* 1976, 56:826–831.

Jones, N. L., Campbell, E. J. M., Edwards, R. H. T., et al. *Clinical Exercise Testing.* Philadelphia: W. B. Saunders, 1975.

Kass, I., Dyksterhuis, J. E., Rubin, H., et al. Correlation of psychophysiologic variables with vocational rehabilitation outcome in patients with chronic obstructive pulmonary disease. *Chest,* 1975, 67:433–440.

Kimbel, P., Kaplan, A. S., Alkalay, I., et al. An inhospital program for rehabilitation of patients with chronic obstructive pulmonary disease. *Chest,* 1971, 60:6S-10S.

Klaustermeyer, W. B., and Hale, F. C. Respiratory mechanics during daily and alternate day corticosteroid therapy in asthma. *Ann Allergy,* 1976, 37:87–90.

Klein, R. C., Salvaggio, J. F., and Kundur, V. G. The response of patients with "idiopathic" obstructive pulmonary disease and "allergic" obstructive bronchitis to prednisone. *Ann Intern Med,* 1969, 7:711–718.

Klock, L. E., Miller, T. D., Morris, A. H., et al. A comparative study of atropine sulfate and isoproterenol hydrochloride in chronic bronchitis. *Am Rev Respir Dis,* 1975, 112:371–376.

Kreukniet, J., and Bangma, P. J. The course of pulmonary function in patients with chronic non-specific lung disease (CNSLD). *Scand J Resp Dis,* 1966, 47:173–181.

Laros, C. D., and Swierenga, J. Rehabilitation program in patients with obstructive-destructive lung disease. Proposition for the selection of the most promising candidates. *Respiration,* 1972, 29:344–358.

Lertzman, M. M., and Cherniack, R. M. State of the art: Rehabilitation of patients with chronic obstructive pulmonary disease. *Am Rev Respir Dis,* 1976, 114:1145–1165.

Levison, H., and Cherniack, R. M. Ventilatory cost of exercise in chronic obstructive pulmonary disease. *J Appl Physiol,* 1968, 25:21–27.

Livingstone, J. L., and Gillespie, M. The value of breathing exercises in asthma. *Lancet,* 1935, 2:705.

Lopez, M., Lowell, F. C., and Franklin, W. A controlled study of disodium cromoglycate in the treatment of bronchial asthma. *J Allergy Clin Immunol,* 1969, 44:118–121.

Lorin, M. I., and Denning, C. R. Evaluation of postural drainage by measurement of sputum volume and consistency. *Am J Phys Med,* 1971, 50:215–219.

Lourenco, R. V., First, M. V., Chung, S. Y. K., et al. Administration of corticosteroids in the form of aerosol. In *Integration in Medicine,* B. Rose (Ed.). Amsterdam: Excerpta Medica Foundation, 1967, p. 249.

Lowell, F. C. The total eosinophil count in obstructive pulmonary disease. *N Engl J Med,* 1975, 292:1182–1183.

Lustig, F., Haas, A., and Castillo, R. Clinical and rehabilitation regime in patients with chronic obstructive pulmonary disease. *Arch Phys Med Rehabil,* 1972, 35:315–322.

Mages, E. N., and Kershaw, R. A. Long continued treatment with tetracycline and prednisolone in chronic bronchitis: A controlled trial. *Lancet,* 1957, 2:1187.

March, H. Appraisal of postural drainage for chronic obstructive pulmonary disease. *Arch Phys Med Rehab,* 1971, 52:528.

McFadden, E. R., Jr., Kiser, R., and DeGroot, W. J. Acute bronchial asthma: Relations between clinical and physical manifestations. *N. Engl J Med,* 1973, 288:221–225.

McKinley, H., Gersten, J. W., and Speck, L. Pressure-volume relationships in emphysema patients before and after breathing exercises. *Arch Phys Med and Rehab,* 1961, 42:513–517.

McNeill, R. S., and McKenzie, J. M. An assessment of the value of breathing exercises in chronic bronchitis and asthma. *Thorax,* 1955, 10:250.

Mellins, R. B. Pulmonary physiotherapy in the pediatric age group. *Am Rev Respir Dis,* 1974, 110(Suppl):137–142.

Mendez, C. *Book of Bodily Exercise.* Transl. by F. Guerra, ed. by F. G. Kilgore. New Haven, Conn.: Elizabeth Glick, Publisher, 1960. (Originally published 1553.)

Mertens, D. J., Shephard, R. J., and Kavanaugh, T. Long-term exercise therapy for chronic obstructive lung disease. *Respiration,* 1978, 35:96–107.

Methison, D. A., Condemi, J. J., Lovejoy, F. W., et al. Cromolyn treatment of asthma: Trials in corticosteroid-dependent asthmatics. *JAMA,* 1971, 216:1454–1458.

Miller, W. F. A physiologic evaluation of the effects of diaphragmatic breathing training in patients with chronic pulmonary emphysema. *Am J Med,* 1954, 17:471–477.

Miller, W. F. Physical therapeutic measures in the treatment of chronic bronchopulmonary disorders. Methods for breathing training. *Am J Med,* 1958, 24:929–940.

Miller, W. F. Rehabilitation of patients with chronic obstructive lung disease. *Med Clin N Amer,* 1967, 51:349–361.

Miller, W. F. Aerosol therapy in acute and chronic respiratory disease. *Arch Intern Med,* 1973, 131:148–155.

Miller, W. F., and Geumei, A. Respiratory and pharmacologic therapy in COPD. In *Chronic Obstructive Pulmonary Disease,* ed. by T. Petty. New York: Marcel Dekker, 1978, pp. 63–105.

Miller, W. F., Johnston, F. F., and Tarkoff, M. P. Use of ultrasonic aerosols with ventilatory assistors. *J Asthma Res,* 1968, 5:335–354.

Miller, W. F., Taylor, H. F., and Jasper, L. Exercise training in the rehabilitation of patients with chronic obstructive lung disease: The role of oxygen breathing. *South Med J,* 1962, 55:1216–1221.

Miller, W. F., Taylor, H. D., and Pierce, A. K. Rehabilitation of the disabled patient with chronic bronchitis and pulmonary emphysema. *Am J Public Health,* 1963, 53:18–24.

Mintz, S., Broder, I., Davies, G., et al. A double-blind cross-over study of beclomethasone dipropionate in asthmatic patients with and without chronic bronchitis. *Post-grad Med J,* 1975, 51(suppl 4):76–79.

Mitchell, R. S., Webb, N. C., and Filley, G. F. Chronic obstructive bronchopulmonary disease. III. Factors influencing prognosis. *Am Rev Respir Dis,* 1964, 89:878–896.

Mitenko, P. A., and Ogilvie, R. I. Bioavailability and efficacy of a sustained-release theophylline tablet. *Clin Pharmacol Ther,* 1974, 16:720.

Modrak, M. *Better Living and Breathing: A Manual for Patients.* St. Louis, Mo.: C. V. Mosby, 1975.

Morehouse, L. E., and Gross, N. J. *Total Fitness in 30 Minutes a Week.* New York: Simon & Schuster, 1975.

Morgan, W. K. C., and Rusche, E. A controlled trial of the effect of steroids in obstructive airway disease. *Ann Intern Med,* 1964, 61:248–254.

Morris, H. G., and Jorgensen, J. R. Recovery of endogenous pituitary-adrenal function in corticosteroid-treated children. *J Pediatr,* 1971, 79:480–488.

Motley, H. L. Effects of slow deep breathing on the blood gas exchange in emphysema. *Am Rev Respir Dis,* 1963, 88:484–492.

Mueller, R. E., Petty, T. L., and Filley, G. F. Ventilation and arterial blood gas changes induced by pursed-lip breathing. *J Appl Physiol,* 1970, 28:784–789.

Murray, J. F. Review of the state of the art in intermittent positive pressure breathing therapy. *Am Rev Respir Dis,* 1974, 110(Suppl):193–199.

Naughton, P., Hellerstein, H. K. *Exercise Testing and Exercise Training in Coronary Heart Disease.* New York: Academic Press, 1973.

Nicholas, J. J., Gilbert, R., Gabe, R., et al. Evaluation of an exercise therapy program for patients with chronic obstructive pulmonary disease. *Am Rev Respir Dis,* 1970, 102:1–9.

Oppenheimer, E. A., Rigatto, M., and Fletcher, C. M. Airways obstruction before and after isoprenaline, histamine, and prednisolone in patients with chronic obstructive bronchitis. *Lancet,* 1968, I:552–557.

Paez, P. N., Phillipson, E. A., Masangkay, M., et al. The physiologic basis of training patients with emphysema. *Am Rev Respir Dis,* 1967, 95:944–953.

Pepys, J. Disodium cromoglycate in clinical and experimental asthma. In *Asthma, Physiology, Immunopharmacology, and Treatment,* K. F. Austen and L. M. Lichtenstein (Eds.). New York: Academic Press, 1973, pp. 279–294.

Peterson, E. S., Essmann, V., Honcke, P., et al. A controlled study of the effect of treatment on chronic bronchitis: An evaluation using pulmonary function tests. *Acta Med Scand,* 1967, 182(F-3):293–305.

Petty, T. L. *Intensive and Rehabilitative Respiratory Care.* Philadelphia: Lea & Febiger, 1971.

Petty, T. L. Pulmonary rehabilitation. *Basics of RD,* 1975, 4:1–6.

Petty, T. L. (Ed.). *Chronic Obstructive Pulmonary Disease.* New York: Marcel Dekker, 1978.

Petty, T. L., Brink, G. A., Miller, M. W., et al. Objective functional improvement in chronic airway obstruction. *Chest,* 1970, 57:216–223.

Petty, T., and Neff, L. *For Those Who Live and Breathe, A Manual for Patients with Emphysema and Chronic Bronchitis,* 2nd ed. Springfield, Ill.: Charles C Thomas, 1972.

Pfeiffer, V. R., Wilson, N. L., and Wilson, R. H. Breathing patterns and gas mixing in patients with pulmonary emphysema. *J Am Phys Ther Ass,* 1964, 44:331–338.

Pham, Q. T., Peslin, R., Puchelle, E., et al. Respiratory function and the rheological status of bronchial secretions collected by spontaneous expectoration and after physiotherapy. *Bull Physiopathol Respir* (Nancy), 1973, 9:293–314.

Piafsky, K. M., Sitar, D., Rangno, R. E., et al. Theophylline disposition in patients with hepatic cirrhosis. *N Engl J Med,* 1977a, 296:1495–1497.

Piafsky, K. M., Sitar, D. S., Rangno, R. E., et al. Theophylline kinetics in acute pulmonary edema. *Clin Pharmacol Ther,* 1977b, 21:310–316.

Pierce, A. K., and Sanford, J. P. Treatment and prevention of infections associated with inhalation therapy. *Mod Treatm,* 1966, 3:1171–1174.

Pierce, A. K., Taylor, H. F., Archer, R. K., et al. Responses to exercise training in patients with emphysema. *Arch Intern Med,* 1964, 113:28–36.

Powell, J. R., Thiercelin, J. F., Vozeh, S., et al. The influence of cigarette smoking and sex on theophylline disposition. *Am Rev Respir Dis,* 1977, 116:17.

Reimer, L. G., Morris, H. G., and Ellis, E. F. Growth of asthmatic children during treatment with alternate day steroids. *J Allergy Clin Immunol,* 1975, 55:224–231.

Renzetti, A. D., Jr., McClement, J. H., and Litt, B. D. The Veterans Administration

cooperative study of pulmonary function: III. Mortality in relation to respiratory function in chronic obstructive pulmonary disease. *Am J Med,* 1966, 41:115–129.
Ruff, F., Boutaric, P., Antoinette, S., et al. A 2-state clinical assessment of beclomethasone dipropionate aerosols. *Postgrad Med J,* 1975, (Suppl. 4):54.
Rusk, H. A. *Rehabilitation Medicine,* 3rd ed. St. Louis: C. V. Mosby, 1971.
Sackner, M. A., Silva, G., Banks, J. M., et al. Distribution of ventilation during diaphragmatic breathing in obstructive lung disease. *Am Rev Respir Dis,* 1974, 109:331–337.
Schutz, K. Respiratory and physical exercises. *Wein Klin Wchnschr,* 1935, 48:392.
Sharp, J. T., Danon, J., Druz, W. S., et al. Respiratory muscle function in patients with chronic obstructive pulmonary disease: Its relationship to disability and to respiratory therapy. *Am Rev Respir Dis,* 1974, 110(Suppl.):154–167.
Shatz, M., Patterson, R., Kloner, R., et al. The prevalence of tuberculosis and positive turberculin skin tests in a steroid-treated asthmatic population. *Ann Intern Med,* 1976, 84:261–265.
Shephard, R. J. On the design and effectiveness of training regimens in chronic obstructive lung disease. *Bull Europ Physiopathol Respir,* 1977, 13:457–469.
Siegel, R. R., Luke, R. G., and Hellebusch, A. A. Reduction of toxicity of corticosteroid therapy after renal transplantation. *Am J Med,* 1972, 53:159–169.
Sinclair, J. D. Effect of breathing exercises in pulmonary emphysema. *Thorax,* 1955, 10:246.
Soyka, L. F. Alternate day corticosteroid therapy. *Adv Pediatr,* 1972, 19:47–70.
Spangler, D. L., Kalof, D. D., Bloom, F. L., et al Theophylline bioavailability following oral administration of six sustained-release preparations. *Ann Allergy,* 1978, 40:6–11.
Stein, M. *New Directions in Asthma.* Sweden: Rahms, 1975.
Storms, W. W., DoPico, G. A., and Reed, C. E. Aerosol Sch 1000, an anticholinergic bronchodilator. *Am Rev Respir Dis,* 1975, 111:419–422.
Streeten, D. H. P. Cortisteroid therapy. II. Complications and therapeutic indications. *JAMA,* 1975, 232:1046–1049.
Tecklin, J. S., Halsclaw, D. S., Jr. Evaluation of bronchial drainage in patients with cystic fibrosis. *Phys Ther,* 1975, 55:1081–1084.
Tecklin, J. S., and Halsclaw, D. S., Jr. Bronchial drainage with aerosol medications in cystic fibrosis. *Phys Ther,* 1976, 56:999–1003.
Thoman, R. L., Stoker, G. L., and Ross, J. C. The efficacy of pursed lips breathing in patients with chronic obstructive pulmonary disease. *Am Rev Respir Dis,* 1966, 93: 100–106.
Toogood, J. H., Lefcoe, N. M., Wonnacott, T. M., et al. Cromolyn sodium therapy: Predictors of response. *Adv in Asthma Allergy,* 1978, 5:2–15.
Tucker, D. H., and Sieker, H. O. Effect of change in body position on lung volumes and intrapulmonary gas mixing in patients with obesity, heart failure, and emphysema. *Am Rev Respir Dis,* 1960, 82:787–791.
Vachon, L., and Rich, E. S., Jr. Visceral learning in asthma. *Psychosom Med,* 1976, 38:122–130.
Vale, J. R. Effect of exercise and O_2 breathing on gas exchange in chronic bronchitis and in diffuse, restrictive pulmonary disease. *Scand J Respir Dis,* 1970, 51:316–332.
Vlagopoulos, T., Townley, R. G., Ghanzanshahi, S., et al. Comparison of the bronchodilating effects of Sch 1000 with isoproterenol in patients with bronchial asthma. *Ann Allergy,* 1976, 36:223–230.
Vyas, M. N., Banister, E. W., Morton, J. W., et al. Response to exercise in patients with chronic airway obstruction. I. Effects of exercise training. *Am Rev Respir Dis,* 1971, 103:390–400.
Watanabe, S., Renzetti, A. D., Bigler, A. Bronchodilator and corticosteroid effects on

regional and total airway resistance in patients with asthma, chronic bronchitis, and chronic pulmonary emphysema. *Am Rev Respir Dis,* 1972, 106:392–403.

Weinberger, M., Hudgel, D., Spector, S., et al. Inhibition of theophylline clearance by troleandomycin. *J Allergy Clin Immunol,* 1977, 59:228–231.

Weiss, E. B., and Segal, M. S. *Bronchial Asthma.* Boston: Little, Brown, 1976.

White, A., Donaldson, A., and Gandevia, B. A therapeutic regimen for the emphysematous patient in hospital. *Austr J Physiother,* 1963, 9:68–86.

Williams, M. H., Jr., and Kane, C. Effect of simulated breath sounds on ventilation. *J Appl Physiol,* 1964, 19:233–235.

Williams, M. H., Kane, C., and Shim, C. S. Treatment of asthma with triamcinolone acetonide delivered by aerosol. *Am Rev Respir Dis,* 1974, 109:538–543.

Woolf, C. R., and Suero, J. T. Alterations in lung mechanics and gas exchange following training in chronic obstructive lung disease. *Dis Chest,* 1969, 55:37–44.

Wu, N., Miller, W. F., Code, F., et al. Intermittent positive pressure breathing in patients with chronic bronchopulmonary disease. *Am Rev Tuberc,* 1955, 71:693–703.

Zohman, L. R., Rehabilitation of patients with pulmonary problems. In *Rehabilitation and Medicine,* ed. by S. Licht. New Haven, Conn.: Elizabeth Licht, 1968.

14
Sensory Disabilities

HILDE S. SCHLESINGER, M.D.
MARGARET LEE, PH.D.

Sensory impairment of the ear or eye is often not easily discernible to individuals or to society. The impairment may be so slight as not to interfere with significant functions or enjoyable activities that hearing and vision provide to persons without any impairment. A large segment of this population, however, has impairments of varying degrees which, in turn, produce a disability that interferes with certain areas of functioning and/or performance—communication in the case of hearing impairment and mobility in the case of visual impairment. These disabilities can, to a large extent, be overcome, and the deaf and blind child can become a competent adult, psychologically healthy and vocationally successful, living up to his or her given potential. Too frequently, however, attitudes about disability are reflected in encounters of disabled individuals with parents, educators, employers and others who, unknowingly and unwittingly, interfere with the normal growth processes within the family unit (familial relationships), within the school environment (educational achievement), and within the world of work (vocational success). The disability then becomes a handicap. The following chapter stresses the steps along the way for each deaf or blind individual who will either maximize or minimize abilities or disabilities.

"America handicaps disabled people. And because that is true, we are handicapping America itself" (Bowe, 1978, p. vii). Although it is true that America handicaps its disabled people less than other cultures have done in the past, much remains to be achieved. There are an estimated 36 million Americans who have some physical, mental, or emotional disability, millions of which are sensory in nature. Sensory disabilities may be only a nuisance, an inconvenience, or they may interfere significantly with functioning or performance in one or more of the areas of human endeavor—particularly mobility and communication. The impact of the disability, however, and its transformation into a handicap is often influenced, blatantly or subtly, by the intricate relationship of the individual and his or her encounters with parents, peers, teachers, employers, and society itself.

How many individuals have sensory disabilities? How many of these become handicapped? What are the encounters with parents, the world of learning, the world of work, and society? What are the characteristics of those who have become handicapped? How can the handicapping process be prevented, reversed, or attenuated? Deafness and blindness will be the two main areas covered in this chapter (with a separate section on the deaf-blind disabled).

What is known is that Sign is a language that bears some resemblance to one of its ancestors, French, and that it possesses a highly complex and regular syntax, still under investigation by linguists (Bornstein, Woodward, & Tully, 1976). Furthermore, it appears at present to be the preferred method of communication among the deaf community. Language is always an improtant feature of the ego, and feelings about language are rampant. There seems to be a tendency on the part of Americans to label some languages good and some bad, instead of conceiving of one language *as more appropriate,* under certain circumstances, than another.

In any case, deaf children, the majority of whom are not exposed to Sign, or to any of the other languages on the continuum of manual language, do reach adulthood with linguistic competencies. Some have competence in Sign, others in English; some are competent in both, some in neither. A survey of entering students at Gallaudet, perhaps the best-known school for the deaf (Bornstein & Kannapell, 1969) indicated that 13 percent had learned Sign from parents, 63 percent from friends, and 37 percent from school staff (some from more than one group). Less than 25 percent learned Sign before they were five years old, and 60 percent before they were ten. Sign, and most of its variants, thus becomes a peer language, except for children of deaf parents, and most hearing parents still continue a process of noncommunication with their deaf children throughout life, at least in the mode usually most effective for deaf persons.

In general, the extent of disability is an important, but not the only, factor for the development of a handicap. The common picture that emerges from this review is that society feels awkward with those who are different, who remind them that bodies and minds are not always intact, that the body ages, that many people are disadvantaged socially and culturally. Those who are different have been pushed aside and prevented from joining the American mainstream. Their encounters with parents, schools, and work, have been restricted, oppressive, fraught with avoidance, rejection, oversolicitude, and so forth. A common picture emerges: individuals who are often unemployable, unemployed, underpaid; who are almost always underemployed; and who often show a great disparity between their potential and their achievement. Psychologically the picture is less clear, and this will be dealt with separately.

DEAFNESS

"Impairment of hearing is the single most prevalent, chronic physical disability in the United States" (Schein & Delk, 1974, p. 1). More than 13 million Americans have some hearing impairment, more than 6 million have significant bilateral hearing impairment, and nearly 2 million are deaf. Of these, 410,522 are prevocationally deaf and 201,625 are prelingually deaf. *Deafness,* according to the latest census definition, is the inability to hear and understand speech. Although there are more specific and sophisticated audiological diagnoses, the above definition is more appropriate for purposes of rehabilitation, since the inability to hear speech—and thus to understand and reproduce it—is the most important factor leading to English language deficits, which in turn leads to academic retardation and vocational difficulties.

Hearing loss, however, is more than a medical and audiological diagnosis. It is a cultural phenomenon in which social, emotional, linguistic, and intellectual patterns and problems are inextricably bound together (Schlesinger, 1969). Although deafness occurs throughout the lifespan and is stressful at any time, the complexities of early prelingual deficit are the most intricate.

There appears to be an increasing proportion of individuals whose deafness occurred prior to three years of age. It is expected, therefore, "that the prevocationally deaf adults in the next decade will mostly be prelingually and congenitally deaf, with the latter predominating (Schein & Delk, 1974, p. 115). Almost one-third of deaf students may be multiply handicapped (Moores, 1978).

What are the encounters of the deaf individual throughout the lifespan that contribute either to successful adaptation or to a massive handicap? Which kinds of encounters are handicapping? It is important to gain some understanding about these encounters to clarify the impact of hearing deficit on academic, psychological, and linguistic skills. Furthermore, early relationships are often reproduced in adulthood, and thus the frustration experienced with parents and teachers may be projected onto the rehabilitation professional.

Encounters with Parents

Most deaf children have hearing parents. The birth of a deaf child into an intact family is in itself a potential life crisis; diagnosis of deafness in a child's early years, however, can precipitate the most normal of parents into crisis. The mourning process that ensues following the realization that the child is not perfect resembles any acute grief reaction. The parents mourn the dream of a perfect child and are beset by a turmoil of thoughts and feelings, tension, anxiety, depression, anger, shame, guilt, and confusion. A mourning process that is permitted to run its course is more promoting of mental health. One that is not resolved early will continue unabated.

Encounters with Experts

Experts frequently have fragmented knowledge about deafness. For example, physicians typically know relatively little about early childhood deafness, prefer a medical condition that they can cure (an unlikely feat with most cases of deafness), and are loath and unskilled in giving out "bad news." Thus it is that most hearing parents do not obtain good professional support from early professional contacts (Meadow, 1968). Furthermore, due to the long, drawn-out controversy about how to deal with deafness (spelled out below), parents are also likely to encounter experts who hold dear professional advice contrary to that of other experts, thus precipitating more conflict for the parents.

Second Stage of Encounters with Parents

Assuming that the initial diagnostic crisis has been traversed successfully, parents must next learn to cope with the alien experience of having a child different from them. The usual experience with child rearing is that children learn to talk easily and acquire language in the same way, in the same stages. The deaf child is different—unable to hear, and thus to process language in the usual way, so that an early deficit of language acquisition occurs. The hearing parents, anxious for usual performance, will search for ways of normalizing the child. They will encounter experts who state that deaf children, if taught early, will learn to hear, to speak normally; if taught early, will learn to read lips like a duck takes to water; will indeed become like a hearing child. Parents clearly yearn for the eventual total normalcy of their hearing-impaired child, a normalcy which is to include normal speech and perfect lipreading. This they desire despite vast clinical experience and research on the relative infrequency of such ideal results. Professionals, either by ignorance or the above-mentioned reluctance to give out "bad news," may encourage such unrealistic pictures. Advice is too often given or perceived by the parents as if they were Old Testament admonitions: "Thou shalt always talk to the deaf child; thou shalt never gesture to the deaf child; thou shalt always praise him and never be angry with him; thou shalt treat him as if he were not deaf; thy lips shall be at eye level for the child; thou, and only thou, are responsible for the outcome, and if thou dost not follow or heed, the child will be lost to thee" (Schlesinger, 1968, p. 349).

Such advice is a heavy burden for parents, and many react by further withdrawal from the child or by an attitude of self-sacrifice and martyrdom for the child. A frequent parental reaction is vacillation between overprotection and overt rejection.

The child, who may have experienced a relatively normal mutuality in infancy, is introduced to the mutuality of linguistic interchange in an atmosphere of conflict, despair, and inability to live up to parental expectations. The child, in turn, may avoid any attempts at communication, develop negativism toward language, and this further diminishes active learning.

The stage is set for the child, unable to learn English as a native tongue, to enter the school system with linguistic retardation. The stage is also set for the child to encounter another modality of language, motoric-manual, rather than vocal. There is a continuum of language from Sign (American Sign Language, AMESLAN or ASL), with its own grammatical constructions and word order, and several other varieties of English reproduced on the hands. Unfortunately, until recently, the deaf child's competence in *any* language was measured only in English (where competence was very low in the majority of children). Competencies of language in the manual mode have not yet been established, although many researchers are searching for ways to establish valid testing.

It has long been known that deaf children of deaf parents show superiority to those of hearing parents in terms of both psychological adjustment and academic achievement, including English language skills (Meadow, 1975). Schlesinger (1978) reports on a group of hearing parents who elected to use manual communication with their deaf infants shortly after diagnosis. The mode typically selected was Bimodal-English by voice and hand. Manual English, resembling spoken English in word order and grammar, was easier for them to acquire, enabled them to speak at the same time, which felt more comfortable, and promoted expectations that the child would also accelerate in both language (English) and speech acquisition. The children reported on in this study, now about thirteen years old, have demonstrated good English skills, use their voices more freely, show more communicative confidence when talking to strangers, and show academic acceleration (Schlesinger, 1978). It is expected that these children will learn Sign as their second language just as other deaf children have learned it as their first language. However, a new controversy is now brewing; the parents in this study used an artificial system of signs that actually extends the continuum of manual languages. Many feel that contrived, artificial languages break linguistic constraints and should not be used, and that the deaf child should be exposed to Sign *first* and learn English as a second language. The author finds a problem with that advice: few hearing people know Sign and could use it competently with deaf infants. The author also feels that linguistic interchange, to be most productive, should occur early, meaningfully, and with the earliest linguistic caretakers, namely, the parents. Furthermore, "teaching" English to deaf younsters, as contrasted to linguistic immersion, has not been particularly successful in the past. How this new controversy will develop and be resolved is an open question.

The rehabilitation professional often encounters the fruits of linguistic retardation and early conflict over language acquisition, and will have to behave differently from the earlier caretakers. He or she must be genuinely respectful of any of the varieties of communication and attempt to acquire competencies in many. If the rapport is good, deaf clients will slow their signing to the skills of the counselor (fast signing is occasionally seen as a form of resistance). A chapter elaborating upon the above can be found in Bolton (1976), with more specific advice about communication with the professional. The professional will also frequently need to involve the parents, who often remain symbiotically attached even to their grown children.

Encounters with the World of Education

Encounters with the world of education can best be summarized by comparison of intelligence test results with educational achievement test results. Vernon (1968) summarized fifty years of research and thirty-seven studies, the compilation of which clearly reveals that deaf individuals have normal intellectual potential. This compares interestingly—and sadly—with fifty years of surveys regarding academic achievement. These latter studies (summarized in Moores, 1978) continue to find serious academic retardation among the deaf, particularly in paragraph reading tests (where grade retardation is eight years) and arithmetic computation (which is one of the highest achievements of deaf children yet still shows a six-year retardation). These findings contribute to demoralization among teachers and frustration among deaf children. It has been said that one-third of deaf youth who leave school each year do not possess the qualifications to continue their education or to become employed (Rice, 1973).

Many deaf youth, even with academic retardation, can continue on to secondary education, and the number of programs available to them is mushrooming. They can attend Gallaudet College (established in

1864 and still the only liberal arts college for the deaf in the world). They can also attend the National Technical Institute for the Deaf (established in 1969) and three regionally funded vocational, technical programs for the deaf—Delgado Vocational-Technical Junior College (in New Orleans), Seattle Community College, and St. Paul Technical Vocational Institute. Furthermore, more than forty regular colleges now have special programs for deaf students (Rawlings, Trybus, Delgado, and Stuckless, 1975). Most of the forty are very small, with the exception of the one at California State University, Northridge. Most of them are also so recent in origin, and their student body so small, that evaluation of the programs has not yet been accomplished.

A special type of secondary education has been established for deaf adults categorized as multihandicapped or low-achieving. These adults tend to have severely limited communication skills, low academic achievement levels, emotional immaturity, secondary disabilities, and poor vocational preparation (Rice, 1973). Earlier in their lives, these same deaf adults might have been considered mentally retarded or multihandicapped. They were often taught by teachers who did not teach them by choice, who felt a lack of training for their function, and who would prefer to teach children without handicaps (Anderson and Stevens, 1969). Such deaf adults are the most seriously handicapped of all deaf individuals.

Many feel that neglect of the educational, social, and psychological needs of the child is the major cause of multiple handicaps in the deaf (Stewart, 1974), and yet even such deaf adults can be successfully habilitated, as the review of studies summarized by Moores (1978) indicates. From 40 to 60 percent of the most disadvantaged of all deaf adults had been gainfully employed following a vast array of support services, including training in communication, living skills, vocational skills, and counseling.

Most researchers feel that early diagnosis, with appropriate intervention, can diminish the huge gap between potential and achievements. There are vitriolic debates, however, about what constitutes appropriate training in the preschool years. Some feel that Oral-Aural training is sufficient, but certain research demonstrates that Oral-Aural preschool training has no future benefits in the areas of speech, speech reading, general achievement, and written language (Vernon and Koh, 1972). More recent philosophical changes encouraging "total communication," wherein the child is exposed to varying manual language systems early, may help to diminish linguistic and academic retardation. The author's view is that parents should be encouraged to use the manual language system that they can most easily learn (or already know, in the case of deaf parents), and to use it competently. That will usually be Signed English or one of the artificial languages for hearing parents, and a combination of Sign and Signed English for deaf parents. Moores (1978, p. 209) states that the most successful school programs include cognitive and academic training, high levels of parental involvement, the use of combined oral and manual communication, and improved utilization of residual hearing. The studies on which these conclusions are based were started in 1970. It remains to be seen whether this superior performance will continue; this author believes it will.

A new trend for the education of the deaf child is the concept of *mainstreaming.* Educators of the deaf point out that mainstreaming has failed in the past and view its new ascendancy with trepidation. If it is to be successful, mainstreaming must have much more careful implementation than planned for heretofore. Some skeptics feel that "we seem to be in an era of simplistic solutions to complex problems" (Brill, 1975, p. 377), citing mainstreaming as a possible example.

Encounters with the Handicap Itself

Some deaf individuals acquire deafness postlingually or even postvocationally. These individuals have developed normal language competencies in English and will not have experienced the diagnostic crisis period with their parents. They too, however, will go through a mourning period, mourning the loss of their own sense of hearing. They too will be precipitated into the crisis of grief, followed by the coping crisis. A study of sudden hearing loss among the war-deafened showed that "the most significant feeling tone from sudden deafness was loneliness; the most common single fear, that of being stupid; and the most keenly felt anxiety, insecurity in social situations" (Levine, 1960, pp. 71–72). However, once the mourning crisis is resolved, these individuals can usually be rehabilitated successfully. The onset of deafness will interact with premorbid personality characteristics, but the reactions are so individualistic that no common trend emerges.

Encounters with the World of Work

Startlingly glowing and startlingly gloomy pictures emerge from research regarding deaf people's encounters with the world of work. It has become clear that deafness need not hinder employability; deaf individuals can be found in all the principal occupations, from professional to domestic. Unemployment figures for the deaf as recently as 1972 (Schein and Delk, 1974) compare favorably with the hearing population (although this does not hold for nonwhites). The rehabilitation rate of deaf individuals compares favorably with those of other handicaps (Schein and Delk, 1974).

Very serious concerns, however, are expressed by several authors (Schein and Delk, 1974; Vernon, 1977). The future may look bleaker than the present insofar as many deaf individuals work in occupations where unemployment figures are rising, such as production of nondurable goods. Many previously lucrative positions for deaf individuals are being phased out through automation. For example, printing, an occupation that once attracted 14 percent of deaf workers, is no longer available due to the replacement of the highly respected and highly paid linotype operator by a phototypesetter of less status and lower income. Similarly, the growing field of employment, such as personal and technical service, has historically been an area of small representation by deaf workers and will require a marked shift in training programs.

Underemployment of the deaf has been the rule, rather than the exception. We find deaf men and women of normal or above-average intelligence everywhere have occupied unchallenging routines (Williams and Sussman, 1971). Employer satisfaction is high, despite many indications of negative attitudes toward deaf workers, summarized by Schein and Delk.

Encounters with the Rehabilitation Process

As the youth proceeds from the school setting to the world of work, the rehabilitation professional may require a psychological evaluation of the client, including a measure of intelligence, an evaluation of personality structure, a measure of educational achievement, an appraisal of communication skills and aptitude, and vocational interest testing. A guide carefully describing the usefulness and pitfalls of tests for the deaf was prepared by Vernon (1967). Another useful work for rehabilitation work with the deaf is Bolton (1976), elaborating much of what has been summarized here.

Encounters with the Model State Plan

Schein (1977), in collaboration with The Council of State Administrators for Vocational Rehabilitation and The National Association for the Deaf, has published a small pamphlet describing a Model State Plan for vocational rehabilitation of deaf clients. The plan was first distributed in 1973; it is very concise and difficult to summarize further. The plan stresses the need for better diagnosis in terms of audiological and ophthalmological testing, improved psychological testing, a more prolonged period of training to help meet individual clients' potential, more effective secondary school programs, and considerably greater consumer involvement. It further spells out training requirements for personnel, with specific emphasis on the need for sign language skills throughout the rehabilitation process, as well as administrative changes at the state level wherein one professional would be nominated to be the State Coordinator for Deaf Services.

Schein, Gentile, and Delk (n.d.) make it clear that the Model State Plan has had an effect. Vocational rehabilitation agencies are undertaking vigorous programs to serve their clients in terms of increasing the number of special counselors for the deaf, requiring more training of them, providing supervision by a qualified state coordinator for deaf services, and so forth. A new, more comprehensive model state plan is now under preparation.

Encounters with Technology

The technological advances that benefit individuals with hearing impairment fall into three broad areas: (1) medical advances that either prevent or lessen the severity of the impairment; (2) communication aids, used for either direct communication or aids that bring mass media to the deaf; and (3) aids that substitute for hearing in terms of making environmental cues available to the deaf.

Medical Technology

Medical advances have influenced the area of deafness both directly and indirectly. As effective treatments and cures for various diseases have been discovered, the causes of deafness have dramatically changed. Advances in the area of prevention and diagnosis of deafness have also been made, such as special X-ray machines (the Polytome, available since 1968) that provide radiographs (tomographs) of the temporal bone. Earlier diagnosis has also been explored through experimenting with techniques developed in the early 1960s to assess the hearing sensitivity of newborns and young infants. These techniques relied on behavioral observances of newborns utilizing an approach called Behavioral Observation Audiometry, or BOA. However, mass screenings were found to produce an unacceptable amount of false positives. The need for early detection then led to a focus on determining "high risk" factors, to be followed by in-depth audiological evaluation. Study of techniques for mass screening continues, and the trend is toward programs that reduce reliance on observer judgment. One program that is being developed is the "Crib-O-gram," which automatically monitors the responses of infants through motion-sensitive transducers attached to isolettes. Early diagnosis allows for early intervention, with the primary goal the provision of early language to the deaf child. The realization of this goal would profoundly change the needs of the deaf community and the function of supportive services (Glasscock, 1976; Lloyd & Dahle, 1976).

In the past twenty years, there have also been dramatic changes in the area of treatment of hearing loss. In the 1950s surgical procedures for mobilizing the stapes, and then for its removal altogether (stapectomy), were developed for treatment of otosclerosis. Also in the 1950s, a procedure for repairing a perforated eardrum (tympanopasty) was developed. The underlying technology that has allowed for these advances includes the operating microscope and new microinstrumentation. Currently, most conductive hearing loss in children is amenable to surgery.

One area of treatment that is potentially exciting, but only in its early stages of development, is the use of electronics in otology. This includes hearing aids implanted in the middle ear that couple directly to the stapes, cochlear implants, and direct electrical stimulation of the brain. Although several dozen deaf individuals have undergone cochlear implantation, the technology at this point involves a single-wire type that does not allow for differentiation between one pitch and another. Single-wire implants permit the deaf person to discern environmental sounds and, by transmitting some rhythmic aspects of speech, function as an aid to lipreading. Multichannel implants that would allow for the necessary discrimination of pitch to understand speech are thought to be ten to twenty years in the future. Even further in the future is the possibility of transmitting sound directly to the brain, bypassing the cochlea and auditory nerve. Experimentation in this area has begun, but this will markedly affect the deaf community probably in the next century.

A second area of advance in technology involves devices that improve communication. This is the area that in the past has had the greatest impact on the deaf person's life. The hearing aid is the most widespread device used by deaf persons. Although this aid was considered reasonably acceptable a decade ago, dramatic improvements have been made during the past ten years. The result is smaller, more reliable aids (e.g., fewer power dropouts) and, therefore, an increase in the use of ear-level aids over the more cumbersome body aids (Lybarger, 1976). Currently, two-thirds of the hearing aids being sold are behind-the-ear aids. With the development of the electret microphone, there has also been an increase in the use of in-the-ear aids during the past few years (Lybarger, 1976).

Another technological device that has opened vast new avenues of communication to the deaf is the telecommunications typewriter (TTY). This development has greatly expanded opportunities for deaf persons to communicate socially, on the job, and as a member of the community able to respond to emergencies and so on. The first TTY was developed in 1964 by Robert Weitbrecht, but it did not really catch on until 1968. Unfortunately, this device is still not available to the average deaf person because of its prohibitive price, varying from $600 to $1,200. In addition to the initial investment, telephone rates are high for distance calling due to the slowness of a typed conversation. As yet, telephone companies have not changed these rates for deaf customers. Despite such problems, increased use of the TTY has resulted in development of many adjunct services: directory assistance; emergency numbers for TTY users; public pay-TTY services; TTY numbers for AMTRAK and Sears & Roebuck catalog departments; various TTY news centers, and so on. The direction of advances in TTY has already been toward smaller, more portable machines offering the choice of paper copy or electronic word scanning. Future developments may include miniaturized, all-electronic TTY machines, TTY machines that can interface with educational computer systems, regular captioned TV programs (but visible only on specially equipped receivers); TV phones with picture and word capacities, and typewriters that convert the printed word into speech. One hopes that the TTY will also be made more available to the average deaf person; that adjustments in TTY call rates will be forthcoming; and that TTY hookups to various facilities and resources will continue at an ever-expanding rate (Bellefleur, 1976).

Various other developments have helped bring the world to the deaf person. These include signed news programs and TV commercials, and captioned films. These services seem more related to an increase in the public's awareness of the deaf, and to the effect the deaf community's "speaking out" has had, rather than to technological advances per se. This is also true for the babytender, lights attached to doorbells and phones, and for the use of "hearing dogs." The technology has existed for a long time, but the growing awareness of the public and the more "vocal" deaf community alluded to above have been the major forces instigating both new product appearance and acceptance by deaf individuals. It is an unfortunate fact that despite these developments, many of the newly available fruits of technology remain unavailable by reason of their prohibitive expense.

Up-to-date information about agencies for the deaf can be obtained from: The National Association of the Deaf, 814 Thayer Avenue, Silver Spring, Maryland 20910.

BLINDNESS

A total of 90 million Americans have some visual deficits. Many of these persons can be or have been restored through corrective lenses or surgery. Many others cannot, and will bear the label of "legally blind" or "individuals with severe visual limitations." The most accepted definition of blindness is that of a visual acuity of less than 20/200, in the better eye with the use of a correcting lens, or with such limitation of the visual field that the widest diameter subtends an angle no greater than twenty degrees. Severe visual limitation is the inability to read newsprint even with the best correction (MacFarland, 1973). A more functional definition is now being sought, since functional visual efficiency is more important than the visual acuity (Lowenfeld, 1973; Rusalem, 1972).

Incidence figures vary from one in 292,000 to 1 million (Kahn & Moorhead, 1970). The usual figure seems to be one in 300,000. Prevalence figures are said to be 225 per 100,000 individuals (Hatfield, 1973). Prevalence figures are higher in the higher age groups, with only 13 percent of blindness occurring prevocationally (Kahn & Moorhead, 1970). Seven out of ten cases of blindness are in women (Scott, 1966). There are an estimated 20,000 to 60,000 individuals with visual limitations in the labor market (Link, 1975). There are said to be about 13,000 blind children in school settings and, of these, more than 50 percent may be classified as multiply handicapped (Lowenfeld, 1968). Note that all statistical figures are estimates. No national census has been conducted, as with the deaf (Schein & Delk, 1974). The closest to a national census for the blind is the model reporting area for blindness statistics, involving sixteen states (Kahn & Moorhead, 1970). It appears that the incidence of all blindness is increasing (Rusalem, 1972), as is prenatal influence on subsequent blindness.

Encounters with Parents

There are very few congenitally blind infants, in contrast to the case for deafness. Parental encounter with blind infants does parallel, in some ways, the analagous encounter with deaf children, especially in terms of the diagnostic crisis. There are differences, however, in the relatively lower incidence of blindness in childhood and the consequent earlier diagnosis, in part due to the more apparent nature of the deficit. Moreover, the coping crisis is vastly different. Blindness in infancy, under the most favorable circumstances, can result in "good ego development, with stability in human object relations, demonstrably good speech, good adaptive hand behavior, free mobility, and a stable concept of self and of 'I'." Ideal circumstances are rare, however, and many congenitally blind children (about twenty-five percent of them) have "... no significant human ties. Language, if present at all, is echolalic, there is no definition of body boundaries, there are motor stereotypes of trunk and hands, and decreased mobility" (Fraiberg, 1976, p. 264). The largest percentage of blind infants falls somewhere between these two extremes. Their parents must be taught adaptive behavior for their own infants—and they have been taught to do so successfully under the most adverse circumstances (Fraiberg, 1977).

Most of the studies of congenital blindless (Parmelee, 1955; Norris et al., 1957; Fraiberg, 1977) describe very similar patterns of development, and most researchers feel that gross abnormalities in certain blind children appear to be associated with total or nearly total blindness from birth *and* a history of inadequate emotional stimulation in the early months of life.

A later onset of blindness does not impact on conceptual development, but it does have a massive effect on mobility and its associated control over the environment (Neu, 1975). But even with later onset, it appears that "the child's functioning was usually closely related to the opportunities which he had for experiences appropriate to his level of development" (Norris, Spaulding & Brodie, 1957, p. 24). Parents of blind infants need to learn what restrictions blindness imposes and what restrictions are imposed by society in order to attempt to lessen the impact of each. Blindness itself makes for difficulty in the perception of space. Touch does not replace vision fully since some objects are inaccessible to direct contact, such as objects in motion; very large objects, such as mountains and lakes; and very small objects, such as animals and some flowers. The behavior of others cannot be observed visually. Blindness also imposes some restrictions in getting about, in turn diminishing experiences that must be provided for in a planned setting (Lowenfeld, 1973).

Encounters with the World of Education

The laments expressed are similar to those described for the deaf child in school: that there is an underdevelopment of the personal, social, and vocational skills for blind children and young adults, so prevalent and so serious that many of them can aspire only to marginal employment. They are static in job advancement, job mobility, and earnings (Link, 1975). And again, most workers for the blind feel that this need not be.

Low achievement test scores in school seem to be related to overprotection. Often the blind child has not had normal learning experiences, since in many cases family, friends, and school staff have done so much for the child. Similarly, the blind child has often been excluded from certain courses which are regarded as important learning opportunities for sighted students. Visually handicapped students are excluded from laboratory experiences, physical education, even typing. A third feature which has seriously affected scores of young blind children is a lack of appropriate learning materials. Test scores may be seriously influenced if the child has had no appropriate resources for learning, such as books in large print or recorded books, and tactual materials to parallel picture content in the books of sighted fellow students (Bauman, 1973).

In general, the laments about education of the blind are not so severe as those for the deaf, and most researchers feel that if the blind child is given adequate opportunities early, the educational process can equal that of sighted peers. Education for the blind has made tremendous strides. In 1900, residential schools for the blind remained practically the only educational provision for the blind in America. From then on, public schools began to provide education for visually handicapped children. At the present time, more than 60 percent of visually handicapped children registered with the American Printing House for the Blind attend public schools, while only 40 percent are placed in residential schools (Lowenfeld, 1973). Furthermore, thousands of blind students presently attend hundreds of colleges (Rusalem, 1972).

Encounters with the World of Work

Again, as for deaf individuals, there are both glowing and gloomy reports. Blind individuals have been successful as far back as the fourth century. Nevertheless, in 1932 it was noted that there were only five major areas in which blind persons were finding employment: music, handicrafts, selling, piano tuning, and white-collar occupations such as teaching and massage (French, 1932). These five areas increased to sixteen by 1936 (Rusalem, 1972). In 1962, no rehabilitation counselors were themselves blind. That has since changed, and in fact the areas of possible employment are now so numerous that listing them is no longer feasible (Rusalem, 1972). At least 600 visually impaired persons are now employed in the computer sciences, 500 teachers, 400 lawyers in government, and 1 medical student. Job opportunities abound in medical transcription, technical writing, chemistry, electronic engineering, management analysis, personnel, and other fields. However, there is now increasing competition due to unemployment. There is also an insufficient number of workshops for the blind (6,000 are served, compared to an estimated 30,000 in need of such services, according to Link, 1975).

Schein and Delk (1974) make an interesting comparison: Although there are 388 deaf persons to every 100 blind persons, 7,364 blind individuals and only 5,915 deaf individuals were rehabilitated in 1970. Thus it would seem that the budget is not distributed in proportion to the size of the population. These statistics are interpreted as requiring more effort on behalf of the deaf, not less for the blind.

Encounters with the Rehabilitation Process

The initial reaction of shock followed by depression has been documented in numerous articles and books dealing with the psychological adjustment to blindness. Cholden (1967) believes that the onset of blindness is such a blow to the psychic system that the ego initiates a protective reaction which, for a time, renders the person incapable of feeling the tremendous psychological pain: "A period of protective emotional anaesthesia which is available to the human organism under such stress" (p. 73). This emotional anesthesia is followed by a period of depression in which the patient feels a tremendous sense of loss and mourning for the lost eyesight. What steps can the rehabilitation professional take in this situation? First, he or she should be informed of the medical situation in order to ensure that it is indeed without current hope for improvement. There is also a need to make sure that a competent professional diagnosis was made. Secondly, visual aids may still help. Again, the counselor needs to ascertain that appropriate professional consultation is available in order that the client may regain a measure of function through technology. Ongoing contact with the patient appears necessary in order to explain any visual aid and to facilitate effective usage of it. Such follow-up has been known to change the statistics from 80 percent discard of an aid to 90 percent active usage. If there is no hope of improvement and no opportunity to regain some visual function with visual aids, the counselor can offer a combination of "1) his own unemotional acceptance of blindness (he may be the first person to whom the client has spoken who did not immediately show great pity and anxiety—a healthy new experience for the client); 2) formal or informal instruction in procedures which make it easier to live as a blind person; 3) realistic planning for the future; 4) understanding, patience, and a gentle persistence which keeps the counselor available until the client and his family are able to reorient themselves to the future, instead of clinging to the past" (Bauman & Yoder, 1966, p. 160).

Following the initial period of shock and depression, an evaluation of the rehabilitation client may be necessary. Initial impressionistic evaluations can provide only partial and tentative data. It is difficult to know how long a blind client will require to adapt to the psychological and physical aspects of the new deficit. Standardized measuring instruments may help in making this determination. Most of the intelligence, personality, manual aptitude and vocational interest tests used for the blind client are adaptations of standardized tests for the sighted. Since such tests yield numerical scores of doubtful direct relevance for blind clients, heavy reliance needs to be placed upon the observations of skilled, experienced examiners. Standardized tests must be augmented by findings on the part of physicians, psychologists, low-vision specialists, audiologists, psychiatrists, and others to ascertain current status and possibilities for improved functioning. Although agencies vary in the evaluation and training areas they use, several areas are widely accepted: personal and social adjustment (this includes appropriate dress, proper grooming, acceptable personal appearance, good personal hygiene, elimination of troublesome mannerisms, pleasing speech, suitable social and table etiquette, proper behavior in public places, normal interpersonal relationships with family, peers, supervisors, and others) and a constructive attitude toward blindness and toward achieving independence in self-direction, orientation, and mobility. The latter area of training includes awareness of the environment, purposefulness and safety of movements, and relatedness to the physical and social cues that inform blind persons about the world in which they live. Other areas involve the skills of daily living—meals, shopping techniques, clothing, personal records, daily routines, handling money, using the telephone, other sensory abilities, and mastery of electronic and other aids and devices (Rusalem, 1972, pp. 156–157).

A Personal Achievement Skills package for use with the blind has been prepared by Roessler and Means (1977), and a number of devices can be obtained from the American Foundation for the Blind. The major categories listed in the foundation's catalog are Braille-writing equipment, clocks, watches, games, geographical aids, kitchen aids, mathematical aids, music equipment, scales, sewing aids, thermometers, tools and instruments, travel aids, writing and drawing aids, and other miscellaneous devices.

Encounters with the Handicap

Blindness evokes such strong emotional reactions that many persons, both blind and sighted, avoid using the word *blind.* Attitudes of others express so much fear, anxiety, and repugnance that the blind person is frequently preoccupied with personal feelings instead of with constructive activities. Shock, withdrawal, and depression tend to follow new blindness, persisting for varying periods of time. Without professional intervention, premature fixation at one or another of these levels may occur, thereby retarding rehabilitation (Rusalem, 1972). There are no identifiable psychological reactions that set the experience of blindness apart from other crisis experiences (Rusalem, 1972). There is, however, more of a cataclysmic effect, arousing feelings of extreme helplessness and despair. A number of studies have been performed on adjustment to blindness (summarized in Rusalem, 1972). It appears that the most stressful areas are the following: the shock reaction; imitation of the sighted; anxiety, dependency, and segregation from the physical and social world.

Encounters with Technology

The technological advances that benefit individuals with visual impairments can also be broken down into three broad areas: (1) medical advances that either prevent or correct the impairment; (2) mobility aids; and (3) aids that enhance vision or substitute alternative sensory input for activities commonly associated with vision.

Loss of mobility is frequently cited as the major impact on a visually impaired individual (especially if the individual is adventitiously blind). Traditionally, both the cane and the seeing-eye dog have been employed to allow the visually impaired person independent mobility. A major drawback of the cane (and the seeing-eye dog) is the very limited nature of environmental feedback received. Many devices have been developed in the past fifty years which provide increased feedback, either by enlarging the area that can be detected or increasing the amount of information about objects that is received by the individual. The surge in development of these devices is a result of the refinements and advances in the field of electronics, particularly during and after World War II. At least twenty electronic guidance devices have been developed; however, only a few remain in use today (Mims, 1973). The reasons for this appear to be availability, cost, and the fact that visually impaired persons have been slow to adopt such devices. Both the Lasercane and the Pathsounder are expensive and hard to use. The Lasercane costs $2,000, and only about 200 are now in use. The Pathsounder may have some value for orthopedically visually impaired persons; however, only 50 are in use at this time. The Sonic-Guide, at a cost of $2,400 has a wider distribution; however, its complex auditory feedback of the environment has been found to interfere with the environment's natural auditory cues, thus confounding an important channel of information (Scione, 1978). Currently there is continued research to refine the use of electronic feedback to increase its utility. There has been some study of the use of these devices as aids in concept development for congenitally blind children; however, there is no widespread application of this sort at present.

Devices that improve vision or substitute for vision, such as reading machines and high-powered magnifying glasses and Braille wrist watches, probably have had a greater impact in the last decade on the lives of the visually impaired than either medical advances or developments in the area of mobility.

The majority (70 to 80 percent) of visually impaired persons have some functional vision. Advances in the area of optics have influenced the lives of many of this majority. High-powered magnifying glasses have been refined and are readily available; closed-circuit TV magnifiers are popular and allow for reading at home. For those who cannot rely on vision, two groups of devices seem to play an important part. The first is the relatively unsophisticated (technologically) aid provided by the availability of objects coded in Braille: Braille watches, kitchen equipment, sewing aids, games and raised outline maps, and others. These devices have recently become more readily available, and have probably had a broader impact than the more dramatic devices on technology.

Another group of devices that had already had a major impact is reading devices that convert printed material into alternative sensory input. The Optacon, on the market since 1971, converts visual information into tactile sensations "read" by the fingertips. There are now 5,000 in use. Although the device is expensive ($2,800), many foundations have helped blind individuals purchase them. The units have also been available through the Veterans Administration, various school districts, and employers. Persons using the Optacon feel the device to be very valuable, but it is seen as an adjunct to Braille, tapes, and readers rather than a replacement for them. The major problem is the limited reading speed (30 to 60 wpm) possible with the Optacon (Goldish & Taylor, 1964). On the horizon are computer-based reading machines that can convert printed material into a spoken word output at rates of up to 250 wpm. One, the Kurzwile Reading Machine, is already available; however, only about 50 are actually in use at the current time. The price of $20,000 at this point limits its availability to an obviously select group. This machine does, however, hold promise for those who might have access to it through government, agency, or industrial channels that might make the machine available to employees or clients through institutional purchase. A more portable model is currently under development. Apart from the aforementioned drawbacks (limited portability and high price), the machine has a further limitation in that it can read only printed material (i.e., it cannot read handwritten copy).

As more devices become available, the variety of performance/limitation tradeoffs will increase and the choice among tools may then be based upon individual requirements (vocational, social, recreational).

For the foreseeable future, an ideal machine, able to do all the eye can do—even within the more realizable constraints imposed by visual tasks involving a stationary field—will not be available.

Medical Advances

Advances in medicine have resulted both in refinements of existing techniques and in the development of some major treatment modalities during the past decade. The advent of microsurgery has been of particular importance in the treatment of visual impairments. Some of the refinements made in treatment in the last decade include the use of new machines in removal of cataracts, resulting in the restoration of sight the day following surgery (the process is called phaco-emulsification); corneal transplants using plastic implants; and the use of the endoscope to search for foreign objects in the eye.

Treatment of visual impairments caused by diabetes has been particularly aided by two new procedures developed in the past decade. One procedure, vitrectomy, uses microsurgery to remove opacity from the eye; recently, the laser has been employed to "burn out" small hemorrhages in the eye, to perform trabeculotomy to relieve excess intraocular pressure, and to "weld" detached retinas back into place.

One further development holding great promise for treatment of glaucoma is the development of the drug Tomorol.

As in the area of the hearing-impaired, the future may include direct stimulation to the visual cortex in the brain through implanted electrodes connected to a camera which "sees" the environment. Research is currently underway in this area; however, the feasibility of such prostheses is as yet undemonstrated in this infant field of research (Dobelle, 1977).

Up-to-date information about agencies for the blind can be obtained from: The American Foundation for the Blind, 15 West 16th Street, New York, New York 10011.

DEAF-BLIND PERSONS

Incidence

Peter Salmon, in July 1970 (quoted in Spar, 1973), indicates that "we do not know how many deaf-blind people there are in the United States, and we will never know until service is available to them. Estimates of the numbers seem to center around 4,000 or 5,000; but we dare say that there may be twice as many as this" (p. 501). At least 48 percent of deaf-blind individuals also have handicaps other than deafness or blindness.

Encounters with Parents and Society

These encounters are even more traumatic than for individuals with deafness or blindness alone. Throughout history, deaf-blindness has almost universally been perceived as a condition rendering the person vocationally helpless. Although there is wide fear and guilt regarding deaf-blind individuals, it has frequently been found that personal contacts result in genuine acceptance and often lead to conviction and enthusiasm about them as human beings; such events can have important and extensive spillover effects for the disabled person (Spar, 1973). The double deprivation usually results in severe functional limitations in educational, vocational, social, and psychological activities. In the absence of specialized programs, most deaf-blind programs have been neglected by service agencies for both the deaf and the blind.

Encounters with Work and Rehabilitation

Organized rehabilitation services for deaf-blind adults in the United States came into being in 1920, when the Industrial Home for the Blind accepted its first deaf-blind vocational rehabilitation client (Rusalem, 1972). In 1947, the Industrial Home for the Blind opened a structured program for deaf-blind people, launched by an inspiring speech delivered by Helen Keller. Despite the grim prognosis usually held for most deaf-blind individuals, it was found that in an evaluation of 142 successive deaf-blind clients, 92 percent became fully independent in self-care; 73 percent did not need a sighted guide in outdoor areas near their homes; 49 percent did not need a sighted guide in outdoor areas away from their homes; 22 percent read Braille regularly and 11 percent occasionally; and, in terms of present status, 59 percent were employed in industry or sheltered workshop, were homeworkers, or were in some form of training. Also, 5 percent were still receiving rehabilitation, 12 percent had retired because of age, and only 24 percent were not employed in some useful pursuit (Rusalem, 1972).

One of the most important areas for the rehabilitation professional serving deaf-blind clients is the acquisition of skills in one or more of the basic communication techniques used by members of this group. These include Sign language, the manual alphabet, Braille, and some electronic devices. In 1967, the Industrial Home for the Blind received a contract from the Rehabilitation Services Administration to operate a National Center for Deaf-Blind Youth and Adults. This new and exciting program offers direct services, such as:

1. Services in the client's home community for initial assessment.
2. Services in the home communities of clients preparing to enter the center.
3. Multidisciplinary evaluative services to determine the rehabilitation potential of each deaf-blind client at the center.
4. Medical, surgical, psychiatric, and other treatment services.
5. Social casework.
6. Residence at the center and transportation for clients.
7. Transportation for family members and close friends, when necessary.
8. Direct placement and placement consultation services to obtain suitable employment in their home communities or elsewhere.
9. Referral for suitable education or vocational placement.
10. Recreational and social activities at the National Center and consultation for such activities in home communities.
11. Referral to rehabilitation centers prepared to offer any rehabilitation services, and consultation to ensure success of such services.
12. Referral, consultation, and long-term follow-up services to assist in the resettlement of deaf-blind persons in their home communities or, when necessary, in other communities.
13. Distributions to clients in the National Center—and to interested deaf-blind individuals throughout the country—of publications in both Braille and large type to provide them with a means of keeping up with current events and of receiving other new information on as nearly a current basis as possible.

Another main function of the National Center is providing training for professional workers, volunteers, and paraprofessional workers (Spar, 1973).

Encounters with Technology

Devices for deaf-blind persons are typically those developed initially for individuals having only the one disability, although some work is underway to create technology specifically geared to the unique needs of this population. Technology for deaf and for blind persons has already been described.

Up-to-date information about agencies for the deaf-blind can be obtained from: The Helen Keller National Center for Deaf-Blind Youths and Adults, 111 Middle Neck Road, Sands Point, New York 11050.

SUMMARY AND CONCLUSIONS

As physicians and audiologists make diagnoses and prescribe interventions, as educators devise strategies, the ability rather than the disability of the individual must be kept in mind. Higher expectations foster higher performance, and the literature still indicates that optimal intervention is not yet a reality for most disabled people.

As engineers, medical researchers, and inventors create and refine technology and devices, the consumer must always be kept in mind. The needs of the deaf and the blind vary, depending upon type of impairment, age of onset, and other factors too numerous to list here. As devices and interventions become available to the public, it is crucial that answers to the questions "who can benefit?" and "what are the benefits?" be clearly demonstrated via thorough testing and feedback from users. In many cases, such as with cortical electrode implants, choice of this intervention for a particular individual will most probably depend on very careful screening by doctors, surgeons, and mental health and other professionals. In addition to determining the best treatment/aid for a particular individual with special needs, all devices need to be thoroughly researched so that the benefits claimed are realistic. An example of sensationalism overriding realistic presentation of a new technique occurred when acupuncture was announced to be a "cure" for deafness. This inspired many deaf individuals to consult the nearest acupuncturist. The failure of acupuncture as a cure for deafness led to needless disappointment.

One of the critical issues delineated in the first part of this chapter involved economics—the need for aids to be cost-accessible to the consumer. Several suggestions have been mentioned above, such as adapting telephone rates to accommodate the use of the TTY or the MCM. One further suggestion is to provide the consumer with information about the relative prices and relative quality of items on the market. This could be done by devoting an issue of a publication like *Consumer's Union* to aids for the disabled (blind, deaf and deaf-blind, and other disabilities.) In addition to providing the consumer with information, this could also encourage competitive marketing. The benefit to the consumer is obvious; however, the manufacturer could also benefit by increasing the number of consumers.

The status of deaf, blind, and deaf-blind individuals has markedly improved through the centuries. The improvement rate is now accelerating, due to legislation since 1920 designed to help disabled persons. This legislation has become more inclusive for both the level of the disability, the age of the disabled person, and nonvocationally oriented rehabilitation. These high-impact legislative acts have also influenced favorably the general societal attitude toward disability (Rives, 1972). Remaining problems for rehabilitation include: delayed diagnoses, especially in nonwhite populations; inadequate schooling; under-employment; inadequate (although now much improved) involvement of consumers in the service process; and often inimical stances on the part of service professionals (as typified by the long-drawn-out battle that Braille—a blind man—had in gaining acceptance of the writing that bears his name, as well as the battle of the deaf community for full acceptance of sign language).

There is cause for optimism and reason to be pessimistic.

REFERENCES

Anderson, R., & Stevens, G. Qualifications of teachers of mentally retarded deaf pupils in residential schools for the deaf. *Special Education in Canada.* 1969, *43,* 23–32.

Bauman, M. K. Psychological and educational assessment. In B. Lowenfeld (Ed.), *The visually handicapped child in school.* New York: John Day, 1973.

Bauman, M. K., & Yoder, N. Y. *Adjustment to Blindness—Re-viewed.* Springfield, Ill.: Charles C. Thomas, 1966.

Bellefleur, P. A. TTY Communication: Its history and future. *Volta Review,* 1976, *78,* 107.

Bolton, B. *Psychology of deafness for rehabilitation counselors.* Baltimore, Md.: University Park Press, 1976.

Bornstein, H., & Kannapell, B. M. New signs for instructional purposes. Final report OE 6-1924. Washington, D.C.: Gallaudet College Press, 1969.

Bornstein, H., Woodward, J. C., Jr., & Tully N. Language and communication. In B. Bolton (Ed.), *Psychology of deafness for rehabilitation counselors.* Baltimore, Md.: University Park Press, 1976.

Bowe, F. *Handicapping America: Barriers to disabled people.* New York: Harper & Row, 1978.

Brill, R. Mainstreaming: Format of quality? *American Annals of the Deaf,* 1975, 120, 377–381.

Cholden, L. *A psychiatrist works with blindness.* Second Printing. New York: American Foundation for the Blind, 1967.

Dobelle, W. H. Current status of research on providing sight to the blind by electrical stimulation of the brain. *Visual Impairment and Blindness,* 1977, *71:7,* 290–297.

Fraiberg, S. Intervention in infancy: A program for blind infants. In E. Rexford, L. Sander, & J. Shapiro (Eds.), *Infant psychiatry.* New Haven: Yale University Press, 1976.

Fraiberg, S. *Insights from the blind.* New York: Basic Books, 1977.

French, R. S. *From Homer to Helen Keller.* New York: American Foundation for the Blind, 1932.

Glasscock, M. E., III. Medical intervention. *Volta Review,* 1976, *78,* 2–5.

Goldish, L. H., & Taylor, H. E. The optacon: A valuable device for blind persons. *The New Outlook,* February 1964, *68,* 49–55.

Hatfield, E. M. Estimates of blindness in the United States. *The Sight-Saving Review,* 1973, *43,* 69–80.

Kahn, H. A., & Moorhead, H. B. *Statistics on blindness in the model reporting area, 1969–1970.* Department of Health, Education and Welfare (DHEW) Publication No. (NIH), 1970, 73–427.

Levine, E. *The psychology of deafness.* New York: Columbia University Press, 1960.

Link, H. J. Placement and employment of the visually impaired: State of the art and identification of unmet needs. *The New Outlook,* September 1975, 69:7, 320–324.

Lloyd, L. L., & Dahle, A. J. Detection and diagnosis of a hearing impairment in the child. *Volta Review,* 1976, *78,* 12.

Lowenfeld, B. *Multihandicapped blind children in California.* Sacramento: California State Department of Education, Division of Special Services, 1968.

Lowenfeld, B. *The visually handicapped child in school.* New York: John Day, 1973.

Lybarger, S. F. Personal hearing aids. *Volta Review,* 1976, *78,* 113.

MacFarland, D. C. The blind and the visually impaired in J. F. Garrett & E. S. Levine (Eds.), *Rehabilitation practices with the physically disabled.* New York: Columbia University Press, 1973.

Meadow, K. P. Parental response to the medical ambiguities of congenital deafness. *Journal of Health and Social Behavior,* 1968, *9:4,* 299–309.

Meadow, K. P. The development of deaf children. In E. M. Hetherington, J. W. Hagen, R. Kron, and A. H. Stein (Eds.), *Review of child development research, Vol. V.* Chicago: University of Chicago Press, 1975, 439–506.

Mims, F. M. Sensory aids for blind persons. *The New Outlook,* November, 1973, 407–414.

Moores, D. F. *Educating the deaf—psychology, principles, and practices.* Boston: Houghton Mifflin, 1978.

Neu, C. Coping with newly diagnosed blindness. *American Journal of Nursing,* December 1975, *75:12,* 2161–2163.

Norris, M., Spaulding, P. J., & Brodie, F. H. *Blindness in children.* Chicago: University of Chicago Press, 1957.

Parmelee, A. H. Developmental evaluation of the blind premature infant. *AMA Journal of Children's Diseases,* 1955, *90,* 135–140.

Rawlings, B., Trybus, R., Delgado, G., & Stuckless, E. (Eds.). *A guide to college/career programs for deaf students: Revised 1975 edition.* Washington, D.C.: Gallaudet College; and Rochester, N. Y.: National Technical Institute for the Deaf, 1975.

Rice, B. *A comprehensive facility program for multiply handicapped deaf adults.* Fayetteville: Arkansas Rehabilitation Research and Training Center, 1973.

Rives, L. H. History of Federal Vocational Rehabilitation as it affects the blind. In R. E. Hardy & J. G. Cull (Eds.), *Social and rehabilitation services for the blind.* Springfield, Ill.: Charles C. Thomas, 1972.

Roessler, R., & Means, B. *Personal achievement skills for the visually handicapped.* Fayetteville: Arkansas Rehabilitation Research and Training Center, 1977.

Rusalem, H. Coping with the unseen environment. New York: Teachers College Press, 1972.

Schein, J. D. *Model state plan for vocational rehabilitation of deaf clients: Revised.* Silver Spring, Md.: National Association for the Deaf, 1977.

Schein, J. D., & Delk, M. T., Jr. *The deaf population of the United States.* Silver Spring, Md.: National Association of the Deaf, 1974.

Schein, J. D., Gentile, M. A., & Delk, M. T. *Implementation of the model state plan for vocational rehabilitation of deaf clients.* Silver Spring, Md.: National Association for the Deaf, n.d.

Schlesinger, H. S. The deaf pre-schooler and his many faces. In G. T. Lloyd, (Ed.), *International Research Seminar on the Vocational Rehabilitation of the Deaf.* S. R. S.—HEW, 1968.

Schlesinger, H. S. Beyond the range of sound. *California Medicine,* 1969, *110,* 213–217.

Schlesinger, H. S. The acquisition of bimodal language. In I. M. Schlesinger & L. Namir (Eds.), *Sign language of the deaf.* New York: Academic Press, 1978.

Scione, M. W. Electronic sensory aids in a concept development program for congenitally blind young adults. *Visual Impairment and Blindness,* 1978, *72:3,* 88–93.

Scott, R. A. *Final Report of the Russell Sage Foundation.* New York: The New York Association for the Blind, 1966.

Spar, H. J. The deaf-blind. In J. F. Garrett & E. S. Levine (Eds.), *Rehabilitation practices with the physically disabled.* New York: Columbia University Press, 1973.

Stewart, L. *Multiply handicapped deaf people.* Keynote address, Conference on multiply handicapped deaf people. Brainerd, Minn.: October 1974.

Vernon, M. A guide for the psychological evaluation of deaf and severely hard of hearing adults. *The Deaf American,* May 1967, *19:9.*

Vernon, M. Fifty years research. *Journal of Rehabilitation of the Deaf,* January 1968, *1:4.*

Vernon, M. The employment picture, deafness and mental health. *Rehabilitation Literature,* June–July 1977, *38:6–7.*

Vernon, M., & Koh, S. Effects of oral preschool compared to manual communication on education and communication in deaf children. In E. Mindel & M. Vernon (Eds.), *They Grow in silence.* Silver Spring, Md.: National Association of the Deaf, 1972.

Williams, B. R., & Sussman, A. E. Social and psychological problems of deaf people. In A. E. Sussman & L. G. Stewart (Eds.), *Counseling with deaf people.* New York: Deafness Research and Training Center, New York University, 1971.

NOTES ON THE CONTRIBUTORS

THOMAS E. BACKER, Ph.D., is a psychologist whose major professional interests are in knowledge utilization, organizational consultation, psychometrics, and psychology and the arts. He is Senior Research Scientist, Human Interaction Research Institute, Los Angeles; Consulting Psychologist, Edward Glaser & Associates, Los Angeles; and is a private consultant in the arts. Dr. Backer has conducted applied research projects for the Rehabilitation Services Administration, National Institute of Mental Health, National Institute of Education, and U.S. Department of Labor; he is the author of more than fifty books, journal articles, and research reports. He also is a consultant to a number of rehabilitation organizations, and teaches psychology and the arts at the University of California, Los Angeles. He received his Ph.D. in psychology from UCLA.

LINDA BARRETT, M.H.A., is a Senior Staff Member of Berkeley Planning Associates, where she and Susan Shea recently completed a two-year effort to refine the performance standards to be used for assessing vocational rehabilitation programs. Most recently, she and Ms. Shea completed an evaluation of the program's response to new provisions of the vocational rehabilitation legislation, particularly the requirements for priority to the most severely handicapped and individualized written rehabilitation programs for clients. Ms. Barrett has several years of previous experience in planning and analysis of public affairs programs. She holds a B.A. from Whittier College and a master's degree in Health Services Administration from Antioch College.

JOHN R. BARRY, Ph.D., is Professor of Psychology and Coordinator of Graduate Education in Psychology at the University of Georgia. He was previously the Consultant for Research to the Georgia State Rehabilitation Agency and Director of the Regional Rehabilitation Research Institute at the University of Florida. He is the author of many journal articles and other publications in rehabilitation, program evaluation, and consultation.

JAMES A. BITTER, Ed.D., is Professor of Special Education and Director of the Regional Rehabilitation Continuing Education Program at the University of Northern Colorado. He has held service, teaching, and research positions in special education and rehabilitation since 1961. Dr. Bitter received his professional education at Marquette University (B.A.), the University of Wisconsin—Milwaukee (M.S.), the University of Northern Colorado (Ed.D.), and the University of Missouri—Columbia (postdoctoral fellow). He has contributed many articles to the professional literature and is the author of the textbook *Introduction to Rehabilitation,* published in 1979.

FRANK BOWE, Ph.D., is Director, American Coalition of Citizens with Disabilities, Inc. (ACCD), the nation's strongest advocate for disabled people. A research psychologist, he has done large-scale and experimental research on consumer involvement in rehabilitation and related issues. Dr. Bowe graduated summa cum laude from Western Maryland College in 1969 with a B.A.; he received his M.A. from Gallaudet College in 1971 and his Ph.D. in 1976 in educational psychology from New York University. Dr. Bowe is author of *Handicapping America, Rehabilitating America,* and about 100 other books and articles on disability.

JEROLD D. BOZARTH, Ph.D., is Professor and Chairperson of the Department of Counseling and Human Development Services, University of Georgia. Previously he was Director of Research, Arkansas Rehabilitation Research and Training Center—University of Arkansas; Director of Research and Continuing Education, Iowa Mental Health Authority, University of Iowa; and Chairperson, Department of Rehabilitation Counseling, University of Florida. He received the Ph.D. degree from the University of Iowa in Rehabilitation Counseling and Mental Health Counseling. Dr. Bozarth received two national research awards from the American Rehabilitation Counseling Association in 1973–1974. His publications include 2 books, 5 book chapters, and about 75 journal articles and government publications.

GARRY S. BRODY, M.D., is Chief of the Plastic and Reconstructive Surgery Service and the Burn Rehabilitative Services at Rancho Los Amigos Hospital, Downey, California. He is also Clinical Assistant Professor of Surgery (Plastic Surgery), University of Southern California School of Medicine. He obtained his medical degree at the University of Alberta, Canada, in 1956, and also holds an M.S. degree in experimental surgery from McGill University in Montreal, Canada.

HERBERT DORKEN, Ph.D., is Adjunct Professor and Research Psychologist, Langley Porter Institute, and member of the graduate group in Health Psychology, University of California, San Francisco. He is also Health Services Consultant to the California State Psychological Association. A graduate of McGill University (M.Sc. '47) and the University of Montreal (Ph.D. '51), he was from 1970 to 1975 on the American Psychological Association's Committee on Health Insurance (Chair 1974 and 1975) and editor-author of *The Professional Psychologist Today: New Developments in Law, Health Insurance and Health Practice* (Jossey Bass, 1976).

FREDERICK A. FAY, Ph.D., is Director of Research for Tufts Rehabilitation Institute's Rehabilitation Research and Training Center. He supervises research in the areas of independent living and rehabilitation engineering as well as consumer involvement in rehabilitation. Dr. Fay has served as Vice-President of the American Coalition of Citizens with Disabilities and as Senior Research Associate at the Urban Institute on the Comprehensive Needs Study. His B.S. in Psychology, M.S. in Rehabilitation Counseling, and Ph.D. in Psychology are from the University of Illinois. Dr. Fay was selected as one of the "Ten Outstanding Young Men of America" by the United States Jaycees for 1978.

ROBERT R. HUMPHREYS, LL.B., is Commissioner of the Rehabilitation Services Administration, where he directs the state-federal Vocational Rehabilitation program. He was previously Special Counsel to the U.S. Senate Committee on Human Resources, where he served as the principal draftsman of the Rehabilitation Act of 1973 and the Randolph-Sheppard Act Amendments and was a major contributor to the development of some 50 other measures relating to labor, handicapped people, aging, health, employment, drug abuse, children and youth, and volunteer programs. Mr. Humphreys is a graduate of the University of Washington in Seattle, where he received his B.A. degree in political science in 1959. In 1965 he received his LL.B degree from the George Washington University Law School in Washington, D.C.

MARK A. JOHNSON, Ph.D., is Clinical Psychologist, Administrative Offices, Child and Youth Service, Orange County Mental Health Service, and Assistant Professor, Department of Psychology, California State University at Los Angeles. Previously he was Clinical Psychologist with the Burn Service, Rancho Los Amigos Hospital, Downey, California. He obtained his doctorate in psychology from the University of Southern California in 1977.

MARGARET LEE, Ph.D., is a clinical psychologist at the Research and Training Center on Mental Health and Deafness at the University of California, San Francisco. She completed her training as a child psychologist specializing in work with the deaf and received her Ph.D. from California School of Professional Psychology in 1978. Her dissertation involved research on the relationship between maternal interaction styles and language development in deaf children.

WILLIAM F. MILLER, M.D., is Professor of Medicine at the University of Texas Southwestern Medical School and Director of the Pulmonary Division at the Methodist Hospital at Dallas. He has served on committees and as a consultant to numerous health organizations. His present professional appointments include consultant to the National Heart, Lung, and Bladder Institute, Pulmonary Disease Section; *Associates of Respiratory Care,* official journal of the American Association of Respiratory Therapy; and consultant to the Joint Review Committee on Respiratory Therapy Education Programs of the American Medical Association, Council of Medical Education. Dr. Miller has written over 130 articles and chapters on pulmonary topics.

JANET A. MINCH, M.A., is Director of the Consumer Involvement Core Research Area at the Tufts Rehabilitation Institute's Rehabilitation Research and Training Center. Ms. Minch is responsible for the design and implementation of the research and training programs in consumer involvement at the R&T Center, and has had other advocacy experience with the Easter Seal Society of Massachusetts. Her B.A. in Economics is from Muskingum College, and her Masters in Urban Affairs is from Boston University.

ELIZABETH PAN, Ph.D., is President of the Institute for Information Studies, a nonprofit organization engaged in technology and information transfer and use. She has been involved in administrative and technical capacities in information retrieval systems in both the scientific and human services areas, and has published numerous papers and reports on these subjects. She has served as project director for a number of studies on the delivery of rehabilitation information. She received her Ph.D. from Rutgers University and previous degrees from the University of Illinois.

JAMES B. RESWICK, Sc.D., is Co-Director of the Rancho Los Amigos Rehabilitation Engineering Center at Rancho Los Amigos Hospital, Downey, California. He holds joint faculty appointments in the University of Southern California Schools of Medicine and Engineering as Professor of Orthopaedics and Professor of Biomedical Engineering, respectively. Dr. Reswick graduated with a B.S. in 1943 and Sc.D. in Mechanical Engineering in 1952 from the Massachusetts Institute of Technology. Author of more than 80 articles on automatic controls, computers, dynamics of machines, engineering education, and biomedical engineering, and co-author of three textbooks, Dr. Reswick also holds ten United States patents.

HILDE S. SCHLESINGER, M.D., is Project Director of the Research and Training Center on Mental Health and Deafness at the University of California, San Francisco. She is a psychiatrist specializing in adult and child deafness and community psychiatry. Her research interests include deafness early language acquisition and its relationship to mental health, mother and child interaction, and the relationship of self-esteem and work performance. She is the author of several chapters and articles relating to deafness and mental health including *Sound and Sign, Childhood Deafness and Mental Health,* co-authored with Kathryn P. Meadow. In 1975 she held the Powrie V. Doctor Chair of Deaf Studies at Gallaudet College.

SUSAN SHEA, M.C.P., is Senior Staff Member of Berkeley Planning Associates, where she and Linda Barrett recently completed a two-year effort to refine the performance standards to be used for assessing vocational rehabilitation programs. Most recently, she and Ms. Barrett completed an evaluation of the program's response to new provisions of the vocational rehabilitation legislation, particularly the requirements for priority to the most severely handicapped and individualized written rehabilitation programs for clients. Ms. Shea earlier won the ARCA research prize for her development of methods for estimating the need for VR services (the "Ridge Methodology") and has directed several studies evaluating VR and other social service programs, including those for runaway youth and families' experiences in child abuse and neglect programs. She holds a B.A. from Wellesley College and a master's degree in City and Regional Planning from the University of California, Berkeley.

SUSAN STODDARD, M.C.P., Senior Analyst with Berkeley Planning Associates, is a candidate for the Ph.D. in Planning from the University of California, Berkeley. She served as consultant and research evaluator for the Center for Independent Living (CIL) in Berkeley, California, and has authored publications on independent living and planning. Ms. Stoddard serves on the faculties of the University of California Extension at Berkeley and Antioch College/West.

ROBERTA B. TRIESCHMANN, Ph.D., is National Consultant to rehabilitation centers on the problems of the physically disabled. Her past appointments include: assistant professor of Rehabilitation Medicine at the University of Washington; chief psychologist at the Southwest Regional System for Treatment of Spinal Injury at Good Samaritan Hospital in Phoenix, Arizona; chief psychologist and associate professor of Rehabilitation Medicine and Psychology at the University of Cincinnati; and project director of the Spinal Cord Injury Research Program at the Easter Seal Society of Los Angeles County. Dr. Trieschmann received the B.S. degree with High Honors in Psychology from the University of Wisconsin in 1961 and the Ph.D. in Clinical Psychology from the University of Minnesota in 1966. She has authored over 20 research articles and chapters in edited volumes, is author of a forthcoming book entitled *The Adjustment to Spinal Cord Injury,* serves on the editorial board of *Rehabilitation Psychology,* and is a consultant to the Rehabilitation Services Administration.

CAROLYN L. VASH, Ph.D., has extensive experience as a clinical psychologist, administrator, and educator, and is former Chief Deputy Director of the California State Department of Rehabilitation. She previously developed a comprehensive vocational rehabilitation program which included a sheltered workshop program at Rancho Los Amigos Hospital in Downey, California. The author of many papers and articles, she also serves on the advisory boards of several rehabilitation projects and commissions. Dr. Vash received the Ph.D. in Psychology from the University of California, Los Angeles, in 1964. She is currently in private practice as a consulting psychologist and lectures at the University of Southern California and California State University at Los Angeles.

INDEX